TEXTBOOK OF
FACIAL REJUVENATION
The art of minimally invasive
combination therapy

TEXTBOOK OF FACIAL REJUVENATION

The art of minimally invasive combination therapy

Editor

Nicholas J Lowe MD FRCP
Cranley Clinic for Dermatology
London
UK
and
Southern California Dermatology, Laser and
Psoriasis Center
Santa Monica, CA
USA

Co-editors

Alastair Carruthers FRCP
Jean Carruthers MD FRCS(C) FRC(OPTH)
Zoe Diana Draelos MD PA
Christopher EM Griffiths MD FRCP
Richard D Glogau MD
Arnold W Klein MD
Gary P Lask MD

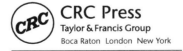

CRC Press
Taylor & Francis Group
Boca Raton London New York

CRC Press is an imprint of the
Taylor & Francis Group, an **informa** business

CRC Press
Taylor & Francis Group
6000 Broken Sound Parkway NW, Suite 300
Boca Raton, FL 33487-2742

First issued in paperback 2019

© 2002 by Taylor & Francis Group, LLC
CRC Press is an imprint of Taylor & Francis Group, an Informa business
Typeset by Scribe Design, Gillingham, Kent, UK

No claim to original U.S. Government works

ISBN-13: 978-1-84184-095-6 (hbk)
ISBN-13: 978-0-367-39600-8 (pbk)

Visit the Taylor & Francis Web site at
http://www.taylorandfrancis.com

and the CRC Press Web site at
http://www.crcpress.com

Contents

Contributors

Andrew Blitzer MD DDS FACS
Professor of Clinical Otolaryngology
College of Physicians and Surgeons of
Columbia University
New York
USA

Eileen Bradbury
The Alexandra Hospital
Cheadle
Cheshire
UK

Douglas Canfield
Canfield Scientific Inc.
Fairfield
New Jersey
USA

Alastair Carruthers FRCP
Carruthers Dermatology Centre Inc
Vancouver
British Columbia
Canada
and
Clinical Professor
Division of Dermatology
University of British Columbia
Canada

**Jean Carruthers MD FRCS(C)
FRC(OPTH)**
Carruthers Dermatology Centre Inc
Vancouver
British Columbia
Canada
and
Clinical Professor
Division of Ophthalmology
University of British Columbia
Canada

**Brian A Coghlan MD FRCS FRCS
(Plast)**
Consultant Plastic, Aesthetic and
Reconstructive Surgeon
London
UK
and
Department of Plastic Surgery
Chelsea & Westminster Hospital
London
UK

Kim K Cook
Coronado Skin Medical Center, Inc
Coronado
California
USA

William R Cook, Jr
Coronado Skin Medical Center, Inc
Coronado
California
USA

Zoe Diana Draelos MD PA
High Point
North Carolina
USA

Daniel Fleming MD
Cosmetic and Laser Surgery Institute of
Australia
Brisbane
Australia

Jerome M Garden MD
Northwestern University Medical School
Department of Dermatology
Evanston
Illinois
and
Children's Memorial Hospital
Division of Dermatology and Plastic
Surgery
Chicago
Illinois
USA

Richard D Glogau MD
San Francisco
California
USA

Christopher EM Griffiths MD FRCP
Dermatology Centre
Hope Hospital
Salford
UK

Suzanne Kafaja MD
Clinical Research Fellow
Clinical Research Specialists
Santa Monica
California
and
UCLA School of Medicine
Los Angeles
California
USA

Roland Kaufmann MD
Professor and Chair of Dermatology
Medical Director of Frankfurt University
Hospital
Zentrum der Dermatologie und
Venerologie
Klinikum der JW Goethe-Universität
Frankfurt am Main
Germany

Arnold W Klein MD
Professor of Dermatology/ Medicine
UCLA
Beverly Hills
California
USA

Gary P Lask MD
UCLA School of Medicine
Los Angeles
California
USA
and
Clinical Research Specialists
Santa Monica
California
USA

Jean Luc Levy MD
Medical Director, Centre Laser
Dermatologique, Marseille
Co-director of European University Board
of Lasers
Consultant, Laser Department Hospital
Red Cross Clinic
Marseille
France

Pamela S Lowe NCSP
Senior Administrator
Cranley Clinic
London, UK
Southern California Dermatology, Laser
and Psoriasis Center
Santa Monica, CA
USA

Philippa Lowe MD ChB
Cranley Clinic for Dermatology
London
UK

Gary D Monheit MD
Dermatology Associates
Birmingham
Alabama
USA

Joseph Niamtu, III MD
Richmond
Virginia
USA

Sue Nicholl BSc
University College London Hospital NHS
Trust
Department of Medical Physics and
Bioengineering
London
UK

Adeline de Ramecourt MD
Electrology Consultant
Paris
France

Teresa T Soriano MD
Division of Dermatology
University of California
Los Angeles
USA

Dow B Stough MD
The Stough Clinic
Hot Springs
Arkansas
USA

Beverley Westwood RN MSc
PS Research
Chichester
UK

Jeffrey M Whitworth MD
Passaic
New Jersey
USA

Dina Yaghmai MD
Chicago
Illinois
USA

Paul S Yamauchi MD PhD
UCLA School of Medicine
Los Angeles
California
USA
and
Clinical Research Specialists
Santa Monica
California
USA

Acknowledgements

I am grateful to my colleagues and teachers for developing new concepts and details of therapy that have transformed my patient practice over the last few decades, and to my patients for their loyalty and understanding.

This is an exciting, continuously evolving medical and surgical arena that is attracting increasing professional as well as public interest as novel facial rejuvenation treatments are introduced, refined, and some, appropriately, discarded!

It is essential that for the safe and satisfactory outcome of patient treatment in the cosmetic field that physicians and surgeons are thoroughly trained and specialised. I would like to thank my co-editors and co-authors of this book who have brought their outstanding skills, innovation and insight to print and who have contributed so much to the specialties of dermatologic and cosmetic surgery. Thank you for giving yet more of your precious time in contributing to the book.

I would like to thank the publisher Martin Dunitz and his editorial staff for encouraging me and refining the book. I hope many will find it of use.

Finally, I would like to thank my wife and sage advisor, Pamela, my beautiful daughters Nichola and Philippa for tolerating me, my many faults and preoccupations. I have been able to take time away from family commitments to complete this book and other projects that would have been impossible without their patience and support.

1. Introduction

Nicholas J Lowe

Facial aging is perceived by some to be an inevitable outward sign of the aging process. However, it is felt by others to be an event that should be delayed or prevented if possible. Treatments that enable them to remain looking as youthful as possible may offer social, personal and professional advantages.

The many treatment choices currently available are the subject of this book. Over the last decade numerous new treatment modalities have emerged which allow the use of minimally invasive and often non-surgical approaches to rejuvenate the aging face. In addition, new topical and photoprotective agents have become available to enable us to protect the skin from UV damage, along with maintenance treatments to retain the most youthful possible skin appearance, and to reduce premature or accelerated skin aging. The development of different novel types of lasers leading to non-ablative and resurfacing laser skin rejuvenation, often in combination with vascular and pigment specific lasers, enable the skilled practitioner to offer realistic (both with regard to result and cost) non-surgical techniques to rejuvenate the face.

Rightly or wrongly, there are associations between perceptions of youth and age. The younger people appear, the more attractive they appear, presenting great promise for the future, being 'cool' and having the potential for fun, whereas the older-looking individual tends to be ignored and discounted with limitations and low expectations placed on their potential.

There is, in addition, a common denial by the individual of their own aging process. Facial aging, in particular wrinkles, solar lentigo and other pigment changes, and telangiectasia are felt by many to be leading indicators of age. Of interest is that up to 70% of 30–50 year olds say that they look younger than their actual age and feel that they have fewer signs of facial aging than their contempories. Statistically, of course, this is impossible, but it remains a common misperception.

While it is true that beauty is only skin deep and that it is the person inside who matters most, we know that we are being judged constantly, if only because we know that we judge others on how they look and dress. Many people, particularly those in competitive social and professional scenarios, want to look as youthful as possible for as long as possible because they feel that their prospects are significantly higher if they look young and that they will be more successful both socially and professionally.[1]

There is a growing trend in many countries of the acceptability of cosmetic procedures.[a] 60% of women overall feel that they would be interested in having a procedure if it can be done safely, and if the results would be subtle enough that it would not be obvious that a procedure had been carried out. Compared to just five years ago, 30–50 year olds are less likely these days to accept that they should allow nature to take its course and not consider defying it. Today, it is more likely that people will do whatever they can to slow down the aging process.

Perceived facial age is often the key to presumed chronological age. Patterns still exist, however, and it

---

[a]2001 Procedural Statistics American Academy of Cosmetic Surgery, Chicago. Website: www.cosmetic-surgery.org/Media_Center/media_center.html.

remains more socially acceptable for women to undergo cosmetic surgery than men. Part of this may be that some existing surgical techniques, for example, face lifting, can be much more difficult to disguise in men than in women because of factors such as hairline and length. In addition, some of the older hair transplantation techniques used for men gave the most unattractive and sometimes disfiguring result of tufting. The most recent hair transplantation techniques give a much more natural look whereby the casual observer cannot tell that a procedure has been performed. Thus, in the future it may be that men are less hesitant to try such a procedure.

The popular demand for facial rejuvenation has expanded dramatically over the last decade. One potential reason for this may be the so-called 'baby boomer' generation who are reaching 35–60 years of age, noticing their facial aging and wishing to reverse and improve realistically their appearance. They have also witnessed their parents' premature facial aging and want to avoid this if at all possible. It has been estimated that the baby boomers born between 1944 and 1964 make up approximately 30% of the US population, which gives a number of almost 80 million people in this age range in the US alone.[b]

This book is intended to provide important information for the medical and surgical specialists who deal with demand for facial rejuvenation about the different treatment options and how these may be successfully selected and combined.

Many maturing people resist the concept of aging. The American Association of Retired People reports that when many people reach the age of 50, there is an inner conflict and a reluctance to let go of the illusion of youth.

Often erroneously, it is thought that men get better with age, while women just get older. This is not necessarily true and, indeed, men can show the ravages of time just as much as women. As a result, increasing numbers of men are now seeking to rejuvenate their appearance with minimally invasive procedures in combination with maintaining their body health with exercise and lifestyle changes. As

with women, it is often important for those in many competitive careers to remain youthful-looking.

For good or bad, the trend to remain as attractive and youthful as possible for as long as possible is upheld by a proportion of the population of the developed world. There are many new procedures that were not available even 5–10 years ago that now allow us to offer treatments that are largely undetectable or become rapidly undetectable with time and yet lead to a more youthful appearance.

It has been well established that exposure to sunlight is the most significant cause of accelerated skin aging and there is now data to support the use of sun protection against skin aging.[2,3]

There are many non-specialist (and indeed many non-medical) practitioners who enter the field of facial rejuvenation and offer some of the treatments discussed in this book. To them I advocate reflection on patient safety and recognition of professional limitations.

The concept for this book arose out of the present author's experiences with many of the more recent treatment options and the need for a book that discusses these options and places them in the context of individual patient needs.

References

1. Etcoff N. Survival of the Prettiest: The Science of beauty. New York: Doubleday, 1999.

2. Fisher GJ, Wang ZQ, Datta SC et al. Pathophysiology of premature skin aging induced by ultraviolet light. N Engl J Med 1997;337:1419–28.

3. Meyers DP, Lowe NJ, Scott IR. Exposure to low levels of ultraviolet light B or ultraviolet light A induces photodamage in human skin. In: Lowe NJ, Shaath N, Pathak M. Sunscreens: Development, evaluation and regulatory aspects, 2nd ed. New York: Marcel Dekker, 1997.

4. Kligman LH, Kligman AM. Ultraviolet radiation induced skin aging. In: Lowe NJ, Shaath P, Pathak M. Sunscreens: Development, evaluation and regulatory aspects, 2nd ed. New York: Marcel Dekker, 1997.

---

[b]Selected Social Characteristics of Baby Boomers 26 to 44 years old. US Census Bureau, February 1996. Website: www.census.gov/population/www/socdemo/age.html#bb.

2. Photoprotection*

Nicholas J Lowe

Sunlight-induced skin aging has been established as a major cause of accelerated skin aging; in addition, the incidence of melanoma and non-melanoma skin cancer has shown a well-documented increase in several continents over the last several years.[1]

Many authorities are recommending primary prevention programs to reduce this incidence of cutaneous photodamage and skin carcinogenesis. An integral component of these programs is the use of protective clothing,[2] as well as hats and effective sunscreens.[3,4]

Most modern sunscreens have highly efficient absorption or reflecting capabilities throughout the ultraviolet (UV) B spectrum; their protective effects against UVA and infrared (IR) wavelengths are more variable. Over the last few years, more efficient sunscreening ingredients have been developed for improved protection.[5–8] See also figure 8.3.

SOLAR RADIATION

The solar spectrum

Solar radiation encompasses the electromagnetic spectrum from short, high-energy cosmic, gamma, and X-rays to the longer, lower energy UV, visible, IR, microwaves, and radio waves. Much solar radiation, including most shorter UVC and UVB wavelengths, is absorbed in the atmosphere by the ozone layer.[9] High-energy radiation (wavelength <10 mm) displaces electrons from incident tissue to form ions. Therefore, radiation in this category, including gamma and X-rays, is termed ionizing radiation. Since they lack the energy to do this, UV, visible, and shorter IR waves are categorized as non-ionizing irradiation.

The radiation striking the earth is approximately 50% visible (wavelengths 400–800 nm), 40% IR (wavelength 1300–1700 nm), and 10% UV (10–400 nm). The UV spectrum is divided, for convenience, into UVA (320–400 nm), UVB (290–320 nm), UVC (100–290 nm), and vacuum UV (10–100 nm). The human eye cannot detect wavelengths other than those in the visible range. Vacuum UV, UVC, and the shortest UVB rays are screened by the ozone layer, which essentially eliminates all UV radiation (UVR) < 290 nm; little UVA is filtered in the atmosphere. The remaining UV that reaches the ground is about 10% UVB and 90% UVA at midday. UVB intensity declines from the noontime apex, but UVA intensity remains relatively constant throughout the day.[9]

Human skin and acute solar overexposure (sunburn)

Erythema, the most familiar manifestation of UVR exposure, occurs in a biphasic manner.[10] The early portion of this reaction, also known as immediate pigment darkening (IPD), is mediated by UVA and lasts

---

*Parts of this chapter have been modified from Lowe NJ, Shaath N. Sunscreens: development, evaluation and regulatory aspects, 2nd edition. New York: Marcel Dekker, 1996.

13–30 minutes; UVA-induced erythema is marked in some individuals while it is undetectable in others. Delayed erythema, a function primarily of UVB dosages, begins 2–8 hours after exposure and reaches a maximum 24–36 hours later, with erythema, pruritus, and pain in the sun-exposed areas.[11] This reaction resolves over a 3–5 day period and initiates increased melanogenesis, which reaches a peak after 2–3 weeks.[10]

A typical minimal erythema dose (MED) for an individual who burns easily and tans slightly (skin type II) is 15 minutes at midday in midsummer in Southern California (NJ Lowe, personal observation). An exposure of 5 MED produces painful sunburn; after 10 MED, edema, vesiculation, and bullae formulation often occur. Skin necrosis leading to scarring and uneven pigmentation may result. Depending on the area involved, severe sunburn can cause the systemic symptoms of 'sun poisoning', including fever, nausea, vomiting, severe headache, prostration, and even shock.[9]

Microscopically, changes are detectable as early as 30 minutes after UVR exposure. Epidermal changes include intracellular edema, vacuolization and swelling of melanocytes, and the development of characteristic 'sunburn cells'.[12] In the dermis, UVR initially leads to interstitial edema and endothelial cell swelling.

Later, there is perivenular edema, degranulation and loss of mast cells, a decrease in the number of Langerhans cells, neutrophil infiltration, and erythrocyte extravasation. This reaction reaches its apex after 24 hours, resolving over 3–5 days.[9,10]

Sunburn cells are dyskeratotic keratinocytes with pyknotic nuclei and homogeneous eosinophilic cytoplasm.[9] Sunburn cell formation is maximal at 18–24 hours postexposure and resolves in 3–7 days. They occur in proportion to the amount of the skin's UVB exposure; UVA is less effective in the development of sunburn cells.[9,10]

Later changes include hyperkeratosis (increased scale), acanthosis (epidermal thickening), disorganization and misalignment of keratinocytes, dermal vascular ectasia, and mononuclear perivascular infiltration (Figures 2.1 and 2.2).[13]

Chronic effects of solar radiation on the skin

There are two major adaptive responses in the skin initiated by UVR exposure: melanogenesis (tanning)

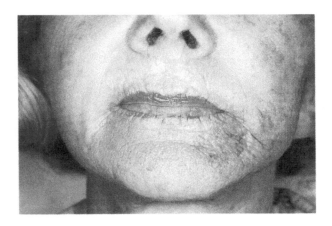

Figure 2.1 *The face of a patient showing more marked accelerated skin aging on the side of her face most exposed to sunlight through her driving-side car-window for at least 30 minutes.*

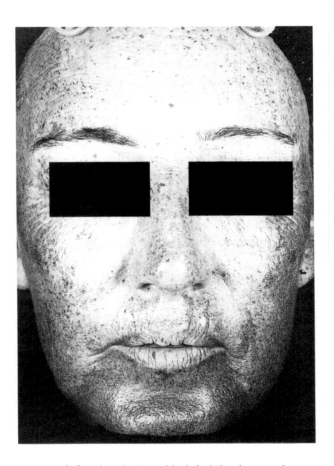

Figure 2.2 *Filtered UVA ('black light') photography is useful to highlight facial dyspigmentation and rhytides induced by repetitive sun exposure (see further Chapters 8 and 26).*

and thickening of the stratum corneum. Tanning occurs as a result of de novo production of melanin in melanocytes. Interestingly, UVB actually induces melanocyte proliferation in both exposed and covered areas of the body.[13]

Melanin is produced from tyrosine through several enzymatically controlled reactions. The initial, rate-limiting step is the conversion of tyrosine into dihydroxyphenylalanine (DOPA). The melanin, incorporated into organelles called melanosomes, is then distributed to surrounding keratinocytes. Some melanosomes remain intact in the keratinocytes as they keratinize and migrate to become the stratum corneum. This amorphous melanin undergoes oxidation in the IPD reaction when exposed to UVA radiation.[14]

Melanin absorbs, reflects and scatters UVR, and also acts as a free-radical trap. Although persons of all skin types have approximately the same number of melanocytes, black-skinned persons have approximately 400 melanosomes per basal epidermal cell, a fourfold increase over the typical pale Caucasian. This difference reduces the UVA and UVB penetration into the dermis by a factor of five in Blacks as compared with Caucasians, and is believed responsible for the 30-fold increase in the typical MED value for Blacks.[13]

Tanning induces a sun-protection factor (SPF) increase of between 2 and 4 against further UVR exposure. Even with a 'protective tanning base', Caucasians are susceptible to a significant amount of UVR-induced damage.

Solar radiation and photoaging

Human skin changes in grossly and microscopically detectable ways over the lifetime of an individual. However, exposure to excessive amounts of solar radiation greatly increases the rate at which skin ages. Dermatoheliosis ('photoaging') is the wrinkled, leathery skin seen in persons chronically exposed to the sun. Photoaging is induced by chronic exposure to all portions of the solar spectrum, including UVA, UVB, and IR.[15]

Grossly photoaged skin appears wrinkled and atrophic with mottled pigmentation. Superimposed are hypopigmented macules as well as hyperpigmented lentigines ('liver spots' or 'sunspots'), telang-

iectasia and raised, roughened, precancerous actinic keratoses.

Microscopically, as skin ages normally, the epidermis atrophies, the dermis becomes hypocellular, the vasculature remains intact, and collagen forms a stable, increasingly crosslinked, matrix. By contrast, the epidermis of photoaged skin becomes acanthotic (thickened), the dermis hypercellular (due to fibroblast and mast-cell proliferation), and the vessels tortuous and dilated. Elastic fibers degenerate into a thickened, amorphous mass displacing the normal collagen in a process termed elastosis. These changes are detectable in most Caucasians before the age of 30. Shorter UVA in the 320–40 nm range is probably responsible for the bulk of UVA-induced photoage.[15]

Chronic exposure to solar radiation also has dramatic effects on the life span of fibroblasts and keratinocytes. It is well documented that human fibroblasts in vitro will only divide a limited number of times before they die. Although the mechanism remains unclear, the number of times they do replicate correlates with the age of the subject from which the fibroblasts are obtained. More recent studies have demonstrated that fibroblasts and keratinocytes from a given individual will replicate more times if obtained from an unexposed area of the body as compared with those derived from more chronically sun-exposed tissue.[16] This implies that solar radiation exposure decreases the regenerative capacity of human skin and thus hastens skin aging.

Solar radiation and cancer

Solar radiation-induced local immune suppression may induce or promote non-melanoma skin cancer (NMSC); UVR definitely induces NMSC in mice. Transformation of normal cells into malignant cells probably occurs as a result of UVR-initiated DNA mutation. Patients with xeroderma pigmentosum (XP), who lack the usual reparative enzymes for damaged DNA, have a greatly increased risk of developing NMSC.[16] Although cumulative UVB appears to be more closely linked to NMSC development, UVA also plays a role. Both can induce thymine dimer formation which may be an initiating step in cell transformation. Also, UVA has been demonstrated to augment the development of UVB-induced NMSC in hairless mice.[13]

Epidemiological studies of cumulative sun exposure and the incidence of NMSC in normal humans are also extremely strong. The risk of basal cell carcinoma in Atlanta, GA, is five times greater than that seen in Minneapolis, MN. The age-adjusted risk for squamous cell carcinoma in Atlanta is four times that seen in Minneapolis. The mutagenicity of 1 J/cm^2 of UVB at 300 nm is 1000 times that of 1 J/cm^2 of UVA at 330 nm. The carcinogenic effects most likely correlate with the mutagenicity, and thus UVB can be assumed to be many-fold more carcinogenic than UVA.[3]

The data on malignant melanoma (MM) are not clear-cut. Nevertheless, MM is probably induced and/or promoted in some way by UVR exposure. Recent trends have shown an alarming rise in the development of MM. Risk factors for the development of MM are complex and do not correlate with cumulative UVB exposure. However, intermittent intense sunlight exposure may correlate with the development of MM.[17] As mentioned earlier, UVB actually induces melanocyte proliferation in both exposed and covered areas of the body. This may explain why MM sometimes occurs in areas without significant prior sun exposure.[13]

Garland et al. postulate that the broader utilization of sunscreens, which primarily protect against UVB wavelengths, encourages susceptible individuals to spend more time in the sun.[17] These persons receive larger cumulative doses of solar radiation outside the UVB range. Increased exposure to non-UVB solar radiation has been suggested to promote the development of MM. Further scientific study of this question is needed to justify this hypothesis.

PHOTOPROTECTION WITH CLOTHING AND SUNSCREENS

Sunscreens

History and development
In 1928, the world's first commercial sunscreen, an emulsion of benzyl salicylate and benzyl cinnamate, was developed in the United States. In the 1930s, a 10% solution of phenyl salicylate appeared on the Australian market. In 1935, lotions of quinine oleate and quinine bisulfate were available in the US. In 1943, para-aminobenzoic acid (PABA) was patented, introducing this popular agent and subsequently its derivatives. The US military utilized red petrolatum, a physical blocking agent, as a sunblock during the Second World War. Their efforts also led to the popularization of other UV-filtering agents including glycerol-PABA, 2-ethyl-hexyl salicylate, digalloyl trioleate, homomenthyl salicylate, and dipropylene glycol salicylate.[18] Most of the early agents were directed towards UVB, the portion of the sun's spectrum responsible for the most palpable and distressing effect, i.e. the familiar sunburn.

Parasol 1789 (avobenzone or 4-t-butyl-4′-methoxydibenzoylmethane), an agent broadly effective in the UVA spectrum, is now marketed in combination with UVB-blocking agents. These formulations provide broad-spectrum chemical sun protection to the US consumer.[19,20] A new subclass of physical blockers, micronized reflecting powders, have recently been made available from a variety of manufacturers. Unlike traditional physical blockers, micronized reflecting powders are less visible yet provide broad-spectrum protection against UVR. These should prove useful in UVR-sensitive patients resistant to older physical blockers for cosmetic reasons; an additional benefit is that they do not cause photosensitization.[21 28]

Future trends in the development of sunscreens include products with efficacy against UVC (which may become more important with further erosion of the ozone layer) and agents directed against IR, because of the concerns about IR-induced photoaging (Tables 2.1 and 2.2).

Substantivity
Substantivity is the characteristic of a sunscreen which reflects how effectively the advertised degree of protection is maintained under adverse conditions, including repeated water exposure or sweating. According to the US Food and Drugs Administration, a sunscreen is declared water resistant if it can maintain its original SPF after two 20-mm immersions. A sunscreen is very water resistant if it retains its protective integrity after four 20-mm immersions.[30] Substantivity is of enormous importance, since sunscreens are used outdoors in settings where

Table 2.1. *US Food and Drugs Administration approved sunscreen ingredients (2000)*

Chemical	Approved (%)
UVA absorbers	
Oxybenzone	2–6
Sulisobenzone	5–10
Dioxybenzone	3
Methyl anthralinate	3.5–5
Avobenzone	3
UVB absorbers	5–15
para-Aminobenzoic acid (PABA)	1–5
Amyl dimethyl PABA (Padimate A)	1–3
2-Ethoxyethyl p-methoxycinnamate	8–10
Digalloyl trioleate	2–5
2-Ethyl 4-bis (hydroxypropyl) aminobenzoate	1–5
2-Ethylhexyl-2-cyano-3,3-diphenylacrylate	7–10
Ethylhexyl p-methoxycinnamate	2–7.5
2-Ethylhexyl salicylate	3–5
Glyceryl aminobenzoate (glyceryl PABA)	2–3
Homomenthyl salicylate	4–25
Lawsome with dihydroxyacetate	0.25% with 3%
Octyl dimethyl PABA (Padimate 0)	1.4–8
2-Phenylbenzimidazole-5-sulfonic acid	1.4
Thethanolamine salicylate	5–12
Physical blockers	
Red petrolatum	30–100
Titanium dioxide	2–25

Table 2.2. *EC permitted and provisionally approved UV filters (adapted from reference 29)*

Chemical	Approved (max. %)
Permitted	
para-Aminobenzoic acid (PABA)	5
N,N,N-trimethyl-4-(2-oxoborn-3-ylidenemethyl) anilinium methyl sulphate	6
Homomenthyl salicylate	10
Oxybenzone	10
3-(Imidazol-4-yl) acrylic acid and its ethyl ester	2 (expressed as acid)
2-Phenylbenaimidazole-5-sulfonic acid and its potassium, sodium and triethanolamine salts	8 (expressed as acid)
Provisionally approved	
2-Ethyl-4-bis (hydroxypropyl) aminobenzoate	5
Ethoxylated para-aminobenzoic acid	10
Glyceryl aminobenzoate (glyceryl PABA)	5
2-Ethylhexyl 4-dimethylaminobenzoate	8
2-Ethylhexyl salicylate	5
Amyl 4-methoxycinnamate	10
2-Ethylhexyl 4-methoxycinnamate	10
Mexenone	4
Sulisobenzone and sulisobenzone sodium	5 (expressed as acid)
Alpha-(2-Oxoborn-3-ylidene) toluene-4-sulfonic acid	6 (expressed as acid)
3-(4-Methylbenzylidene) bornan-2-one	6
3-Benzylidenebornan-2-one	6
1-p-Cumenyl-3-phenylpropoane-1,3-dione	5
4-Isopropylbenzyl salicylate	4
1-(4 tert-Butylphenyl)-3-(4-methoxyphenyl) propane-1, 3-dione	5

abundant sweating and repeated immersion in water is common.

Active sunscreen ingredients

Protectants against UVB

PABA. PABA has been available since 1943 and was popular in the 1950s and 1960s. Nowadays, PABA is utilized infrequently as a sunscreen for a variety of reasons. Its absorption peak at 296 nm is relatively far from the UVB-induced erythema peak at 307 nm.[18] It is poorly soluble in water and must be used as a 5–15% solution in alcohol. After application, PABA penetrates the stratum corneum effectively, where it

is trapped and remains bonded via hydrogen bonding to epidermal proteins. This greatly enhances its substantivity but also increases the risk for contact or photocontact dermatitis.[31] Sensitivity of this sort is seen in up to 4% of the population.[32] PABA can cause a stinging sensation when applied, and stains both cotton and synthetic fabrics. After photo-oxidation, this can leave a permanent yellow discoloration.

PABA derivatives. PABA esters are created by addition of hydrocarbon groups to the PABA molecule. Many of these molecules are an improvement over PABA in that they are water soluble and do not penetrate the stratum corneum. The most widely utilized of the PABA derivatives is Padimate 0, or octyl dimethyl PABA. Its absorption peak is more desirable at 300 nm in non-polar solvents, ranging to 316 nm in polar solvents.[18] Padimate A (amyl-dimethyl PABA) is similar to Padimate 0 and is also used in combination with other agents. Neither ester stains clothing, although both can cause stinging when applied.

Another derivative, glycerol PABA, has frequently been implicated as the etiological agent in both contact and photocontact dermatitis. However, after careful testing, it appears that contaminating impurities, including benzocaine, may actually have been responsible.[33]

Salicylates. These agents are ortho-distributed aromatic compounds with a peak absorption around 300 nm. Two compounds of this type, octyl salicylate and homomenthyl salicylate (homosalate), are currently approved in the US. Although not very effective as sunscreens, they have the benefit of being exceptionally stable, essentially non-sensitizing and water insoluble, leading to high substantivity. They are also useful as solubilizers of other poorly soluble sunscreen ingredients such as the benzophenones.[18] They are used commonly in 'PABA-free' products.[33]

Cinnamates. 2-Ethylhexyl p-methoxycinnamate (Parsol MCX) (absorption maximum 310–11 nm), 2-ethoxyethyl p-methoxycinnamate, and octylmethoxinnamate are available in the US. These are effective in blocking UVB but have poor substantivity and are generally found in combination with other agents.[8] Cinoxate is the cinnamate most often seen with other cinnamates, found in balsam of Peru, balsam of Tolu, coca leaves, and cinnamon oil.[33]

Protectants against UVA

Benzophenones. Benzophenones are aromatic ketones that absorb predominantly in the UVA portion of the spectrum between 320 and 350 nm. For example, oxybenzone has an absorption maximum of 326 nm in polar solvents compared with 352 nm in non-polar solvents. Benzophenone-3, sulisobenzone and dioxybenzone are also approved for the US market.[18] Oxybenzone is frequently impli-

cated as the etiological agent in photocontact allergy, although reactions have also been reported with dioxybenzone.[33]

Dibenzoylmethanes. Dibenzoylmethanes are substituted diketones which undergo keto–enol tautomerism on absorption of UVR. The keto form of the dibenzoylmethanes has a UV absorption maximum of 260 nm while the enol form absorbs > 345 nm. Parasol 1789 (avobenzone or 4-t-butyl-4'-methoxy-dibenzoylmethane), with an absorption maximum at 355 nm, is the only agent of this class available in the US. Although these compounds are capable of a high degree of UV absorption, they are unstable and can undergo photoisomerization to compounds which are not protective.[19] Parasol 1789 has been shown to have a loss of protective power as high as 36% due to photodegradation.[18]

Physical blockers. Physical blocking or reflecting agents such as zinc oxide, titanium dioxide, iron oxide, kaolin, ichthamnol (ichthyol), red veterinary petrolatum, talc ($MgSiO_x$), and calamine (FeO_2) are composed of particles of a size that scatter, reflect, or absorb solar radiation in the UV, visible, and even IR ranges. Twenty per cent zinc oxide, 20% titanium dioxide and 1% iron oxide have been spectrophotometrically demonstrated to reduce transmittance in the UVA and visible ranges to a maximum of approximately 20%. However, a combination of the zinc and iron oxides together is synergistic, effectively reducing transmittance in the UVA and visible ranges to as low as 1.5%. These data were confirmed in vivo in a hematoporphyrin derivative-sensitized guinea pig model.[6]

Older physical blockers had the disadvantage that they were comedogenic, had to be applied in a relatively thick layer, and melted in the sun, staining clothing. They were opaque and therefore visible, making them cosmetically undesirable for many individuals. These formulations found a market in young people who apply brightly pigmented products in limited areas. Because of their efficacy and broad-spectrum coverage, physical blockers are potentially important for persons with certain photosensitivity disorders.

Recently developed micronized preparations, now available in the US, provide an excellent option within this class of sunscreens. Micronized physical blockers are suspensions of finely ground material, such as titanium dioxide, which reflect at wavelengths shorter than the visible spectrum. Since they do not reflect in the visible spectrum, they are invisible and thus more cosmetically acceptable. Micronized titanium dioxide is chemically stable and does not cause any photoallergic or contact dermatitis.

Micronized sunscreens are more effective at the shorter UV wavelengths. A major difficulty in formulating micronized sunscreens is in preventing agglomeration of the particles. If this occurs, the portion of the spectrum reflected will shift into the visible range and the product will have characteristics of traditional opaque physical blockers.

Newer sunscreen filters

Most of the impetus for new sunscreens comes from Europe – notably France and Germany. This is probably because the regulatory authorities in Europe are more flexible towards new sunscreen ingredients than in the US, where these agents are classified as over-the-counter drugs rather than as cosmetic ingredients. Full investigations of new ingredients in the US following new drug applications are taking much time and investment.

A recent trend in Europe has been the filter Mexoryl SX, produced by the French company L'Oréal. This has excellent broad-spectrum UVA absorption and seems more photostable and versatile in formulation compared to avobenzone. Mexoryl is currently not available in the US.

Newer ingredients are being developed that may have greater flexibility in formulation and combination with other sunscreen filters. These are important developments because of the established importance of UVA in skin photoaging.

Sunscreen vehicles

The choice of vehicle for a sunscreen is important for several reasons. First, the proper vehicle can enhance a sunscreen's substantivity or ability to remain on the skin, and therefore its effectiveness. Second, the wrong vehicle can act as a skin irritant, induce a phototoxic or photoallergic reaction, or may be comedogenic. Finally, a solvent may modify the sunscreening agent because of its polarity and thereby dramatically shift the absorption spectrum of the agent towards or away from the desired range.[7]

Sun protection

Sun protection for normal skin

It is well established that chronic exposure to UVB leads to deleterious effects on human skin, including photoaging and NMSC. Application of a UVB-blocking sunscreen does decrease the risk for development of NMSC. Therefore, the author recommends that patients utilize sunscreens depending on their skin phototype (Table 2.3).

Table 2.3. *Skin types and suggested sunscreen protection factors*

Skin type	Characteristic	Examples	Suggested SPF	
			Routine day	Outdoor activity
I	Always burns easily, never tans	Celtic or Irish extraction, often blue eyes, red hair, freckles	15	25–30 (waterproof)
II	Burns easily, tans slightly	'Fair skinned' individuals; often have blond hair	12–15	25–30 (waterproof)
III	Sometimes burns, then tans gradually and moderately	Most Caucasians	8–10	15 (waterproof)
IV	Burns minimally, always tans well	Hispanics and Asians	6–8	15 (waterproof)
V	Burns rarely, tans deeply	Middle Easterners, Indians	6–8	15 (waterproof)
VI	Almost never burns, deeply pigmented	Blacks	6–8	15 (waterproof)

Additionally, all individuals should be encouraged to stay indoors or seek shade during the peak hours of solar radiation flux from 10am to 2pm; a hat or a sun visor is a useful addition. Patients with pale complexions should be reassured that 'fair' skin is attractive. Those who insist on darker skin should use a self-tanning lotion containing dihydroxyacetone (DHA). Tanning salons should be avoided, since intense UVA exposure provides limited protection and induces photoaging and photoallergic responses.[34-39]

Individuals who spend a significant amount of time outdoors, particularly in areas of high solar flux, should be cautious about the acute and chronic risks from UV exposure and should be advised as to how to properly protect themselves. Included in this list of individuals are naturalists, skiers, hikers, bicyclists, fishermen, mountain climbers, gardeners, as well as members of certain professions (e.g. farmers and farm workers, lifeguards, and postal delivery persons).

Sun protective clothing

Although UV radiation is partially reflected by clothing, some lightweight fabrics typically worn in the summertime do not even provide an SPF of 15. Once damp from sweat or water, the SPF of some fabrics falls. The weave of some fabrics does appear to affect the flux of solar radiation through garments. Solumbra™, a maker of sun-protective wear, manufactures clothing that has been demonstrated in vivo to provide an SPF of > 30, regardless of textile, color, or moisture content.[2] Such special fabrics are useful for some photosensitivity sufferers. Practitioners should be aware that some fabrics provide protection via an applied coating which may lose efficacy over time. Formal protection standards for sun-protective clothing need to be developed.

Other barriers

Window glass effectively blocks UVR below 320 nm, thus providing solid protection against UVB. Tinted windows and the plastic interleaf found in auto windshields effectively block nearly all UVA.[40,41] However, front and side window tinting sufficient to protect individuals with UVA sensitive skin is illegal in many states in the US because of concerns about reduced driver visibility and limited ability for law enforcement officers to see what is happening inside such a vehicle.

CONCLUSIONS

Current understanding of the effects of sun on the skin continues to evolve. A relationship between UVB exposure and the development of basal cell and squamous cell carcinoma has been documented. It appears likely that high-dose exposure to UVR increases the risk for the development of malignant melanoma. Chronic exposure to either UVA or UVB increases the rate of skin aging.

Development of new, highly effective sunscreens, both of the traditional chemical kind as well as newer micronized physical blockers, continues. More effective UVB-blocking formulations may lead to increased cumulative sun exposure and thus increased UVA exposure. However, only time will delineate the impact this will have on the rates of skin cancer and skin aging. Meanwhile, physicians may most benefit their patients by discouraging sun exposure, and encouraging prudent and frequent use of sunscreens.

Patients who are seeking advice about treating their aging faces are, in the author's opinion, wasting their time and money if they do not start to use, or continue using, a broad-spectrum sunscreen. This is especially important if skin resurfacing procedures are performed, or if tretinoin or alpha-hydroxy acid creams are applied, as there is a potential increase in UV damage to skin not protected by effective sunscreens.

References

1. Scotto J, Fears TR, Fraumeni JF. Incidence of non-melanoma skin cancer in the United States. Washington, DC: US Dept of Health & Human Services Publication; 1983:82–2433.

2. Sayre RM, Lowe NJ. Scientific poster presentation at the American Academy of Dermatology Meeting, December 1992.

3. Stern RS. Sunscreen use and non-melanoma skin cancer. In: Lowe NJ, Shaath N, editors. Sunscreens: development, evaluation and regulatory aspects. New York: Marcel Dekker; 1990:85–92.

4. Thompson SC, Jolley D, Marks R. Reduction of solar keratoses by regular sunscreen use. N Engl J Med 1993;329:1147–51.

5. Kaidbey KH. The photoprotective potential of the new superpotent sunscreens. J Am Acad Dermatol 1990;22:449–52.

6. Roelandts RJ. Which components in broad spectrum sunscreens are most necessary for adequate UVA protection? Am Acad Dermatol 1991;25:999–1004.

7. Lowe NJ, Weingarten D, Wortzman M. Sunscreens and phototesting. Clin Dermatol 1988;6(3):40–9.

8. Luftman DB, Lowe NJ, Moy RL. Sunscreens: update and review. J Derm Surg Oncol 1991; 17:744–6.

9. Roberts J. Exposure to the sun. In: Auerbach P, editor. Management of wilderness and environmental emergencies, 2nd edition. St Louis: Mosby Inc; 1989.

10. Epstein JH. Biologic effect of sunlight. In: Lowe NJ, Shaath N, editors. Sunscreens: development, evaluation and regulatory aspects. New York: Marcel Dekker; 1990:43–54.

11. Lowe NJ. Sun protection factor: comparative techniques and selection of UV sources. In: Lowe NJ, Shaath N, editors. Sunscreens: development, evaluation and regulatory aspects. New York: Marcel Dekker; 1990:379–94.

12. Garmyn M, Sohrabvand N, Roelandts R. Modification of sunburn cell in 8-MOP-sensitized mouse epidermis: method of assessing UVA sunscreen efficacy. J Invest Dermatol 1989;93: 642–5.

13. Kaplan LA. Suntan, sunburn and sun protection. Wilderness Med 1992;3:173–96.

14. Harber LC, DeLeo VA, Prystowsky JH. Intrinsic and extrinsic photoprotection against UVB and UVA radiation. In: Lowe NJ, Shaath N, editors. Sunscreens: development, evaluation and regulatory aspects. New York: Marcel Dekker; 1990:359–78.

15. Kligman LH, Kligman AM. Ultraviolet radiation-induced skin aging. In: Lowe NJ, Shaath N, editors. Sunscreens: development, evaluation and regulatory aspects. New York: Marcel Dekker; 1990:55–72.

16. Kraemer KH. Heritable diseases with increased sensitivity to cellular injury. In: Fitzpatrick TB, editor. Dermatology in general medicine, 3rd edition. New York: McGraw-Hill; 1987:1791–811.

17. Garland CF, Garland FC, Gorham ED. Rising trends in melanoma: an hypothesis concerning sunscreen effectiveness. AEP 1993;3(1):103–10.

18. Shaath NA. Evolution of modern sunscreen chemicals. In: Lowe NJ, Shaath N, editors. Sunscreens: development, evaluation and regulatory aspects. New York: Marcel Dekker; 1990:3–36.

19. Lowe NJ, Dromgoole SH, Sefton J, et al. Indoor and outdoor efficacy testing of a broad spectrum sunscreen against ultraviolet A radiation in psoralen-sensitized subjects. J Am Acad Dermatol 1987;17:224–30.

20. Lowe NJ. UVA photoprotection. In: Lowe NJ, Shaath N, editors. Sunscreens: development, evaluation and regulatory aspects. New York: Marcel Dekker; 1990:459–68.

21. Gotlieb A, Bourget T, Lowe NJ. Sunscreens: effects of amounts of application of sun protection factors. In: Lowe NJ, Shaath N, editors. Sunscreens: development, evaluation, and regulatory aspects. New York: Marcel Dekker; 1990:441–6.

22. Cole C, VanFossen R. Measurement of sunscreen UVA protection: an unsensitized human model. J Am Acad Dermatol 1992;26:178–84.

23. Kaidbey KH, Barnes A. Determination of UVA protection factors by means of immediate pigment darkening in normal skin. J Am Acad Dermatol 1991;25:262–6.

24. Agin PP, Stanfield JW. Letter in J Am Acad Dermatol 1992;27:136–7.

25. Chardon A. Immediate pigment darkening. Presented at the 4th Congress of the European Society for Photobiology, September 1–6, 1991.

26. Diffey BL, Robson JJ. A new substrate to measure sunscreen protection factors throughout the ultraviolet spectrum. Soc Cosmet Chem 1989;40: 127–33.

27. Roelandts R, Sohrbvand N, Garmyn M. Evaluating the UVA protection of sunscreens. J Am Acad Dermatol 1989;21:56–62.

28. Sayre RM, Agin PP. A method for the determination of UVA protection for normal skin. J Am Acad Dermatol 1990;23:429–40.

29. Janousek A. Regulatory aspects of sunscreens in Europe. In: Lowe NJ, Shaath N, Patnak MA, editors. Sunscreens: development, evaluation and regulatory aspects, 2nd edition. New York: Marcel Dekker; 1996:227–40.

30. Kaidbey KH. Substantivity and water resistance of sunscreens. In: Lowe NJ, Shaath N, editors. Sunscreens: development, evaluation and regulatory aspects. New York: Marcel Dekker; 1990:405–10.

31. Fisher AA. Sunscreen dermatitis: para-aminobenzoic acid and its derivatives. Cutis 1992;50:190–2.

32. Dromgoole SH, Maibach HI. Contact sensitization and photocontact sensitization of sunscreening agents. In: Lowe NJ, Shaath N, editors. Sunscreens: development, evaluation and regulatory aspects, 2nd edition. New York: Marcel Dekker; 1996:313–40.

33. Dromgoole SH, Maibach HI. Sunscreening agent intolerance: contact and photocontact sensitization and contact urticaria. J Am Acad Dermatol 1990;22:1068–78.

34. Mosher DB, Fitzpatrick TB, Ortonne JP, et al. Disorders of pigmentation. In: Fitzpatrick TB, editor. Dermatology in general medicine, 3rd edition. New York: McGraw-Hill; 1987.

35. Fusaro RM, Johnson JA. Topical photoprotection for hereditary polymorphic light eruption of American Indians. J Am Acad Dermatol 1991;24: 744–6.

36. Bickers DB, Pathak MA. The porphyrias. In: Fitzpatrick TB, editor. Dermatology in general medicine, 3rd edition. New York: McGraw-Hill; 1987;1666–715.

37. Bernhard JD, Pathak MA, Kochevar E, et al. Abnormal reactions to ultraviolet radiation. In: Fitzpatrick TB, editor. Dermatology in general medicine, 3rd edition. New York: McGraw-Hill; 1987:1481–506.

38. Roelandts RJ. Chronic actinic dermatitis. J Am Acad Dermatol 1993;28:240–9.

39. Callen JP, Roth DE, McGrath MA, Dromgoole SH. Safety and efficacy of a broad spectrum sunscreen in patients with discoid or subacute cutaneous lupus erythematosus. Cutis 1991;47: 130–6.

40. Stern RS, Weinstein MC, Baker SG. Risk reduction for non-melanoma skin cancer with childhood sunscreen use. Arch Dermatol 1986; 122:537.

41. Johnson JA, Fusaro RM. Broad spectrum photo-protection: the role of tinted auto windows, sunscreens and browning agents in the diagnosis and treatment of photo-sensitivity. Dermatology 1992;185:237–41.

3. Topical retinoids for the ageing face

Christopher EM Griffiths

INTRODUCTION

Although cosmeticians, dermatologists and entrepreneurial New World explorers have sought and occasionally claimed to have discovered the 'fountain of youth' this is still for the most part fantasy. The sole reason that fantasy is not absolute is because of the discovery made almost 20 years ago that topical retinoids have the ability to repair photoaged skin. Surprising as these first observations were, subsequent rigorously controlled clinical, biochemical and molecular studies, particularly by researchers at the University of Michigan, USA, have underscored the ability of topical retinoids to both repair and prevent photoageing. The major part of this work has focused on the role of all-trans retinoic acid (tretinoin) in this process but other retinoids possess similar properties.

As alluded to in other chapters, the title of this book is an acknowledged misnomer. More than 90% of therapies used for rejuvenation are in fact treatments for photoageing. Wrinkles and actinic lentigines (age spots) are mainly a legacy of cumulative, chronic sun exposure and to the general public (and many of the medical profession) are synonymous with senility. Intrinsic ageing of the skin is for the most part a subtle process unlikely to produce any major histological or clinical changes until the subject is over the age of 70 years. Indeed, intrinsic ageing is more likely to result in functional impairment whereas extrinsic ageing, e.g. sun exposure, produces the main cosmetic or appearance-related changes. The remit of this book is to provide advice for clinicians performing topical rejuvenation, i.e. a clinical textbook. However, retinoids may in themselves be a key factor in determining intrinsic ageing of human skin and the moniker 'premature ageing' sometimes used to describe photoageing or photodamage may not be entirely misplaced. Overall, the history of the use of topical retinoids to treat photoageing and perhaps ultimately ageing skin is fascinating and exemplifies the key attributes of clinical research, i.e. bench to bedside.

RETINOIDS

The parent molecule of all natural retinoids is vitamin A or all-trans retinol, an important fat-soluble vitamin (Figure 3.1). Vitamin A has pleiotypic effects on cell function most particularly differentiation and proliferation. The term retinoid is traditionally applied to vitamin A and its metabolites, i.e. first-generation retinoids.[1] Nowadays synthetic retinoids such as adapalene and tazarotene are entering the marketplace; although structurally dissimilar to all-trans retinol they have retinoid-like effects by virtue of their ability to bind to nuclear retinoid receptors, including the retinoic acid receptors (RAR) and retinoid X receptors (RXR).[2] These new drugs are known as third-generation retinoids.[1]

Perhaps the most important and potent metabolite of vitamin A is all-*trans* retinoic acid (tretinoin) produced via oxidation of retinol (Figure 3.1). Tretinoin has two important stereos-isomers: 13-*cis*-retinoic acid (isotretinoin), best known for its use in treating acne and 9-*cis*-retinoic acid that has important

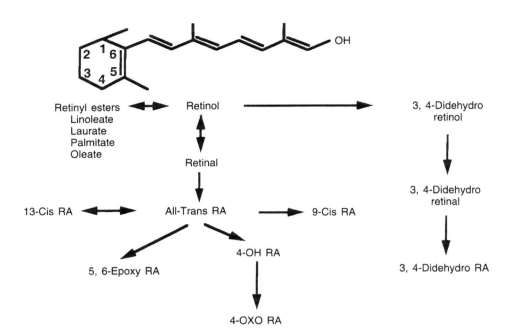

Figure 3.1 *Vitamin A (all-*trans *retinol) and its major metabolites.*

pharmacological properties currently under investigation for efficacy in the treatment of acne. Tretinoin is itself further metabolized, in a process dependent on retinoic acid 4-hydroxylase (a member of the cythochrome p450 family of enzymes).[1] The main products of tretinoin hydroxylation are the polar metabolites 40H and 40X0 retinoic acid, both of which, in mouse skin at least, have some retinoid activity as assessed histologically.[3] An interesting extension of the observation that retinoic acid 4-hydroxylase is a key step in the metabolism of tretinoin is that liarozole (an imidazole compound) will selectively inhibit this enzyme.[4] Consequently, orally administered liarozole has been found to have efficacy in the treatment of psoriasis.

As previously mentioned, retinoids only have an effect on cells following binding to cognate nuclear receptors (RAR and RXR) that belong to the steroid thyroid family of ligand-dependent nuclear transcription factors. This is an important family, particularly in the world of dermatological therapy, containing receptors for glucocorticosteroid, vitamin D and thyroid hormone amongst others.[2] Both RAR and RXR exist as three distinct subtypes: α, β and γ. Tretinoin binds solely to RAR, whereas its stereoisomer 9-*cis*-retinoic acid binds to both RAR and RXR. Intriguingly isotretinoin, at present, has no known nuclear receptor. A prerequisite for retinoid activity

in human skin is that epidermal and dermal cells contain RAR and RXR. It is now well established that the predominant nuclear receptors in the epidermis are RXRα and RARγ;[5] RARβ is expressed only in the dermis, but its expression in fibroblasts is further inducible by tretinoin. Tretinoin in topical form was first used for treating acne.[6] Topical tretinoin 0.1% cream obtained licensed approval for treatment of acne in the 1970s. As with many major leaps forward in the management of dermatological disease, the initial observation that topical tretinoin may alleviate facial wrinkling associated with photoageing was serendipitous. Young to middle-aged women using topical tretinoin for treatment of facial acne reported an improvement of fine periorbital wrinkling. As a consequence, Kligman et al., who made this observation, performed ground-breaking work to ascertain that topical tretinoin could indeed efface sun-induced wrinkles.[7] Their experiments used an animal model of photoageing developed by them – the albino *skh*-hairless-1 mouse irradiated with UVB for 10 weeks. Treatment of this photoaged mouse with topical tretinoin for 10 weeks produced a significant 'repair zone' of new papillary dermal collagen, later shown to correlate with wrinkle effacement.[8] This model is still relevant for studies of human photoageing. Subsequently two studies of topical tretinoin to treat human photoageing were made.[9,10]

In 1983, Cordero published a small, vehicle-controlled study on the effects of tretinoin on facial wrinkling.[9] He had observed that the use of tretinoin to treat comedones in Favre-Racouchot Syndrome also appeared to improve wrinkles on adjacent skin. Over the course of a 6-month study he observed that a 0.001–0.05% range of concentrations of tretinoin produced mild to moderate improvement in wrinkles at 6 months and actinic lentigines at 4 months. Kligman et al., following on from their animal studies, used tretinoin 0.05% cream in an open study for 3–12 months on photoaged faces and forearms. It seemed that tretinoin not only produced a clinical improvement in photoageing but that this was accompanied by deposition of reticulin fibres in papillary dermis and new blood vessel formation (angiogenesis) in the dermis. Surprisingly, this study concentrated, for the most part, on histological changes in tretinoin-treated skin with little documentation of clinical improvement.

Based on these observations, it was imperative that the ability of tretinoin to benefit photoaged skin was subject to rigorous vehicle-controlled trials. The first such trial was reported by Weiss et al. 1988.[11] They were able to demonstrate, in a 4-month randomized vehicle-controlled trial, that 0.1% tretinoin cream used once daily could significantly improve fine facial wrinkling. Documented improvement also occurred in coarse wrinkles, sallowness, tactile roughness and actinic lentigines, although the latter did not disappear despite lightening. Up to 92% of subjects using tretinoin in this study reported what is known as a retinoid dermatitis, i.e. erythema, pruritus and scaling, at the site of application. The issue of retinoid dermatitis is an important one: in some subjects it is a limitation to the use of tretinoin and has raised the legitimate question as to whether this 'irritation' is the mechanism underlying retinoid-induced repair. As discussed later, evidence for this is sparse in that topical tretinoin appears to have a specific, non-irritant mechanism of action. Further studies have confirmed these initial observations, whether using 0.05% tretinoin cream continually for 3–6 months[12] or in a dose-escalating fashion starting with 0.01% cream and finishing with 0.05% cream in an attempt to induce tolerance.[13]

As dryness, scaling and pruritus continued to be a problem, a new emollient cream formulation of

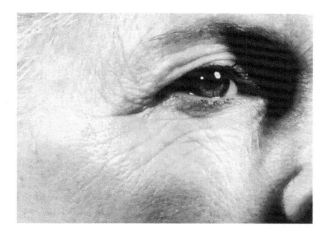

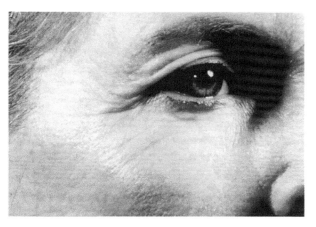

Figure 3.2 *50-year-old woman at baseline and after 40 weeks of treatment with once daily 0.05% tretinoin cream.*

0.05% tretinoin was developed specifically for the indication of Photoageing. This formulation (Renova®, Johnson & Johnson, USA) was trialled in two large multicentre studies to assess its efficacy and safety in the treatment of mild photoageing.[14,15] The number of assessable patients reported in these two studies combined was 547, of whom 393 had received tretinoin in doses ranging from 0.001 to 0.05%, once daily. The main message from these studies is that 6 months use of 0.05% tretinoin emollient cream is an effective treatment for fine wrinkling, mottled hyperpigmentation and skin roughness that are the results of photodamage (Figure 3.2). The ability of 0.01% tretinoin cream to effect such changes is somewhat uncertain: the study by Weinstein et al. was positive;[14]

and that of Olsen et al. was negative, with the 0.001% formulation producing no improvement over the 6 months of use.[15] Further studies have endorsed the efficacy of tretinoin cream for treating photoageing-associated wrinkles, despite initial speculation that assessment of this was a highly subjective process open to bias from the almost inevitably associated dermatitis.[16] The only truly objective methodology, not open to such accusations of bias, for assessing the response of wrinkles to treatment is the use of optical profilometry a technique developed and refined by Grove et al.[17] This method employs silflo replicas, i.e. moulds of the crow's foot area onto silicone rubber, whose ridges and furrows are then assessed by means of light scatter or shadowing from an oblique laser light source.[18] This technique of skin microtopography corroborates the purely observational measures employed in previous studies.

The ability of long term – over 1 year – tretinoin treatment to maintain improvement in photoaged skin has also been reported: Ellis et al. reported the results of 22 months of tretinoin treatment in 16 photoaged subjects.[19] In this study three treatment regimens were employed: all 16 subjects used 0.1% tretinoin once daily for 4 months and then (1) continued with this regimen (three patients) (2) continued with this regimen for 6 months and then changed to alternate day treatment for the last 12 months of the study (8 patients) or (3) used 0.05% tretinoin daily for 5 months (months 6–10 inclusive), and then reduced to alternate day treatment for months 11–22 inclusive. Overall, it appeared that improvement in wrinkling continued until month 10 and was maintained thereafter, despite a return of pretreatment epidermal thickness in this time. This observation infers that wrinkle effacement is a consequence of dermal changes. As a continuation of the large multicentre studies of tretinoin emollient cream,[14,15] patients were randomized to either stop treatment or to continue treatment for a further 24 weeks with 0.05% tretinoin used once or thrice weekly.[20,21] It appeared that thrice weekly treatment with 0.05% tretinoin cream was able to maintain improvement in fine wrinkles better than was achievable if applied only once a week. If therapy was stopped then some clinical deterioration occurred. Advice on how to use tretinoin cream for therapy of photoaged skin and the expected time line of improvement is given in Tables 3.1 and 3.2.

Although the major studies on photoageing took account of the effects of topical tretinoin on actinic lentigines and mottled hyperpigmentation, few trials have made this the primary outcome measure. In the original studies of tretinoin for treatment of photoaged skin there was only passing reference to lightening of lentigines. In both multicentre studies using 0.05% tretinoin lightening of mottled hyperpigmentation and actinic lentigines occurred.[14,15] Interestingly, the only significant histological correlation with improvement of any clinical feature in these studies was with lightening of actinic lentigines.[22] Reduction of epidermal melanin showed a weak

Table 3.1 *How to use 0.05% tretinoin cream in the treatment of photoaged facial skin*

Apply to whole face; initially four pea-sized amounts of cream, one each on the chin, each cheek and the forehead

Apply once daily, at night, following washing of the face

Moisturizer may be applied 20 minutes after application of tretinoin

Sunscreen SPF ≥ 15 applied at least daily prior to going outdoors

If tolerated, increase quantity of tretinoin applied each evening

If dermatitis develops, stop treatment for 1–2 days, apply moisturizer liberally, then restart with small pea-sized amounts of tretinoin

After 6–9 months, treatment can reduce to alternate day use to maintain improvement

Table 3.2 *Time course of improvement in photoaged skin following treatment with 0.05% tretinoin cream*

1–4 weeks	Smoothening
4–8 weeks	First lightening of lentigines
12–18 weeks	First improvement in wrinkles
24 weeks	If no improvement probably will not be of benefit and treatment should be stopped

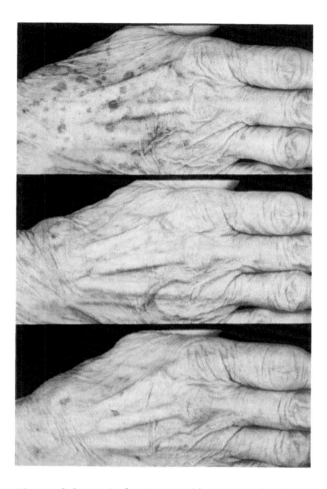

Figure 3.3 Hand of a 70-year-old woman at baseline and after 40 weeks of treatment with once daily 0.1% tretinoin cream and 27 months following cessation of treatment. Reproduced with permission from Rafal ES et al 1992.[23] Copyright © 1992 Massachusetts Medical Society. All rights reserved.

correlation with clinical lightening induced by tretinoin. Four studies have specifically addressed the effects of topical tretinoin in the treatment of actinic lentigines. These studies include different ethnic groups, one each from Caucasian,[23] Japanese and Chinese,[24] Thai[25] and Indonesian[26] subjects. The bias towards Far East Asian subjects reflects the observation that mottled hyperpigmentation and/or actinic lentinges are an important feature of photoageing in these populations.

The present author and co-workers performed a 10-month, vehicle-controlled study on the effects of once daily treatment of 0.1% tretinoin cream on facial and upper extremity actinic lentigines in Caucasians.[23] Eighty-four per cent of tretinoin-treated patients had clinical lightening or clearance of actinic lentigines, compared to 28% of the vehicle-treated group. Lentigines, on the face or upper extremities, responded equally well to treatment, with the first significant lightening observed after 4–8 weeks of treatment. However, the clinical diagnosis of actinic lentigines proved difficult; only 59% of biopsied lesions were histologically consistent with this diagnosis with the other diagnoses being flat, pigmented seborrhoeic keratoses and solar elastosis. Follow-up of these patients off tretinoin treatment (for up to 3 years) revealed that actinic lentigines which had disappeared on treatment remained clear (Figure 3.3). Using the same trial design, it was shown that 'brown spots', mainly actinic lentigines, in Japanese and Chinese people also lightened or cleared using tretinoin treatment (Figure 3.4).[24] An

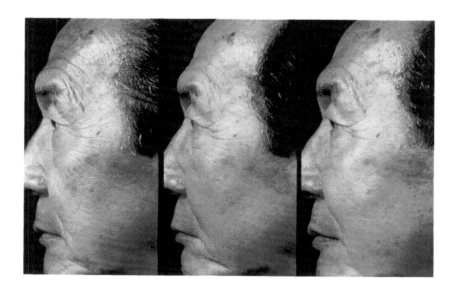

Figure 3.4 Face of a 65-year-old Japanese man at baseline after 24 and 40 weeks of treatment with once daily 0.1% tretinoin cream. Reprinted with permission from reference 24.

objective assessment of skin colour, a colorimeter, was used to measure the colour of individual pigmented lesions. Colorimeters work on the principle of light reflectance and thus provide an accurate, objective measure of clinical response not open to bias. Colorimeter readings correlated well with clinically observed lightening of lentigines. Studies in Thai[25] and Indonesian[26] subjects have confirmed the observation that tretinoin can lighten actinic dyspigmentation in different, skin types.

Consideration of irritation as the mechanism by which topical tretinoin improves photoageing was investigated by comparing the efficacy and irritancy of two concentrations of tretinoin cream, 0.1% and 0.025%, in the treatment of this condition.[16] Used once daily for 48 weeks showed no significant difference in the overall improvement in photoageing produced by the two concentrations but 0.1% tretinoin was significantly more irritating. This observation suggests that irritancy and efficacy can be divorced but it does not entirely exclude low-grade irritancy as a mechanism.

OTHER RETINOIDS

Isotretinoin

Compared with the burgeoning literature on the use of topical tretinoin for the treatment of photoaged skin, there are relatively few studies which assess the capabilities of other retinoids. A 36-week study of once daily isotretinoin 0.1% cream indicated efficacy in the treatment of coarse and fine wrinkles and actinic lentigines.[27] Isotretinoin appears to be less irritating and perhaps less effective than tretinoin; however, this may be because it requires isomerization to tretinoin for activity. Two other studies have reported improvement in fine wrinkles after 36 weeks of treatment, comprising an initial 12-week course of isotretinoin 0.05% cream followed by 24 weeks of a 0.1% formulation.[28,29]

Retinyl esters

The effectiveness of retinaldehyde (retinal) 0.05% cream in the treatment of photoageing has been compared directly with 0.05% tretinoin and vehicle creams over an 18-week period: retinaldehyde appears to produce significant improvements in fine and deep wrinkles, maintained at 44 weeks and confirmed by a second study.[30,31] Retinaldehyde is significantly less of an irritant (23% of subjects) than tretinoin. One randomized controlled trial indicated that a retinol–melibiose–lactose formulation produced significant improvement in fine wrinkles after 12 weeks of treatment.[32] Patch-test assay studies on normal human skin indicate that retinol may be as effective as tretinoin in producing 'retinoid histological changes' (keratinocyte proliferation) in the epidermis but with significantly less irritancy.[33]

There is no evidence that topical retinyl propionate (0.15% cream) is effective in the treatment of photoaged skin.[34]

Third-generation retinoids

Inevitably, the new, synthetic topical retinoids, adapalene[35] and tazarotene,[36] primarily developed and licensed for treatment of acne and psoriasis, respectively, have been investigated for their efficacy in photoageing. Initial studies appear promising for both drugs and it is likely that one or both will eventually be licensed for the treatment of photodamage.

MECHANISM OF ACTION

Considerable resource has gone into establishing how topical retinoids alleviate the clinical features of photoaged skin. When topical tretinoin was demonstrated to be of value in the treatment of photoageing the cellular, biochemical and molecular mechanisms of the photoageing process were poorly understood. On that basis, it is self-evident that any research aimed at unravelling the mechanism(s) of action of topical retinoids is highly dependent on a good working knowledge of the photoageing process. It is not the remit of this chapter, nor this book, to discourse extensively on mechanisms of photoageing. Discussed below is what is known about retinoid-induced smoothening (the first discernible change), lightening/clearance of actinic lentigines and wrinkle effacement.

Smoothness

The first change in skin topography to be reported by subjects using topical retinoids is a distinct smoothness of the treated skin. This change is noticed within the first month, often the first 2 weeks, of treatment. The rapidity of change indicates that skin smoothening results from events occurring in the epidermis due to the rapid turnover of keratinocytes. The smoothness is most probably a combination of compaction of the stratum corneum (from its usual rough, basket-weave appearance) and deposition of mucinous material between keratinocytes.[37] This mucin (glycosaminoglycans[38]) is colloidal, iron positive and testicular hyaluronidase digestible, implying a high content of hyaluronic acid. Hyaluronic acid is hygroscopic and thereby draws water into the epidermis, where it is retained. Furthermore, biochemical assays have demonstrated that epidermis treated with tretinoin assumes features of a wet, mucosal epithelium, e.g. expression of the simple mucin carbohydrate Le^y.[39]

Lightening of actinic lentigines

Biopsies taken from actinic lentigines, both pre- and post-treatment with tretinoin and assessed histologically, have helped confirm, perhaps unsurprisingly, that clinical lightening of these lesions correlates with a reduction in epidermal melanin.[23] How this is achieved is probably a result of several mechanisms: increased turnover and subsequent shedding of melanin-laden keratinocytes; reduced transfer of melanosomes from melanocyte to keratinocyte; and direct inhibition of tyrosinase activity.[40] It is important to note that, unlike hydroquinone, retinoids do not depigment normal skin. In fact, tretinoin treatment can induce melanin production in normal skin thereby producing a 'tanning effect'.[41]

Effacement of wrinkles

Perhaps the most discussed and dramatic effect of topical retinoids is their ability to efface wrinkles. Wrinkles are most probably a consequence of sun-induced deterioration in the extracellular matrix of the papillary dermis. As dermal cells turnover at a

slower pace than those of the epidermis, clinical improvement in wrinkles is slower in onset than the epidermally related lentigines and roughness. Components of the extracellular matrix inevitably make a major contribution to the tensile strength and integrity of human skin. Indeed, it has been shown that synthesis of collagen I,[42] III[43] and VII[44] (anchoring fibrils) are significantly reduced in photoaged skin. Fibrillin, predominantly synthesized by epidermal keratinocytes (as is collagen VII), is a key component of the dermal elastic fibre network providing the 'scaffolding' upon which elastin is laid down.[45] Fibrillin fibrils subjacent to the dermo–epidermal junction are rapidly lost in photoaged skin, thus providing an early histological marker of this process.[45] Accompanying the reduction in collagen synthesis is an increase in matrix metalloproteinase production particularly by the epidermis.[46] Thus, the net loss of collagens, and perhaps fibrillin, is a combined effect of reduced production and increased breakdown.

Treatment of photoaged skin with tretinoin results in increased synthesis of collagen I[42] and VII,[47] and fibrillin,[48] thus evincing repair (Figures 3.5 and 3.6). Moreover, tretinoin treatment of non-photoaged skin prior to irradiation with UVB has a prohibitive effect on subsequent damage.[49] Irradiation with UVB produces a significant rise in matrix metalloproteinases (collagenase, gelatinase) in human skin.[46] Repeat irradiation on this basis would eventually produce breakdown of collagen and the subsequent

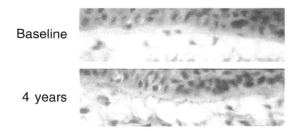

Figure 3.5 Fibrillin staining in photoaged facial skin: pre- and post-long-term (4 years) treatment with once daily 0.05% tretinoin cream. Note tretinoin-induced restoration of candelabra network of fibrillin in papillary dermis.

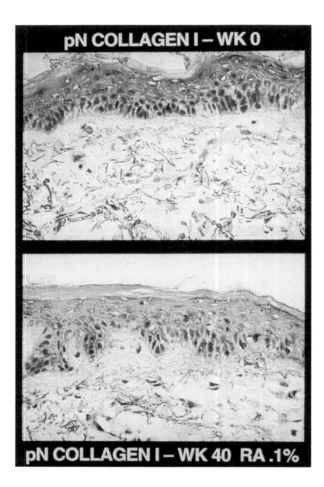

Figure 3.6 Collagen I staining in photoaged skin: pre- and post-48-week treatment with 0.1% tretinoin cream. Reproduced with permission from Griffiths CEM et al 1993.[42] Copyright © 1993 Massachusetts Medical Society. All rights reserved.

appearance of wrinkles. Treatment of skin with tretinoin prior to UVB exposure significantly inhibits metalloproteinase secretion, probably by a process of transrepression whereby the transcription factor NF-κB is blocked.[49]

Thus, topical tretinoin (and probably other retinoids) has a dual effect on the process of photoageing: (1) repair of already photoaged skin; and (2) prevention of further photoageing. These startling findings emphasize the key advantage that chronic tretinoin treatment has over the 'quick-fix' effects of dermabrasion, peels and surgery.

TRETINOIN AND AGEING SKIN

Intrinsic ageing of the skin has, for the most part, been overlooked, particularly in the world of cosmetic rejuvenation. However, the observation that there are, biochemically at least, some similarities between very old (> 70 years) and photoaged skin gives some validity to the statement that photoageing is premature ageing.[50] Indeed, old non-sun-exposed skin are characterized by reduced levels of collagens I and III and increased levels of matrix metalloproteinases.[50] Using a semi-in vivo culture assay of small pieces of adult sun-protected skin and neonatal foreskin it was observed that addition of tretinoin to the assay system induced topical retinoid changes (e.g. epidermal keratinocyte proliferation) in the adult skin but not in the neonatal one.[51] This observation infers that aged skin has enhanced retinoid sensitivity, possibly a consequence of retinoid deficit. Whether retinoid depletion is an effector or a consequence of the ageing process remains to be determined. Kligman et al. demonstrated that topical tretinoin applied for 6 months to sun-protected, chronologically aged skin of women induces a rejuvenated histological phenotype in the treated skin.[52] Further work by Varani et al. demonstrated that the relatively non-irritating retinoid retinol, used under plastic occlusion on aged skin (> 70 years) for 1 week, would restore levels of collagen III mRNA to those seen in skin from subjects half that age. Long-term clinical studies are now being conducted.[53]

CONCLUSIONS

Topical retinoids, and tretinoin in particular, offer the physician a dynamic long-term treatment and prophylaxis of photoageing and perhaps even ageing skin. Their pleiotropic effects are immense and tretinoin can be used in conjunction with most of the rejuvenating procedures currently in use. The main hindrance to use is the problem of irritation but this is only a problem in a few subjects, possibly a consequence of cellular retinoid receptor levels. The discovery of topical retinoid efficacy in the therapy of photoageing has not only provided one of the few truly evidence-based treatment modalities for this condition but the consequent research has provided a better understanding of the photoageing process.

References

1 Orfanos CE, Zouboulis CC, Almond-Roesler B, Geilen CC. Current use and future potential role of retinoids in dermatology. Drugs 1997;53:358–88.

2 Evans RM. The steroid and thyroid hormone receptor family. Science 1988;240:889–95.

3 Reynolds NJ, Fisher GJ, Griffiths CE, et al. Retinoic acid metabolites exhibit biological activity in human keratinocytes melanoma cells and hairless mouse skin in vivo. J Pharmacol Exp Ther 1993;266:1636–42.

4 Dockx P, Decree J, Degreef H. Inhibition of the metabolism of endogenous retinoic acid as treatment for psoriasis: an open study with oral liarozole. Br J Dermatol 1995;133:426–32.

5 Fisher GJ, Talwar HS, Xiao JH, et al. Immunological identification and functional quantitation of retinoic acid and retinoid X receptor proteins in human skin. J Biol Chem 1994;269:20,629–35.

6 Pedace FJ, Stoughton R. Topical retinoic acid in acne vulgaris. Br J Dermatol 1971;84:465–9.

7 Kligman LH, Akin FJ, Kligman AM. Sunscreens prevent ultraviolet photocarcinogenesis. J Am Acad Dermatol 1980;3:30–5.

8 Kligman LH, Chen HD, Kligman AM. Topical retinoic acid enhances the repair of ultraviolet damaged connective tissue. Conn Tiss Res 1984;12:139–50.

9 Cordero A Jr. La vitamina A acida en la piel senile. Actualizaciones Terapeuticas Dermatoligicas 1983;6:49–54.

10 Kligman AM, Grove GL, Hirose R, Leyden JJ. Topical tretinoin for photoaged skin. J Am Acad Dermatol 1986;15:836–59.

11 Weiss JS, Ellis CN, Headington JT. Topical tretinoin improves photoaged skin: a double-blind vehicle-controlled study. JAMA 1988;259:527–32.

12 Leyden JJ, Grove GL, Grove MJ, et al. Treatment of photodamaged facial skin with topical tretinoin. J Am Acad Dermatol 1986;21:638–44.

13 Caputo R, Monti M, Motta S, et al. The treatment of visible signs of senescence: the Italian experience. Br J Dermatol 1990;122(Suppl 35): 97–103.

14 Weinstein GD, Nigra TP, Pochi PE, et al. Topical tretinoin for treatment of photodamaged skin. Arch Dermatol 1991;127:659–65.

15 Olsen EA, Katz I, Levine N, et al. Tretinoin emollient cream: knew therapy for photodamaged skin. J Am Acad Dermatol 1992;26:215–24.

16 Griffiths CEM, Kang 5, Ellis CN, et al. Two concentrations of topical tretinoin (retinoic acid) p cause similar improvement of photoaging but different degrees of irritation. Arch Dermatol 1995;131:1037–44.

17 Grove GL, Grove MJ, Leyden JJ. Optical profilometry: an objective method for quantification of facial wrinkles. J Am Acad Dermatol 1989;21:631–7.

18 English DR, Armstrong BK, Kricker A. Reproducibility of reported measurements of sun exposure in a case-control study. Cancer Epidemiol Baiomarkers Prey 1998;7:857–63.

19 Ellis CN, Weiss JJ, Hamilton TA, et al. Sustained improvement with prolonged topical tretinoin (retinoic acid) for photoaged skin. J Am Acad Dermatol 1990;23:629–37.

20 Olsen EA, Katz HI, Levine N, et al. Tretinoin emollient cream for photodamaged skin: results of 48-week, multicenter, double-blind studies. J Am Acad Dermatol 1997;37:217–26.

21 Olsen EA, Katz HI, Levine N, et al. Sustained improvement in photodamaged skin with reduced p tretinoin emollient cream treatment regimen: effect of once-weekly and three-times-weekly applications. J Am Acad Dermatol 1997;37:227–30.

22 Bhawan J, Gonzalez-Serva A, Nehal K, et al. Effects of tretinoin on photodamaged skin. A histologic study. Arch Dermatol 1991;127:666–72.

23 Rafal ES, Griffiths CEM, Ditre CM, et al. Topical tretinoin (retinoic acid) treatment for liver spots associated with photodamage. N Engl J Med 1992;326:368–74.

24 Griffiths CEM, Goldfarb MT, Finkel LJ, et al. Topical tretinoin (retinoic acid) treatment of

hyperpigmented lesions associated with photoaging in Chinese and Japanese patients. J Am Acad Dermatol 1994;30:76–84.

25 Kotrajarus R, Kligman AM. The effect of topical tretinoin on photodamaged facial skin: the Thai experience. Br J Dermatol 1993;129:302–9.

26 Goh SJ. The treatment of visible signs of senescence: the Asian experience. Br J Dermatol 1990;122(Suppl 35):105–9.

27 Maddin S, Lauharanta J, Agache P, et al. Isotretinoin improves the appearance of photodamaged skin: results of a 36-week, multicenter, double blind, placebo-controlled trial. J Am Acad Dermatol 2000;42:56–63.

28 Sendagorta E, Lesiewicz J, Armstrong RB. Topical isotretinoin for photodamaged skin. J Am Acad Dermatol 1992;27:S15–S18.

29 Armstrong RB, Lesiewicz J, Harvey G, et al. Clinical assessment of photodamaged skin treated with isotretinoin using photographs. Arch Dermatol 1992;128:352–6.

30 Humphreys TR, Werth V1 Dzubow L, Kigman A. Treatment of photodamaged skin with trichloroacetic acid and topical tretinoin. J Am Acad Dermatol 1996;34:638–44.

31 Creidi P, Vienne MP, Ochonisky S, et al. Profilometric evaluation of photodamage after topical reinaldehyde and retinoic acid treatment. J Am Acad Dermatol 1998;39:960–5.

32 Pierard-Franchimont C, Castelli D, Cromphaut IV, et al. Tensile properties and contours of aging facial skin. A controlled double-blind comparative study of the effects of retinol, melibose–lactose and their association. Skin Res Technol 1998;4:237–43.

33 Duell EA, Derguini F, Kang S, et al. Extraction of human epidermis treated with retinol yields retro-retinoids in free retinol and retinyl esters. J Invest Dermatol 1996;107:178–82.

34 Green C, Orchard G, Cerio R, Hawk JLM. A clinicopathological study of the effects of topical retinyl proprionate cream in skin photoageing. Clin Exp Dermatol 1998;23:162–7.

35 Goldfarb M, Kang S, Griffiths CEM, et al. Photographic assessment of the effects of adapalene 0.1% and 0.3% gels and vehicle on

photodamaged skin. J Euro Acad Dermatol Venereol 2000;14:315 (abstract).

36 Sefton J, Kligman AM, Kopper SC, et al. Photodamage pilot study: a double-blind, vehicle-controlled study to assess efficacy and safety of tazarotene 0.1% gel. J Am Acad Dermal 2000;43:656–63.

37 Griffiths CEM, Finkel LT, Tranfaglia MG, et al. An in vivo experimental model for topical retinoid effects on human skin. Br J Dermatol 1993;129:389–94.

38 Fisher GJ, Tavakkol A, Griffiths CEM, et al. Differential modulation of transforming growth factor β_1 expression and mucin deposition by retinoic acid and sodium lauryl sulfate in human skin. J Invest Dermatol 1992;98:102–8.

39 Griffiths CEM, Dabelsteen E, Voorhees JJ. Topical retinoic acid changes the epidermal cell surface glycosylation pattern towards that of a mucosal epithelium. Br J Dermatol 1996;134:431–6.

40 Orlow SJ, Chakraborty AK, Pawelek JM. Retinoic acid is a potent inhibitor of inducible pigmentation in murine and hamster melanoma cell lines. J Invest Dermatol 1990;94:461–4.

41 Ho KK, Halliday GM, Barnetson RS. Topical retinoic acid augments ultraviolet light-induced melanogenesis. Melanoma Res 1992;2:41–5.

42 Griffiths CEM, Russman An, Majmudar G, et al. Restoration of collagen formation in photodamaged human skin by tretinoin (retinoic acid). N Engl J Med 1993;329:530–5.

43 Talwar HS, Griffiths CE, Fisher GJ, et al. Reduced type I and III procollagens in photoaged adult human skin. J Invest Dermatol 1995;105:285–90.

44 Craven NM, Watson REB, Jones CJP, et al. Clinical features of photodamaged human skin are associated with a reduction in Collagen VII. Br J Dermatol 1997;137:344–50.

45 Watson REB, Griffiths GEM, Craven NM, et al. Fibrillin-rich microfibrils are reduced in photo-aged skin. J Invest Dermatol 1999;112:782–7.

46 Fisher GJ, Wang ZQ, Datt SC, et al. Pathophysiology of premature skin aging induced by ultraviolet light. N Engl J Med 1997;337:1419–28.

47 Woodley DT, Zelickson AS, Briggaman RA, et al. Treatment of photoaged skin with topical tretinoin increases epidermal–dermal anchoring fibrils: a preliminary report. JAMA 1990;263:3057–9.

48 Watson REB, Craven NM, Kielty CM, et al. Effect of retinoic acid treatment on the abundance of fribrillin-rich microfibrils in photoaged skin. Br J Dermatol 2000;142:600.

49 Fisher GJ, Datta SC, Taiwar HS, et al. Molecular basis of sun-induced premature skin ageing and retinoid antagonism. Nature 1996;379:335–9.

50 Varani J, Fisher GJ, Kang S, Voorhees JJ. Molecular mechanisms of intrinsic skin aging and retinoid-induced repair and reversal. J Invest Dermatol Symp Proc 1998;3:57–60.

51 Varani J, Perone P, Griffiths CEM, et al. All-trans retinoic acid (RA) stimulates events in organ-cultured human skin that underlie repair: adult skin from sun-protected and sun-exposed sites responds in identical manner to RA while neonatal foreskin responds differently. J Clin Invest 1994;94:1747–56.

52 Kligman AM, Dogadkinn D, Lavker RM. Effects of tretinoin on non-sun-exposed protected skin of the elderly. J Am Acad Dermatol 1993;29:25–33.

53 Varani J, Warner RL, Garaee-Kermani M, et al. Vitamin A antagonizes decreased cell growth and elevated collagendegrading matrix metalloproteinases and stimulates collagen accumulation in naturally aged human skin. J Invest Dermatol 2000;114:480–6.

COMBINATION TREATMENT (Nicholas J Lowe)

Indications	Potential combination treatments	Chapter reference
Skin surface photodamage	Photoprotection	2
	Topical and physical skin lightening	3
Solar lentigo	Chemical peels	7
	Lasers – pigment	8
Telangiectasia	Lasers – vascular	9
	Lasers – hair removal	22
Skin laxity	Non-ablative laser rejuvenation	12
	Laser skin resurfacing	10,11
	Periorbital surgery	23
	Endoscopic surgery	24
	Fillers – temporary	17, 18
	Fillers – permanent	19
	Botulinum toxin	14

4. Other topical agents for the aging face

Zoe Diana Draelos

INTRODUCTION

The aging face is characterized by tissue laxity, dyspigmentation, fine wrinkles, coarse wrinkles, rough texture, and sallow color. There are a variety of surgical and medical procedures that have been developed to address each of these characteristics, yet there exists the need for maintenance of the skin surface and the use of topical agents to enhance antiaging procedures. A better understanding of skin physiology, coupled with advancements in raw materials and finished formulations, have allowed the development of topical agents useful in improving the appearance of the aging face. These topical preparations are more aptly termed cosmeceuticals, since they are cosmetics, yet have documented and intended pharmaceutical activity.[1] This concept was developed by Albert M Kligman to describe products falling somewhere between cosmetics and drugs.[2] The concept of cosmeceuticals was embraced by the cosmetics industry in 1961, when Reed published the guidelines for cosmeceuticals presented in Table 4.1.[3]

Table 4.1. *Reed concept of cosmeceuticals*

1. A cosmeceutical is a scientifically designed product intended for external application to the human body
2. A cosmeceutical produces a useful, desired product
3. A cosmeceutical has desirable esthetic characteristics
4. A cosmeceutical meets rigid chemical, physical, and medical standards

This chapter discusses the currently available substances available for incorporation into products that fall within the cosmeceutical realm. These substances include vitamins, botanicals, and other miscellaneous moisturizing ingredients.

VITAMIN COSMECEUTICALS

The value of oral vitamins in terms of wound healing and skin health is not disputed, but the usefulness of topical vitamin application remains controversial. This discussion examines what is currently known about vitamins commonly used in over-the-counter and prescription antiaging preparations. The vitamins currently formulated into antiaging preparations are: vitamin A, vitamin C, vitamin E, panthenol, niacinamide, essential fatty acids, biotin, and ubiquinone.

Vitamin A

Vitamin A is of primary importance to the survival of human and plant life in an environment rich in oxygen.[4] Vitamin A, and its precursor beta-carotene, are found in yellow, orange, and green vegetables, egg yolk, liver, butter, and fish oils. Plants especially high in vitamin A include spinach, carrots, sweet potatoes, squash, and cantaloupe. In the plant kingdom, vitamin A (retinol) functions as a free-radical scavenger, protecting plants from ultraviolet (UV) radiation damage. To humans, vitamin A is one of a family of natural and synthetic related derivatives collectively known as retinoids.[5] Retinoids are biologic modifiers that produce receptor-specific effects within the body. The naturally occurring retinoids will be discussed first.

Vitamin A is a component of all multivitamins sold for both children and adults. Current recommendations from the US Department of Agriculture and the National Cancer Institute call for a beta-carotene intake of 5.6–6.0 mg per day, either from natural or supplemental sources.[6] This minimum daily oral intake was determined after the review of human studies demonstrating an increased risk of lung cancer in persons with low beta-carotene consumption.[7,8] Vitamin A reservoirs are maintained in the liver; however, systemic toxicity can occur with excessive oral intake. Vitamin A is a known teratogen; however, it remains a component of prenatal vitamins in low concentration. High intake of vitamin A should be avoided during pregnancy.

As mentioned previously, oral vitamin A is an important endogenous antioxidant.[9] Oxidation occurs due to formation of oxygen radical species, such as hydrogen peroxide, superoxide anion, and hydroxy radicals that transfer their energy to living human cells resulting in damage. Cellular proteins, enzymes, DNA, and RNA are damaged, but oxidative damage to the unsaturated fatty acid component of cell membranes is of primary importance. Hydroxy radicals initiate lipid peroxidation in cell membranes to form lipid peroxides that are responsible for accelerated cutaneous aging. One of the primary oxidation products thought to induce aging is malondialdehyde (MDA).[10] Interestingly, MDA is also increased in cells that have undergone carcinogenesis. Oral vitamin A appears to have an effect on this process.

Recently, the use of topical forms of naturally occurring vitamin A in skin-care products has been popularized. Vitamin A can perform several different functions when topically applied. It is a known humectant, meaning that it can attract water from the dermis and viable epidermis to the stratum corneum. This aids skin hydration when the humectant vitamin A is combined with an occlusive agent, such as petrolatum or mineral oil, to prevent water evaporation. Vitamin A can also function as a preservative by preventing oxidation of the lipids in the moisturizer in the form of retinyl palmitate; however, this naturally occurring form of vitamin A has no biological activity.

There is some evidence that naturally occurring forms of vitamin A, such as retinyl palmitate and retinol, can function as topical antioxidants, enhancing functioning of the skin. It is now well recognized that the skin is an enzymatically active organ capable of metabolic alteration of topically applied substances. Retinyl palmitate can become biologically active following cutaneous enzymatic cleavage of the ester bond and subsequent conversion of retinol to retinoic acid. It is this cutaneous conversion of retinol to retinoic acid that is responsible for the biological activity of some of the new stabilized over-the-counter vitamin A preparations.[11] Unfortunately, only small amounts of retinyl palmitate and retinol can be converted by the skin, accounting for the increased efficacy seen with prescription preparations containing retinoic acid (see below).

The vitamin A derivatives that have been discussed up to this point are considered to be nutritional supplements and thus are found in cosmetic preparations. Synthetic vitamin A derivatives – designed to alter the structure and function of the skin – include tretinoin (Retin-A®, Ortho), 13-cis-retinoic acid (Accutane®, Roche), acitretin (Soriatane®, Roche), adapalene (Differin®, Galderma), and tazarotene (Tazorac®, Allergan). The synthetic retinoids, as well as the naturally occurring forms of vitamin A, are difficult to formulate due to their inherent photoinstability. As antioxidants, upon light exposure they degrade immediately to biologically inactive forms. For this reason, oral forms of synthetic and natural vitamin A are packaged in amber bottles to prevent UV radiation exposure and prescription topical retinoids are packaged in opaque metal or plastic tubes. Topical preparations where the retinoid has oxidized turn yellow, an indication that some degradation has occurred.[12]

The remainder of this discussion focuses on the use of topical synthetic retinoids for purposes of decreasing and reversing the signs of cutaneous aging.[13] The use of retinoids in the reversal and prevention of photoaging was discovered by Albert M Kligman, who noted that topical tretinoin improved wrinkling, lentigenes, roughness, and precancerous actinic keratoses.[14] The list of observed retinoid effects is summarized in Table 4.2.[9,15]

The initial effect observed following the first few weeks of topical tretinoin treatment is improvement

Table 4.2. *Cutaneous effects of vitamin A*

Gross dermatologic effects
1. Improvement in fine and coarse facial wrinkling
2. Decreased tactile roughness
3. Reduction of actinic keratoses
4. Lightening of solar lentigenes

Histologic dermatologic effects
1. Reduction in stratum corneum cohesion
2. Decreased epidermal hyperplasia
3. Increased production of collagen, elastin, and fibronectin
4. Reduction in tonofilaments, desmosomes, melanosomes
5. More numerous Langerhans cells
6. Angiogenesis
7. Decreased glycosaminoglycans
8. Reduced activity of collagenase and gelatinase
9. Normalization of keratinization of the pilosebaceous unit

Dermatologic disease
1. Enhanced wound healing
2. Reduction in open and closed comedones
3. Improved appearance of striae distensae
4. Healing of inflammatory cystic acne
5. Improvement in disorders of keratinization
6. Normalization of skin in psoriasis

in tactile smoothness. This is felt to be due to a stratum corneum with a more compact pattern with increased epidermal thickness due to spongiosis.[16] Increased hyaluronic acid is also produced, allowing the water-holding capacity of the skin to increase, also contributing to the early improvement in skin smoothness.[17] Thickening also occurs in the epidermal granular cell layer.[18] The effect of topical tretinoin following 4 months of use is an improvement in fine wrinkles, representing a dermal effect, which is due to an increase in collagen production.[19] Furthermore, it has been demonstrated that tretinoin decreases UVB-induced collagenase activity, thus preventing photoaging.[20] Topical tretinoin does not prevent photoaging by acting as a sunscreen, since it does not reduce UVB-induced erythema. The improvement in skin condition continues with prolonged use and may be seen in both sun-exposed and sun-protected skin.[21,22] Side-effects are consistent with hypervitaminosis A of the skin and include mild

skin irritation (erythema, peeling, burning) and a clinically insignificant burning sensation in the eyes.[23]

Topical tretinoin also appears to have an effect on skin pigmentation as seen by a decrease in cutaneous freckling and lentigenes.[24] It is the irregular grouping and activation of melanocytes that accounts for the dyspigmentation associated with photoaging,[25] but normalization of this change has been histologically demonstrated by Bhawan et al.[26] Improvement in dyspigmentation has also been demonstrated in Oriental and Black skin types.[27,28]

Initial studies also demonstrate that topical tretinoin may improve the appearance of early stretch marks, although the mechanism of action has not yet been elucidated.[29] Topical tretinoin has been anecdotally used on a variety of dermatoses, ranging from keratosis pilaris to oral lichen planus to actinic chelitis. It has been utilized as a penetration enhancer in combination with topical corticosteroids. Large-scale scientific studies have not been performed for these indications. It is certain that the role of topical retinoids in dermatology will become increasingly important as new synthetic derivatives are developed.

Vitamin C

Vitamin C, another of the antioxidant vitamin family, is vitally important to the proper functioning of the skin. The biologically active form of vitamin C is L-ascorbic acid, which functions as an antioxidant by scavenging and quenching free radicals, and by regenerating vitamin E from its radical form.[30,31] However, vitamin C can also act as an oxidant when in the presence of transition metal ions such as iron. Thus, its function is dependent on the hydrophilic cellular milieu in which it resides.

Vitamin C is a water-soluble vitamin found in vegetables and citrus fruits. Due to its water solubility, no toxic effects have been observed in populations taking more than 100 times the recommended daily dose of 60 mg/day. Oral consumption of vitamin C is necessary for wound healing, since it is a necessary cofactor for lysyl and prolyl hydroxylase, which stabilize the triple helical structure of collagen. Deficiency of endogenous vitamin C, known as scurvy, results in fragile tissues, bleeding gums, and characteristic corkscrew hairs. While the necessity of oral vitamin C ingestion is undisputed, the value of topical supplementation remains controversial.

The dermatology literature contains a few published reports of the topical effects of vitamin C which are worth reviewing. Darr et al. demonstrated enhanced cutaneous vitamin C levels following topical application of 10% L-ascorbic acid.[32] This work was completed in a porcine model and corresponding human data have not been published. Further work by Murray et al. demonstrated a decrease in the minimal erythema dose and less erythema following UVB exposure in human subjects treated with topical 10% L-ascorbic acid.[33] At the time of writing, vitamin C is not an approved photoprotectant in the US.

Even though the preliminary research on topical vitamin C has shown promise, this vitamin has been slow to enter the mass cosmetic market. This is due to the inherent instability of vitamin C when exposed to light, oxygen, and moisture. Vitamin C-containing products readily discolor on the shelf due to auto-oxidation, rendering them biologically inactive. One attempt to stabilize vitamin C is the development of magnesium L-ascorbyl-2-phosphate, which has enhanced stability and can be enzymatically converted by the skin to active L-ascorbic acid: Kameyama et al. have reported lightening of skin dyspigmentation with this formulation.[34]

Current vitamin C research has focused on methods of enhancing cutaneous reservoirs of vitamin C that are rapidly depleted upon exposure to sunlight. Once the stores are depleted, the body's ability to protect the skin from oxidative damage and ultimate photodamage is decreased. At the time of writing, the best way to deliver vitamin C to the skin is through oral ingestion. Body stores of vitamin C are only 1500 mg, which means that vitamin C deficiency can occur rapidly. Steady, regular consumption of fruits and vegetables is necessary to maintain a constant body reservoir, rather than the use of topical vitamin C preparations.

Vitamin E

The last antioxidant vitamin to be discussed is vitamin E. Vitamin E is a broad group of chemicals which includes the tocopherols and tocotrienols. The only biologically active forms are alpha- and gamma-tocopherol, with alpha-tocopherol possessing greater biological activity than gamma-tocopherol. Vitamin E is found naturally in the membranes of cells and organelles. It prevents oxidation of the polyunsaturated fatty acids of the phospholipids in the membranes by capturing singlet oxygen species,[35] and also stabilizes the membranes against damage by phospholipase A, free fatty acids, and lysophospholipids.[36]

Vitamin E is present in vegetables, oils, seeds, corn, soy, wholewheat flour, margarine, nuts, and some meats and dairy products. It is felt to be safe in doses of up to 3000 mg/day for extended periods of time; however, oral supplementation in the 400–1000 mg/day range is generally recommended in patients with a history of coronary artery disease. In this instance, vitamin E is used to decrease clotting of the blood and to minimize atherosclerotic plaques through its antioxidant effect. Patients who are undergoing surgery must stop oral vitamin E supplements, since it is a potent anticoagulant and can increase postoperative bleeding; it may also cause increased bruising.

The antioxidant capabilities of alpha-tocopherol are due to its ability to function as a lipid-radical scavenger able to terminate lipid-radical chain reactions. In this reaction, a low-energy tocopheroxyl radical is formed; however, this radical cannot function further as an antioxidant. Regeneration can occur in the presence of vitamin C to again allow the vitamin E to function as a radical scavenger.[37] It may also protect membrane proteins containing selenium or sulfur. The vitamin E concentration in the epidermis is about 1.0 nmol/g.[38] Even though its concentration in the body is relatively low, it is the most important lipid-soluble membrane-bound antioxidant in the body.

A variety of claims have been made regarding the topical effects of vitamin E on the skin including improved moisturization, increased softness, and better smoothness. These are cosmetic claims that do not require scientific validation. Medical photoprotective effects have been evaluated for both topical preparations. Topically applied alpha-tocopherol has been shown to inhibit UVB-induced edema and erythema, conferring a sun protection factor (SPF) of 3.[39] This is thought to be due to its ability to marginally absorb light and function as a free-radical quenching, lipid-soluble antioxidant.[40] Oral vitamin E was shown to confer no photoprotective effects.[41]

Vitamin E may also have an anti-inflammatory effect on the skin, due to the inhibition of the production and release of chemical mediators, such as histamine. It may also stabilize the membranes of lysosomes by interacting with eicosanoids to reduce prostaglandin E2 synthesis and increase IL-2 production.[42] This produces both anti-inflammatory and immunostimulatory effects.[43] A survey of elderly individuals found that high plasma tocopherol levels predisposed to a lower incidence of both infection and cancer.[44]

Vitamin E is lipophilic and can be incorporated into products for both the skin and hair in the form of vitamin E acetate, the stable esterified form of vitamin E, and vitamin E linoleate. One report lists vitamin E linoleate as a source of allergic contact dermatitis in a body lotion, probably due to improper formulation.[45] Vitamin E linoleate can enter into the epidermal lipids providing enhanced moisturization. It should be formulated at a pH of between 4.5 and 8.0 to enhance stability, in the presence of ascorbyl palmitate, BHA, and BHT.

Alpha-tocopherol is used as an antioxidant preservative in formulations to prevent the rancidity of fats, particularly unsaturated fatty acids and their derivatives. It is a more potent antioxidant when combined with ascorbyl palmitate, inhibiting the production of nitrosamines. There are some preliminary data, however, suggesting that alpha-tocopherol may be enzymatically metabolized during skin permeation, negating any antioxidant activity.[46]

Panthenol

The prior discussion has focused on the antioxidant vitamins A, C, and E, which are biologically active in skin physiology. There are other vitamins that are incorporated into topical formulations for their ability to function as actives, without biological relevance. An important topical vitamin in this regard is panthenol. Panthenol is the biologically active alcohol form of pantothenic acid, also known as vitamin B5, and is enzymatically converted to pantothenic acid in the skin. It is widely used topically as a skin- and hair-conditioning agent in moisturizers, shampoos, hairsprays, hairstyling aids, etc. Its function is best characterized as a humectant, since it can both hold and attract water, which is important since water is the plasticizing agent naturally found in both skin and hair.

There are four forms of panthenol utilized in hair- and skin-care products: d-panthenol, the dextrorotatory isomer, dl-panthenol, the racemic form, d-calcium pantothenate, and ethyl panthenol. The physiological activity of the racemic form is 50% less than that of the dextrorotatory isomer.[47] d-Panthenol is a colorless liquid and dl-panthenol is white crystalline powder, but both are oil insoluble. Aqueous solutions are most stable between pH 4 and 7. Panthenol can be used to control viscosity, maintain water content in the formulation, increase spreadability, act as a plasticizer, impart better glide, and improve the clarity of gel formulations. In skin preparations it is usually found at a concentration of 5%.

Many vitamin-enriched moisturizing creams and lotions contain panthenol at a concentration of 5%, which has been shown to enhance wound healing. As a humectant ingredient, it is able to attract water from the viable epidermis and dermis to the stratum corneum, where it must be trapped by an occlusive ingredient if the barrier to transepidermal water loss is impaired. Under conditions where the ambient humidity exceeds 70%, panthenol could also draw water from the environment. Panthenol is an important ingredient in many moisturizer formulations, since water that is applied to the skin in the absence of a humectant is rapidly lost to the atmosphere.[48] Humectants may also allow the skin to feel smoother by filling voids between the corneocytes through swelling.[49] Thus, panthenol functions not only to enhance the water-holding capacity of the skin but also to improve the tactile attributes of rough skin.

Panthenol functions similarly in hair-care products, where humectancy is also important to increase the water content of the hair shaft, thus increasing elasticity. Elasticity prevents hair-shaft breakage by increasing its resistance to trauma. Panthenol functions well in rinse-off products, since it is substantive for hair keratin and can actually penetrate the hair shaft through voids where the cuticle has been disrupted. Panthenol is used in concentrations of 0.75–1% for rinse-off products, such as shampoos, 0.5–0.75% for leave-on products, such as styling gels, and 0.25% for hairsprays. Thus, panthenol imparts increased manageability, better shine, less static electricity, and improved softness to damaged hair.

Niacinamide

Niacinamide, also known as nicotinamide, is the pyridine-3-carboxylic acid amide form of niacin. It is a white crystalline solid that is soluble in water, and stable to both heat and oxygen. It is found in the body in all metabolically active tissues, including the skin.[50] Niacinamide does not produce the flushing experienced with niacin, and nor is it valuable in the treatment of hyperlipidemias. It has no effect on blood pressure, pulse, or body temperature.[51]

Topical niacinamide is an interesting topical vitamin with some rather diverse reported cutaneous effects. Niacinamide has been shown to be of dermatologic benefit in the treatment of papular and pustular acne in a 4% gel.[52] It has also been reported to aid the treatment of bullous pemphigoid[53,54] and necrobiosis lipoidica.[55] Interestingly, niacinamide may be valuable in the antiaging armamentarium of the dermatologist. The antiaging cutaneous effects of niacinamide include the promotion of antitumor characteristics in keratinocytes[56] and the suppression of UVB photocarcinogenesis.[57]

The beneficial cutaneous effects from the topical application of niacinamide, especially the improvement in photocarcinogenesis and its antitumor characteristics, have led to further research as to the usefulness of niacinamide as a moisturizer additive. It is easy to formulate due to its water solubility and stability in the presence of light and oxygen. Niacinamide has appeared in several newly marketed antiaging moisturizers.

Essential fatty acids

Other substances that are traditionally ingested have also found their way into antiaging moisturizers. For example, essential fatty acids (EFA), sometimes referred to as vitamin F in the skin-care industry, are composed of unsaturated linoleic, linolenic and arachidonic acid. These fatty acids are termed essential since they cannot be synthesized by the body, thus requiring oral ingestion. Rodents that are fed diets missing EFA develop skin that is rough and dry in appearance, due to hyperkeratinization.[58] Rubbing sunflower oil onto the skin surface reduces the hyperkeratinization, since this oil is high in EFA; however, dietary intake of the EFA is the recommended treatment. It is difficult for humans to eat a modern diet completely deficient in EFA.

The EFA are very important in maintenance of the barrier function of the stratum corneum. Linoleic acid is found in high concentrations in ceramides, which are a major component of the intercellular lipids filling the spaces between the corneocytes. Topical application of pure linoleic acid is not desirable, since it is a strong cutaneous irritant and is unstable. Vitamin E linoleate is a better choice for topical supplementation of EFA and, for this reason, many barrier repair creams contain vitamin E linoleate.

Biotin

The discussion will now turn to oral supplements that are technically not vitamins but deserve attention due to their popularity in the present marketplace. One oral supplement that has gained modest scientific acceptance in dermatology is biotin. Biotin is a monocarboxylic acid functioning as a coenzyme in carboxylation reactions of fat, carbohydrates, and protein, and is considered to be a conditional B vitamin. It is synthesized by intestinal bacteria. It is mentioned in the context of vitamins, since it has been used as a supplement for preventing cracking in the hooves of thoroughbred race horses. Human oral supplementation has been shown to be effective in improving nail brittleness and nail peeling;[59] however, the beneficial nail effects of topical biotin have not been demonstrated. No standard accepted dose for oral biotin supplemention for nail splitting has been identified.

Ubiquinone

Ubiquinone, also known as coenzyme Q10, is a fat-soluble vitamin-like substance synthesized in all tissues of the body. It is not a true vitamin, since it can be manufactured endogenously from tyrosine. It is available, however, as an oral supplement and is finding its way into topical antiaging moisturizers. It is the 'ubiquitous' nature of this quinone family coenzyme that, in 1957, led Morton to name the substance he isolated from rat liver as ubiquinone. Folker and coworkers at Merck defined its chemical structure, but the first human application for oral ubiquinone was developed by Yamamura to aid in the treatment of congestive heart failure. Ubiquinone is found in mitochondria as part of the electron-transport chain and is felt to aid heart muscle contractility.[60] Medications, such as lovastatin, used to lower cholesterol are HMG-CoA reductase inhibitors and also block ubiquinone synthesis.[61] Oral supplementation with ubiquinone is also used in Japan for patients with periodontal disease and cancer.

Ubiquinone may also function as an antioxidant by providing electrons to oxygen radicals, and, for this reason, it is becoming an additive in many therapeutic dermatologic moisturizers. Since it is an endogenous antioxidant synthesized by the body when a normal solid food diet is consumed, it is unclear how topical supplementation affects the skin.

DERMATOLOGIC ISSUES REGARDING TOPICAL VITAMINS

The prior discussion concerning vitamins has presented the best science that is currently available regarding their usefulness in topical preparations. It is rather amazing that so little is known about the dermatologic benefits of vitamins, despite their large presence in the marketplace. Remember that vitamins are currently unregulated and considered a food supplement. This means that they can be easily added to a variety of skin preparations, without making any specific claim attributed to their functioning or effects. Once claims are made in this manner, the product becomes a drug and not a cosmetic. Thus, few manufacturers really wish to determine the implications of topical vitamin application. Rather, most companies simply state on the label that the product 'contains' a given vitamin, which technically is not a claim but a statement of fact. Nevertheless, the dermatologist needs to carefully assess the value of topical vitamin formulations. This discussion is aimed at providing a logical framework for product analysis.

Proper formulation of topical vitamins is the key to preparing a product with true skin benefit. The requirements for proper formulation are listed in Table 4.3. First, it is of primary importance that the vitamin additive meets the requirements for

Table 4.3. *Considerations for formulating topical vitamin preparations*

1. The vitamin must be non-toxic and of cosmetic grade
2. The vitamin must be bioavailable in the vehicle selected with substantivity for the skin
3. The vitamin must remain in its biologically active form during manufacture, in its final packaging, and under consumer-use conditions
4. The vitamin must reach the target tissue in its biologically active form

Table 4.4. *Vitamin stability*

Vitamin	Oxygen	Light	100°C	Acids	Bases
A	U	U	S	U	S
E	U	U	S	S	S
Niacinamide	S	S	S	S	S
Panthenol	S	S	U	U	U
C	U	U	U	S	U

U, unstable; S, stable

cosmetic-grade ingredients. This means that the raw material is without contaminants, verifying its concentration and purity: cosmetic-grade vitamins are less likely to cause allergic and irritant contact dermatitis. Second, the amount of the vitamin in the product must be sufficient to allow for adequate bioavailability. Also, the vehicle must be carefully selected to maintain the biological activity of the vitamin and promote cutaneous bioavailability. Third, the vitamin must remain biologically active until it is applied to the skin surface. This means that the vehicle must prevent chelation, inactivation, and degradation of the vitamin. Table 4.4 details the oxygen, light, temperature, and acid and base stabilities of some of the vitamins discussed previously. Notice, for example, that vitamin A and vitamin C cannot be combined in their biologically active forms in a moisturizer as vitamin C is an acid and vitamin A is unstable in the presence of acids. Lastly, the vitamin must enter the skin, escape enzymatic degradation, and reach the target tissue in a biologically active form. In some cases this may be the epidermis, which is the active site for the humectant panthenol. In other cases this may be the dermis, which is the site of oxygen-radical formation where antioxidants must reside in order to be biologically effective, and protect collagen and elastin.

In summary, much research remains to be conducted in the area of topical vitamins and their value as part of the cutaneous antiaging armamentarium. New formulations that are forthcoming should provide enhanced efficacy with scientifically documented results.

BOTANICAL COSMECEUTICALS

Another source of cosmeceutical additives to skin-care products, aside from the vitamins previously discussed, are plant extracts, also known as botanicals. Botanicals formed the basis of all early medical treatments. Increased understanding of human physiology, disease processes, and chemistry led to the extraction and synthesis of many medically important substances from these early botanical remedies. Recently, there has been a renewed interest in botanical extracts and their incorporation into cosmeceutical skin-care products.

This section discusses some of the currently popular botanical extracts with their purported value, chemical constituents, and interesting details. Botanical pharmacopeias contain thousands of plants with anecdotal purported skin benefits, unfortunately lacking scientific validation. This discussion focuses on cosmeceutical botanical extracts with the intent of offering antiaging skin benefits.

Ginkgo biloba

Ginkgo biloba is a plant with numerous purported benefits that is a common part of homeopathic medicine in the Orient. The plant leaves are said to contain unique polyphenols such as terpenoids (ginkgolides, bilobalides), flavonoids, and flavonol glycosides that have anti-inflammatory effects. These anti-inflammatory effects have been linked to antiradical and antilipoperoxidant effects in experimental fibroblast models.[62] Ginkgo flavonoid fractions containing quercetin, kaempferol, sciadopitysin, ginkgetin, and isoginkgetin have been

demonstrated to induce human skin fibroblast proliferation in vitro. Increased collagen and extracellular fibronectin were also demonstrated by radioisotope assay.[63] Various unknown ginkgo fractions are added to skin moisturizers for antiaging benefits, even though no controlled trials exist regarding cutaneous benefits.

Green tea

Green tea is another botanical popular in the Orient for both topical application and oral ingestion. Orally, green tea is said to contain beneficial flavonoids that act as potent antioxidants. A study by Katiyar et al. demonstrated the anti-inflammatory effects of topical green tea application on C3H mice.[64] A topically applied green tea extract containing GTP [(−)-epigallocatechin-3-gallate] was found to reduce UVB-induced inflammation as measured by double skin-fold swelling. Future research may result in topical green tea formulations that may reduce photoaging.

Echinacea

Echinacea, also known as black-eyed Susans or American cone flower, is native to Kansas, Nebraska, and Missouri, but can be propagated as an annual in any environment with ample water. It was a common botanical homeopathic remedy used by the American Indians that is currently seeing renewed topical popularity. The American Indians used every part of the plant for medicinal purposes: the fresh leaves were ground to produce an antiseptic and pain reliever for wounds and bites; the juice of the roots was used to bathe burns. Echinacea purpurea species is currently advocated for its antiaging value as an anti-inflammatory in moisturizers designed for mature, sensitive skin.

Prickly pear

Prickly pear, a plant native to the southwestern desert, is a cactus also known as cactus pear, Indian pear, or tuna fig. It is was imported to Europe in the sixteenth century and became a part of a salve designed to soothe cutaneous wounds and burns. The fleshy pad of the prickly pear contains 83% water and

10% sucrose, with small amounts of tartaric acid, citric acid, and other mucopolysaccharides. American Indians would rub the mucilage from the broken pad over the skin surface to act as a sunscreen and moisturizer. An extract of prickly pear is incorporated into some antiaging moisturizers to act as a soothing agent when other irritants, such as glycolic acid exfoliants, are also present.

Jojoba

Jojoba is currently a protected endangered plant in the southwestern United States. The plant is valued for the lightweight oil obtained from its fruit that is highly desirable in the skin-care industry. Jojoba is difficult to domesticate, so it is an expensive botanical additive. Jojoba oil was first used by the American Indians and Mexicans for its ability to soothe and heal wounds. The oil is now finding its way into antiaging moisturizers as a specialty additive, designed to retard moisture loss and improve fine, dehydration wrinkles of the face.

Aloe vera

Probably the most widely used botanical additive in antiaging facial moisturizers is aloe vera. The mucilage is released from the plant leaves as a colorless gel and contains 99.5% water and a complex mixture of mucopolysaccharides, amino acids, hydroxy quinone glycosides, and minerals. Compounds isolated from aloe vera juice include: aloin, aloe emodin, aletinic acid, choline, and choline salicylate.[65] The reported cutaneous effects of aloe vera include increased blood flow, reduced inflammation, decreased skin bacterial colonization, and enhanced wound healing.[66]

In most skin preparations, aloe vera is added as a powder, not as a mucilage. The composition of aloe vera powder may not be the same as that of aloe vera juice that oozes from the freshly broken plant leaf. It is estimated that aloe vera must be present at a concentration of 10% to have a moisturizing effect in products designed to remain on the skin for extended periods of time. Concentration and formulation are important considerations when determining whether or not a botanical additive has an antiaging skin benefit.

Allantoin

Allantoin is a currently popular antiaging botanical extract that is obtained from common comfrey root. It is felt to induce cell proliferation and act as an anti-inflammatory. Most allantoin currently used in skin-care products is not botanically derived, but rather manufactured by the alkaline oxidation of uric acid in a cold environment. It is a white crystalline powder that is readily soluble in hot water, making it easy to formulate in a variety of cosmeceutical moisturizing products.

MISCELLANEOUS COSMECEUTICAL MOISTURIZING INGREDIENTS

There are other active ingredients, besides those of botanical origin, that are found in many cosmeceutical moisturizers. Several substances, such as urea and petrolatum, have been used for many years in dermatology, and yet other ingredients, such as natural moisturizing factor (NMF) and sodium pyrrolidone carboxylic acid (PCA), are chemical entities developed through extraction techniques applied to the stratum corneum. All of these substances aim to increase the water content of the stratum corneum, which is commonly decreased in the aging face.

Urea

Urea is a bioactive ingredient that alters the structure of the stratum corneum. It is a penetrating moisturizer that possesses a high osmotic effect on the skin by diffusing into the outer layers of the stratum corneum and disrupting hydrogen bonding. This chemically exposes the water-binding sites on the corneocytes, allowing enhanced absorption of water. Urea also promotes desquamation and exfoliation by dissolving the intercellular cementing substance between the corneocytes. In this manner, it can also promote the absorption of other topically applied drugs functioning as a penetration enhancer for other actives.[67] Formulation with urea is somewhat difficult, however, since it must be present at an acidic pH or the urea will decompose to ammonia, which is both odorous and irritating. In the past urea has not appeared in moisturizer formulations due to problems with irritancy, but this drawback has been overcome by adsorbing the urea onto talc prior to dispersion into the emulsion. Urea is presently found in many exfoliating facial antiaging formulations that also contain hydroxy acids.

Petrolatum

Petrolatum is the most effective moisturizing ingredient on the market today, reducing transepidermal water loss by 99%. It functions as an occlusive agent to create an oily barrier through which water cannot pass. Thus, it maintains cutaneous water content until barrier repair can occur. Petrolatum is able to penetrate into the upper layers of the stratum corneum and aid in the restoration of the barrier, which is initiated through the production of intercellular lipids. There are three intercellular lipids implicated in epidermal barrier function: sphingolipids, free sterols, and free fatty acids. It has been established that these lipids are necessary for barrier function, since solvent extraction of these chemicals leads to xerosis directly proportional to the amount of lipid removed. Treatment of the skin with petrolatum increases the rapidity with which these lipids are synthesized in the skin.

Petrolatum impacts all phases of skin remoisturization, which is the first step towards barrier repair and wound healing. Remoisturization of the skin occurs in four steps: initiation of barrier repair, alteration of the surface cutaneous moisture partition coefficient, onset of dermal–epidermal moisture diffusion, and synthesis of intercellular lipids. It is generally thought that a stratum corneum containing between 20% and 35% water will exhibit the softness and pliability of normal stratum corneum. Petrolatum allows the water content to rise by decreasing evaporative losses, which creates the moist environment necessary for fibroblast migration leading to wound healing and eventual barrier restoration.

Some dermatologists are concerned that petrolatum is comedogenic. The comedogenicity of petrolatum is somewhat controversial, if standard lists of comedogenic substances are reviewed. It is important to recognize that comedone formation is based on the formation of a follicular plug, not on the oiliness or greasiness of the substance applied to the skin

surface. While oily or greasy substances can occlude the skin surface and the eccrine sweat ducts, resulting in the immediate formation of miliaria, comedone formation is a process requiring prolonged skin contact. Petrolatum is a hydrocarbon and can easily contain impurities if not well manufactured. Poor-quality petrolatum may indeed contain tar impurities and tar is a known comedogen; however, cosmetic-grade petrolatum is devoid of tar impurities and does not cause comedone formation. Perhaps some of the confusion regarding the comedogenicity of petrolatum is due to the comedogenicity of the impurities.

Outside of water, petrolatum is one of the most biologically active substances applied to the aging face. It fits the definition of a cosmeceutical, since it is a cosmetic with pharmaceutical significance. Petrolatum decreases the appearance of dehydration-related fine lines on the face. It functions to reduce itching and mild pain by creating a protective film over exposed lower epidermal and dermal nerve endings. It acts as an emollient by entering the space between the rough edges of desquamating corneocytes, restoring a smooth skin surface. It can also function as an exfoliant by loosening desquamating corneocytes, which are physically removed as the petrolatum is rubbed into the skin. Petrolatum is also an important component of many other cosmeceutical formulations that contain additional actives.

Natural moisturizing factor (NMF)

There are a group of substances reported to regulate the moisture content of the stratum corneum known as the natural moisturizing factor (NMF). The NMF consists of a mixture of amino acids, derivatives of amino acids, and salts. More specifically, the NMF contains: amino acids, pyrrolidone carboxylic acid, lactate, urea, ammonia, uric acid, glucosamine, creatinine, citrate, sodium, potassium, calcium, magnesium, phosphate, chlorine, sugar, organic acids, and peptides.[68] Ten per cent of the dry weight of the stratum corneum cells is composed of the NMF. Skin that cannot produce NMF is dry and cracked;[69] thus, it has been theorized that the addition of this ingredient cocktail to moisturizers may enhance water retention by the stratum corneum and miminize facial xerosis.

Sodium pyrrolidone carboxylic acid

Sodium pyrrolidone carboxylic acid (sodium PCA) is a substance that has been considered by some cosmetic chemists to represent the single ingredient that most mimics the NMF discussed above. It is the sodium salt of 2-pyrrolidone-5-carboxylic acid and experimentally has been shown to be a better moisturizer than glycerol.[70] Sodium PCA is used as a humectant in many cosmetics in concentrations of ⩾ 2%. In this role, it attracts water to the stratum corneum, which is valuable in minimizing the appearance of lines on the face due to dehydration.

SUMMARY

The number of ingredients available for incorporation into cosmeceutical agents is expanding rapidly. This chapter has covered a few of the well-known additives with purported benefits for the aging face. More advanced formulations with better stability and bioavailability promise to offer products with enhanced efficacy in the future. Novel delivery systems will also enter the marketplace as methods of increasing penetration of actives into the skin are improved. It is certain that the next millenium will bring better products for the aging face. This chapter is merely a primer.

References

1. Lavrijsen APM, Vermeer BJ. Cosmetics and drugs: is there a need for a third group: cosmeceutics. Br J Dermatol 1991;124:503–4.

2. Vermeer BJ, Gilchrest BA. Cosmeceuticals. Arch Dermatol 1996;132:337–40.

3. Epstein H. Factors in formulating cosmeceutical vehicles. Cosmet Toilet 1997;112:91–9.

4. Goodman DS. Vitamin A and retinoids in health and disease. N Engl J Med 1984;310(16):1023–31.

5. Garmyn M, Ribaya-Mercado JD, Russel RM, Gilchrest BA. Effect of beta-carotene supplementation on the human sunburn reaction. Exp Dermatol 1995;4:104–11.

6. Lachance P. Dietary intake of carotenes and the carotene gap. Clin Nutr 1988;7:118–22.

7. Ziegler RG. Vegetables, fruits, and carotenoids and the risk of cancer. Am J Clin Nutr 1991;53:2515–95.

8. Shekelle RB, Lepper M, Liu S, et al. Dietary vitamin A and the risk of cancer in the Western Electric Study. Lancet 1981;2:1185–90.

9. Noy N. Interactions of retinoids with lipid bilayers and with membranes. In: Livrea MA, Packer L, editors. Retinoids. New York, NY: Marcel Dekker; 1993:17–27.

10. Osawa T. Plant antioxidants: protective role against oxygen radical species. Cosmet Toilet 1994;109:77–81.

11. Duell EA, Derguini F, Kang S, Elder JT, Voorhees JJ. Extraction of human epidermis treated with retinol yields retro-retinoids in addition to free retinol and retinyl esters. J Invest Dermatol 1996;107:178–82.

12. Tsunoda T, Takabayashi K. Stability of all-trans-retinol in cream. J Soc Cosmet Chem 1995;46:191–8.

13. Kligman LH, Do CH, Kligman AM. Topical retinoic acid enhances the repair of ultraviolet damaged dermal connective tissue. Connect Tiss Res 1984;12:139–50.

14. Kligman AM, Grove GL, Hirose R, Leyden JJ. Topical tretinoin for photoaged skin. J Am Acad Dermatol 1986;15:836–59.

15. Goodman DS. Vitamin A and retinoids in health and disease. N Engl J Med 1984;310(16):1023–31.

16. Weiss JS, Ellis CN, Headington JT, et al. Topical tretinoin improves photoaged skin: a double-blind, vehicle controlled study. JAMA 1988;259:527–32.

17. Fisher GJ, Tavakkol A, Griffiths CEM, et al. Differential modulation of transforming growth factor-beta one expression and mucin deposition by retinoic acid and sodium lauryl sulfate in human skin. J Invest Dermatol 1992;98:102–8.

18. Olsen EA, Katz I, Levine N, et al. Tretinoin emollient cream: a new therapy for photodamaged skin. J Am Acad Dermatol 1992;26:215–24.

19. Woodley DT, Zelickson AS, Briggaman RA, et al. Treatment of photoaged skin with topical tretinoin increases epidermal–dermal anchoring fibrils: a preliminary report. JAMA 1990;263: 3057–9.

20. Fisher GJ, Datta SC, Talwar HS, et al. Molecular basis of sun-induced premature skin ageing and retinoid antagonism. Nature 1996;379:335–9.

21. Goldfarb MT, Ellis CE, Weiss JS, Voorhees JJ. Topical tretinoin therapy: its use in photoaged skin. J Am Acad Dermatol 1989;21:645–50.

22. Kligman AM, Dogadkina D, Lavker RM. Effects of topical tretinoin on non-sun-exposed protected skin of the elderly. J Am Acad Dermatol 1993; 29:25–33.

23. Weiss JS, Ellis CE, Headington JT, Voorhees JJ. Topical tretinoin in the treatment of aging skin. J Am Acad Dermatol 1988;19:169–75.

24. Weinstein GD, Nigra TP, Pochi PE, et al. Topical tretinoin for treatment of photodamaged skin. Arch Dermatol 1991;127:659–65.

25. Gilchrest BA, Blog FB, Szabo G. Effects of aging and chronic sun exposure on melanocytes in human skin. J Invest Dermatol 1979;73:141–3.

26. Bhawan J, Serva AG, Nehal K, et al. Effects of tretinoin on photodamaged skin a histologic study. Arch Dermatol 1991;127:666–72.

27. Griffiths CEM, Goldfarb MT, Finkel LJ, et al. Topical tretinoin (retinoic acid) treatment of hyperpigmented lesions associated with photoaging in Chinese and Japanese patients. J Am Acad Dermatol 1994;30:76–84.

28. Green CK, Griffiths CEM, Finkel LJ, et al. Topical retinoic acid (tretinoin) for melasma in Black patients. Arch Dermatol 1994;130:727–33.

29. Kang S, Kim KJ, Griffiths CEM, et al. Topical tretinoin (retinoic acid) improves early stretch marks. Arch Dermatol 1996;132:519–26.

30. Chan AC. Partners in defense, vitamin E, and vitamin C. Can J Physiol Pharmacol 1993;71: 725–31.

31. Beyer RE. The role of ascorbate in antioxidant protection of biomembranes: interaction with vitamin E and coenzyme Q. Arch Bioeng Biomem 1994;26:349–58.

32. Darr D, Combs S, Dunston S, Manning T, Pinnell SR. Topical vitamin C protects porcine skin from ultraviolet radiation-induced damage. Br J Dermatol 1992;127:247–53.

33. Murray J, Darr D, Reich J, Pinnell S. Topical vitamin C treatment reduces ultraviolet B radiation-induced erythema in human skin (abstract). J Invest Dermatol 1991;96:587.

34. Kameyama K, Sakai C, Kondoh S, et al. Inhibitory effects of magnesium L-ascorbyl-2-phosphate on melanogenesis in vitro and in vivo. J Am Acad Dermatol 1996;34:29–33.

35. Burton GW, Joyce A, Ingold KU. Is vitamin E the only lipid-soluble, chain-breaking antioxidant in human blood plasma and erythrocyte membranes? Arch Biochem Biophys 1983;221:281–90.

36. Kagan VE. Tocopherol stabilizes membrane against phospholipase A, free fatty acids, and lysophospholipids. Ann NY Acad Sci 1989;570: 121–35.

37. Kagan V, Witt E, Goldman R, Scita G, Packer L. Ultraviolet light-induced generation of vitamin E radicals and their recycling. A possible photosensitizing effect of vitamin E in skin. Free Rad Res Commun 1992;16:51–64.

38. Fuchs J, Hufleijt ME, Rothfuss LM, Wilson DS, Carcamo G, Packer L. Acute effects of near ultraviolet and visible light on the cutaneous antioxidant defense system. Photochem Photobiol 1989;50:739–44.

39. Idson B. Vitamins and the skin. Cosmet Toilet 1993;108:769–92.

40. Mayer P, Pittermann W, Wallat S. The effects of vitamin E on the skin. Cosmet Toilet 1993;108: 99–109.

41. Werninghaus K, Meydani M, Bhawan J, Margolis R, Blumberg JB, Gilchrest BA. Evaluation of the photoprotective effect of oral vitamin E supplementation. Arch Dermatol 1994;130: 1257–61.

42. Diplock AT, Xu G, Yeow C, Okikiola M. Relationship of tocopherol structure to biological activity, tissue uptake, and prostaglandin synthesis. In: Diplock AT, Machlin LJ, Paker L, Pryor WA, editors. Vitamin E: biochemistry and health implications. New York, NY: New York Academy of Sciences, 1989:72–84.

43. Meydani SN, Barklund MP, Liu S, et al. Vitamin E supplementation enhances cell-mediated immunity in healthy elderly subjects. Am J Clin Nutr 1990; 52:557–63.

44. Knekt P, Aromaa A, Maatela J, et al. Vitamin E and cancer prevention. Am J Clin Nutr 1991;53: 283S–6S.

45. Perrenoud D, Homberger HP, Auderset PC, et al. An epidemic outbreak of papular and follicular contact dermatitis to tocopheryl linoleate in cosmetics. Dermatology 1994;189:225–33.

46. Lee AC, Tojo K. Metabolism of vitamin E during skin permeation. J Soc Cosmet Chem 1996;47:85–95.

47. Idson B. Vitamins and the skin. Cosmet Toilet 1993;108:79–94.

48. Rieger MM, Deem DE. Skin moisturizers II. The effects of cosmetic ingredients on human stratum corneum. J Soc Cosmet Chem 1974;25:253–262.

49. Robbins CR, Fernee KM. Some observations on the swelling of human epidermal membrane. J Soc Cosmet Chem 1983;37:21–34.

50. Hankes LV. Nicotinic acid and nicotinamide. In: Machlin LJ, editor. Handbook of Vitamins. New York, NY: Marcel Dekker; 1984, pp 329–77.

51. Stratford MRL, Rojas A, Hall DW, et al. Pharmacokinetics of nicotinamide and its effect on blood pressure, pulse and body temperature in normal human volunteers. Radiother Oncol 1992;25:37–42.

52. Ellis CN. Niacinamide in the treatment of acne. Skin and Allergy News 1988;19(8):3.

53. Honl BA, Elston DM. Autoimmune bulous eruption localized to a breast reconstruction site: response to niacinamide. Cutis 1998;62:85–6.

54. Fiverson DP, Breneman DL, Rosen GB, Hersh CS, Cardone S, Mutasim D. Nicotinamide and tetracycline therapy of bullous pemphigoid. Arch Dermatol 1994;13:753–8.

55. Handfield-Jones S, Jones S, Peachey R. High dose nicotinamide in the treatment of necrobiosis lipoidica. Br J Dermatol 1988;118:693–6.

56. Ludwig A, Dietel M, Schafer G, Muller K, Hilz H. Nicotinamide and nicotinamide analogues as antitumor promoters in mouse skin. Cancer Res 1990;50:2470–5.

57. Gensler HL. Prevention of photoimmunosuppression and photocarcinogenesis by topical nicotinamide. Nutrition Cancer 1997;29:157–62.

58. Elias PM, Brown BE, Ziboh VA. The permeability barrier in essential fatty acid deficiency: evidence for a direct role for linoleic acid in barrier function. J Invest Dermatol 1980;75:230–3.

59. Hochman LG, Scher RK, Meyerson MS. Brittle nails: response to daily biotin supplementation. Cutis 1993;51:303–5.

60. Mortensen SA, Vadhanavikit S, Folkers K. Deficiency of coenzyme Q10 in myocardial failure. Drugs Exp Clin Res 1984;7:497–502.

61. Folkers K, Langsjoen PH, Willis R, et al. Lovastatin decreases coenzyme Q levels in humans. Proc Natl Acad Sci 1990;87:8931–4.

62. Joyeux M, Lobstein A, Anton R, Mortier F. Comparative antilipoperoxidant, antinecrotic and scavenging properties of terpenes and biflavones from Ginkgo and some flavonoids. Plant Med 1995;61:126–9.

63. Kim SJ, Lim MH, Chun IK, Won YH. Effects of flavonoids of Ginkgo biloba on proliferation of human skin fibroblast. Skin Pharmacol 1997;10: 200–5.

64. Katiyar SK, Elmets CA, Agarwal R, et al. Protection against ultraviolet-B radiation-induced local and systemic suppression of contact hypersensitivity and edema responses in C3H/HeN mice by green tea polyphenols. Photochem Photobiol 1995;62:855–61.

65. McKeown E. Aloe vera. Cosmet Toilet 1987;102: 64–5.

66. Waller T. Aloe vera. Cosmet Toilet 1992;107: 53–4.

67. Raab WP. Uses of urea in cosmetology. Cosmet Toilet 1990;105:97–102.

68. Wehr RF, Krochmal L. Considerations in selecting a moisturizer. Cutis 1987;39:512–15.

69. Rawlings AV, Scott IR, Harding CR, Bowser PA. Stratum corneum moisturization at the molecular level. Progr Dermatol 1994;28(1):1–12.

70. Wilkinson JB, Moore RJ. Harry's Cosmeticology, 7th edition. New York, NY: Chemical Publishing; 1982:62–4.

COMBINATION TREATMENT (Nicholas J Lowe)

Indications	Potential combination treatments	Chapter reference
Skin surface photodamage	Photoprotection	2
	Topical and physical skin lightening	3
Solar lentigo	Chemical peels	7
	Lasers – pigment	8
Telangiectasia	Lasers – vascular	9
	Lasers – hair removal	22
Skin laxity	Non-ablative laser rejuvenation	12
	Laser skin resurfacing	10,11
	Periorbital surgery	23
	Endoscopic surgery	24
	Fillers – temporary	17, 18
	Fillers – permanent	19
	Botulinum toxin	14

5. Facial rejuvenation: psychological issues

Eileen Bradbury

INTRODUCTION

The face is of profound importance in the psychological and social world of human beings. It is a powerful tool of communication and social interaction, and conveys information about age, gender, ethnicity, family and personal experience. Throughout the history of the human race, men and woman have decorated their faces to modify the effect they have on others. Warriors have painted their faces to look fierce, women have covered their faces with make-up and reddened their lips to look more sexually attractive. People have also hidden their faces through the use of masks, and thus hidden themselves. The face, untouched, reveals all. As human beings, we are sensitively attuned to all the messages a face may send, however subtle.

Given the power of the face, it is not surprising that people should seek to modify aspects of facial appearance and thus manipulate the responses of others. Creating a more youthful appearance has become one of the most popular ways in which facial appearance is modified. This chapter explores the social and psychological factors which influence attitudes towards facial rejuvenation, and describes the process of assessing patients prior to such intervention.

PSYCHOLOGICAL AND SOCIAL ISSUES IN FACIAL REJUVENATION

What are the factors which motivate people to look younger? These are many and varied but consistent themes do emerge.

Attractiveness

This is often the first reason that people put forward to explain their desire to look younger. Of all areas of research in the field of social psychology, some of the most consistent findings come from work into the impact of facial attractiveness. It is not simply a matter of aesthetics. From the times of the Greeks and Romans, physical attractiveness has always been a desirable construct, associated with positive character traits: 'What is beautiful is good' (Sappho, Fragments). Those rated as attractive are judged more positively than others, even by those who know them, and they tend to exhibit more positive behaviours and traits than others.[1]

However, it is not all good news. Attractive young people may find that they do not need to develop a range of social skills and other sources of social confidence. For such people, it is enough to be attractive in order to win attention and gain social popularity. Dating is easy and partners are not difficult to find. In this context, middle age can be a time of crisis, particularly when relationships are disrupted or employment is precarious. They may find they have become socially invisible and can no longer rely on appearance for social power. Those who have built their careers in the media and elsewhere on the basis of physical attractiveness may find that their careers falter as they get older. Thus, for those whose lives have been empowered by physical attractiveness, growing older is a serious threat to their social and economic status.

The underlying assumption of those seeking a more youthful appearance in order to look more attractive is that attractiveness is a construct of youthfulness. The female face most commonly rated as attractive is youthful with smooth skin, large eyes and a symmetrical appearance.[2,3] In fact, symmetry has been found to serve as a cue for youth in old age.[4] Whilst men have a little more leeway, they too are rated on appearance. They are seen as more attractive if they have a smoother skin and an alert and healthy look.[5] It has been found that women are attracted to men with the neotenous features of large eyes, the mature features of prominent cheekbones and a large chin, the expressive feature of a big smile, and high status clothing.[6]

These psychosocial factors are reinforced by dramatic technological changes. Differences between nations are mediated by the global internet village run by young people. Much of humanity in the twenty-first century shares the common experience of a culture dominated by images of beautiful young men and women. These images of beauty are universally images of youth. This is particularly true for women: there are very few older women on film or television and those who do appear are not portrayed as beautiful. Men do not escape unscathed: older men may play romantic leads but they have to be attractive and look young, fit and healthy. Only comedians escape these demands, for the jester has never been required to look attractive. In this common world culture, beauty is inextricably linked to youth. Although it has been found that older faces are less attractive, but more distinctive and memorable than younger appearing faces, people seeking facial rejuvenation are happy to exchange distinction for the advantages of a youthful look.[7]

There is also evidence that biological factors affect perceptions of attractiveness and link this to youth. Preference for attractiveness comes early, with 6-month old babies preferring to look at faces which adults find attractive.[8] There is a universal agreement about what constitutes attractiveness which supersedes cultural differences.[1] In addition, human beings share with animals a preference for the symmetrical face. This preference for a youthful symmetrical face could be linked to perceived reproductive success and the sign of a healthy individual.

Enhancement of social and economic status

Although the literature does reveal clear links between attractiveness and youth, the desire to look younger is more complex than this. In a world of youthful financiers, wealthy young footballers and teenage pop stars, youth is associated with power, status and control. Facial appearance has long been used to signal economic and social status. The white make-up applied to Queen Elizabeth I's face was in stark contrast to the tanned complexions of those of her subjects who worked in the fields. When overseas travel became fashionable for the wealthy, Coco Chanel encouraged a new trend in which a tan indicated that the individual could afford to travel.

Yet despite these vagaries of fashion, a smooth complexion has always conferred status, for both women and men. This links to biological factors described above, a signal that the individual is youthful, vigorous, fertile and economically strong.

Increased self-confidence and self-esteem

Given the powerful psychological, sociological and biological factors described above, there are obvious gains for those who look younger. This is of particular significance for those whose self-confidence is affected by other people's perceptions and judgements of them. The effect is most apparent when the individual is coping with a life crisis in which his or her self-esteem has been diminished. The newly divorced and the unemployed tend to be more vulnerable to other people's judgements.

Generally, those who are physically attractive are advantaged by social responses to them. An increase in attractiveness is often associated with increased levels of social confidence and self-esteem. Studies have demonstrated an association between improved physical appearance and increased self-esteem and interpersonal interactions.[9]

It is also a matter of temperament. Those most vulnerable to the perceived judgements of others will have a sense of being observed critically by others. In a study which examined links between attractiveness and eating disorders, the authors found that attractiveness was positively related to weight preoccupation, perfectionism and a tendency to be anxious and hypercritical.[10] These traits are likely to be reinforced by the ageing process, with the loss of control over facial appearance.

Finding or maintaining a relationship

Family dynamics are changing with great speed. One-third of marriages now end in divorce and 40% of adults live alone. In real terms, this means that many people find that they are on their own in middle age and will be seeking new relationships. In this context, physical appearance is of great importance. It is likely that, in the area of dating, those who are more attractive will be more successful in finding partners. Geneticists suggest that women with a youthful, neotenous appearance signal fertility and the continuation of the species. Bearing in mind the links between attractiveness and youthfulness described above, the search for new relationships is likely to precipitate a desire for facial rejuvenation. In one study it was found that whilst younger subjects rated younger and older attractive faces as equal in social desirability, older male subjects rated only younger attractive faces as socially desirable.[11] This will be of particular significance for older women who do not feel that they are attractive to older men and suggests that women would be at a greater advantage when seeking new relationships if they looked younger.

However, economic development has disrupted traditional social patterns. It may be that older men find younger women socially desirable: they may feel that it signals to others that they can support a younger woman and that they are sexually potent, and they may look to their younger partner as a reflection of their own sense of youthfulness. But times are changing. Younger women in many parts of the world have more economic power and do not necessarily seek an older man for financial security. If they are looking for financial security and economic power from a partner, they can often find it in young men whose high financial status can be achieved early in their careers. Independent young women may well be looking for someone who will be an equal partner. Men may seek younger female partners, but for the woman an older partner is likely to be at the end of his working life and thus lacking economic power, social status and physical vigour.

The older man cannot therefore necessarily attract the younger woman on the basis of age and financial status alone. He then begins to invest in facial treatments and to seek facial rejuvenation surgery to look younger, healthier and more tempting to the younger and more assertive female.

Male homosexual relationships have traditionally placed importance on appearance.[12] A fit and youthful appearance is often very important and those seeking to attract homosexual partners may feel that they need surgery, even at a relatively young age. In terms of gaining a partner, one study compared sexual partner age preferences of heterosexual and homosexual subjects and found that, like heterosexual men, homosexual men preferred a younger partner.[13] Thus the pressures remain.

Youthful appearance is not just an issue for those seeking new relationships. Many people in relationships will feel insecure and uncertain about their ability to hold their partner against the opposition of alternative potential partners.

Finding or maintaining employment

In this new century, public-sector work and traditional manufacturing is giving way to an economy dominated by the media, service industries and the world of the internet; all are types of work associated with the young. Jobs are no longer secure until retirement and the generation which assumed they would be employed for the duration of their working lives now find themselves seeking employment in competition with their children's generation. Those in employment may feel threatened by the younger people around them and fear they are perceived as being less vigorous than their younger colleagues.

Postponement of mortality

The Holy Grail is perpetual youth. Above all, youth represents life and a future. Old age leads inevitably to death. In the context of the twenty-first century consumer society, everything can be purchased and all aspirations are possible, limited only by the number of credit cards individuals can acquire.

It is not surprising that such consumers should seek to purchase the ultimate commodity, i.e. life. Without this, retail therapy is futile. The trap is permayouth – that state of suspended animation where people's faces stay young whilst the rest of their bodies age. Even when breasts are pert and stomachs taut, the back of hands, skin blemishes and general body shape disclose real age. Those unable to face old age who use surgery as a form of denial risk becoming dependent upon the illusion that they will live forever. For such patients, facial rejuvenation can never meet their needs but it allows them to believe that it does.

PREOPERATIVE ASSESSMENT

Despite the social, psychological and economic advantages of looking younger, not everyone benefits from surgery and other forms of treatment. There are some people who should not have surgery at all and others who should only undertake it with supportive preoperative counselling.

It is important for all those engaged in the work of facial rejuvenation to assess whether their patients should proceed, should only proceed with caution and support, or be discouraged from treatment. People seek this treatment in order to feel better about themselves, both psychologically and socially, and this must be an important aim of surgery. If surgical outcome fails to satisfy the patient, it fails completely, and the clinician needs to understand these dynamics in order to understand the responses of the patient following surgery and other forms of treatment.[14]

Patients who will benefit from surgery

Some patients will be clear candidates for surgery and will do well. They will fulfil the following criteria:

- they make a realistic appraisal of what they wish to change;
- they are flexible in their thinking and can modify their expectations in the light of technical information;
- their life situation is reasonably stable and they have established social and family relationships;
- they are sufficiently self-conscious and motivated to tolerate a range of technical outcome and do not demand perfection;

- they are not currently suffering from psychiatric illness.

Contraindications and caution

There are certain patients who should be assessed and treated with caution, described below.

Those in the middle of a life crisis

It is not unusual for people to seek radical change to their appearance when everything in their life appears to be out of control. Such people may be involved in an acrimonious separation, they may have recently lost their jobs, they may have just been through a serious illness or they may have been recently bereaved.

In a time of crisis, people tend to lose their sense of judgement. Decision-making is affected as they develop aims which bear little relationship to the likely outcome of surgery. For example, a woman who has been rejected by her husband for a younger woman may seek a facelift to gain revenge on him, to win him back, to win a younger man or to redirect her energies. She may tell the surgeon that she simply wants to look more attractive. It is conceivable that she might achieve one or all of these aims. However, it is also entirely possible that she will make a rushed decision, that she will not take heed of warnings about possible complications and less than perfect results, that she will be unhappy with any technical outcome because it does not achieve her covert aims. She may then redirect her energies and anger on to the (often male) surgeon.

A man who has been through treatment for cancer may want surgery to enable him to forget that he has this condition, by removing the memory of treatment from his stressed and thinner face. Someone recently bereaved may want surgery to gain some sense of control in a world that has gone out of control. However good the technical outcome, it is unlikely to achieve these aims, leaving the patient dissatisfied. If there are any problems with technical outcome, the tolerance of the patient will be minimal.

When the patient is in this situation, the clinician would be advised to suggest a more cautious approach, postponing any decision-making until things settle down. Some patients would benefit from referral to a counsellor to help them work through their current difficulties prior to any surgical intervention.

Those with a history of significant social and psychological problems

Some people seeking treatment do so as part of a life-long pattern of social and psychological dysfunction. This category includes those with a history of disastrous relationships, those who have suffered from eating disorders and those who have been abused.

For example, a young woman may seek a face lift because she cannot tolerate the way she looks. This comes out during the consultation process when it becomes clear that she wants to look entirely different. On further discussion, a troubled history emerges. Even when there is no active psychopathology at the time of consultation, this woman is profoundly influenced by her sense of low self-worth cultivated by her past history of physical abuse and her eating disorder. The desire for surgery is based on self-rejection and is unlikely to be of benefit to her unless she receives psychological therapy.

For such a patient, the clinician should encourage her to accept a referral for psychological help. Surgery alone is unlikely to solve her problems and may only precipitate more difficulties, especially if it does not go according to plan. She may well eventually benefit from surgical treatment which will improve her appearance, help her to have a fresh start and increase her self-esteem. However, this should only be carried out on the recommendation of the psychologist treating her.

Those suffering from psychiatric illness

People with a range of psychiatric problems can be attracted to cosmetic surgery. Those suffering from clinical depression may want surgery to give them a boost and lift their mood state. There is also a specific psychiatric condition, body dysmorphic disorder, which causes patients to harbour delusional beliefs about their appearance (see below). Whilst most clinicians are attuned to recognizing the depressed patient and the clearly psychotic patient, it is those with dysmorphic problems who may escape detection.

Body dysmorphic disorder (BDD)

This is described in the American Psychiatric Association's diagnostic criteria (DSM-1V, 300.7) as follows:

- preoccupation with an imagined defect in appearance. If a slight physical anomaly is present, the person's concern is markedly excessive;
- the preoccupation causes clinically significant distress or impairment in social, occupational or other important areas of functioning;
- the preoccupation is not better accounted for by another mental disorder (e.g. dissatisfaction with body shape and size as in anorexia nervosa).

It is important to recognize that not all those who are excessively preoccupied with a perceived defect suffer from BDD. They may have been taunted about their appearance by others, they may compare themselves unfavourably to media images of beauty or they may be going through any of the life problems described above. These people are able to discuss such issues and modify their thinking. The trait which characterizes those truly suffering from BDD is a fixed and delusional belief which is *not* amenable to reasoned discussion, and which is causing significant problems in functioning out of all proportion to the actual physical problem, or even the perceived problem.

Thus, a woman with BDD may become preoccupied with perceived loose skin under her eyes and request a blepheroplasty. The surgeon cannot see the problem as she describes it. Even when they both look in a mirror and she is pointing out the problem, the surgeon does not see it. The more they talk and the more resistance the surgeon puts up, the more agitated she becomes. She describes how she cannot get a job because she is so self-conscious and cannot go to interview. She stays at home because any social contact causes her acute distress as she cannot maintain eye contact.

There are other cues which distinguish those with BDD. The average patient who feels his or her appearance is judged critically by others is generally quite specific about external social judgements. Those with BDD refer less to external judgement, struggle to describe other people's perceptions and generally have difficulty empathizing with others. Their preoccupations are likely to be secret. In fact, it is notable how often such patients present as being socially isolated with limited relationships.

Another characteristic of people with BDD is the way they behave if surgery has been refused or delayed. They will frequently contact the clinician and/or the secretary on a regular, often daily, basis; they tend to be persistent because they have few other strategies for coping other than surgery. They also tend to become agitated and hostile when surgery is refused or opposition is put in the way; they plead and they threaten, they say they cannot cope without surgery; they generally refuse a psychiatric referral as they are fixed on a physical solution.

Sometimes, because of a desire to help, or out of fear that the patient will go down the road to a less reputable surgeon or because of the need to stop this patient pestering them (or for all these reasons), the clinician gives in and carries out surgery. Does it work? Phillips and co-workers found that all the BDD patients in their study failed to benefit from surgery.[15] If a patient has been deluded about what the defect looked like before surgery then they are unlikely to make a realistic appraisal of technical outcome. It is also unlikely that the patient will have paid attention to preoperative discussions about complications and scars, and so could be horrified by them. Following surgery, the patient is highly likely to seek further operations, as the first has not served their purpose of correcting the imagined problem. They may well return to the same surgeon, who becomes more and more enmeshed in this desperate enterprise until the patient finally goes to law and sues. The surgeon is then accused of clinical negligence because of operating on a patient who is clearly deluded and suffering from a known psychiatric condition.

There is a more severe type of this condition known as monosymptomatic hypochondriacal psychosis (MSP).[16] This is often associated with delusions about skin infestations or nose shape. For the patient concerned about the nose, it is generally accompanied by olfactory hallucinations. Such patients can become very aggressive and could be a serious threat to the surgeon.

Clinicians need to be alert to the psychiatrically disturbed patient: feeling pressured to carry out treatment against their better judgement is a clear sign that something is wrong. With such patients, trying to understand what they want from a surgical point of view is futile, and the clinician may be drawn into a collusive deluded view as he or she tries to empathize. Reinforcing delusions by 'seeing' defects that are not really there is deeply misguided and inadvisable for either surgeon or patient. Suggesting other areas of the face that may need treatment (even if they do) in such patients is ill-advised, as they will be receptive to the surgeon's expert view and develop a whole new range of problems which they will then demand that the surgeon rectify. This is a nightmare scenario of the surgeon's own making.

Such patients should be gently but firmly discouraged from surgery and encouraged to accept a referral to an experienced psychologist or psychiatrist. If this referral is refused, then there is nothing further the surgeon should offer, however sympathetic and caring. To act is to do harm.

PREOPERATIVE SCREENING PROCESS

Given the potential problems described above, how does the surgeon make a good assessment? This needs to be carried out during the course of the preoperative consultation. As most treatment for facial rejuvenation is privately funded, such a consultation is not subject to the pressures of time imposed by public health clinics. Some surgeons routinely offer two preoperative consultations, allowing the patient time to consider what has been discussed after the first consultation before returning for final preoperative discussions.

For patients who fit into the category of those likely to do well from surgery, then the bulk of the discussion can be taken up with technical issues. A few simple questions can establish the person's life situation. Agreement over what needs to be changed can generally be a straightforward affair. The best-informed and most reasonable patient may have unrealistic expectations based on articles in the media and needs to be clear about likely outcome, without the surgeon trying to be too optimistic or too pessimistic. Patients like to be told the truth and many resist the 'hard sell'. They are cautious and know that the media is full of horror stories about surgery that has gone wrong. However, because cosmetic surgery is frequently advertised at the back of women's magazines, it can be seen by some as a form of beauty treatment with no risks and an assured outcome. Thus, there is a tension in the media between the way cosmetic surgery is portrayed as routine and foolproof, and the scare stories which abound. For the clinician, a reasonable middle ground needs to be forged which acknowledges the potential problems but does not encourage unnecessary fears.

INDICATIONS FOR A PSYCHOLOGICAL OR PSYCHIATRIC REFERRAL

Preoperative assessment

A preoperative assessment is needed when the surgeon has concerns and feels that an opinion about the patient's psychological suitability for surgery would be helpful. This is likely to arise when there are pre-existing problems and/or a psychiatric history, when the patient presents in a way which worries the surgeon or when there have been problems following previous surgery which are not accounted for by poor technical outcome.

Decision-making

Potential patients may need help to reach an effective decision about whether it is advisable to proceed with surgery, or which type of surgery or other treatment they should have. Patients who are undecided generally appreciate the opportunity to explore issues and decide about surgery away from the surgeon's room with someone who understands the psychological and social issues but who does not benefit financially, or in any other way, from a decision to proceed. In a world where cosmetic surgery can be associated with sharp practice and slick salespersonship, it is reassuring to know that time can be taken with a neutral and objective professional to reach a decision, and the potential patient feels that his or her holistic needs are being met.

Psychological therapy

Some patients may have had a troubled history of psychological and social problems, or be suffering from a current psychiatric illness such as clinical depression. Apart from those diagnosed with BDD (see above), this does not preclude the individual

from surgery. Even those with schizophrenia have been found to have good psychological outcome from surgery if it is carried out in conjunction with a psychiatrist. However, it would be unwise to offer surgery unless in conjunction with psychological treatment. Generally, the psychologist will suggest that surgery be delayed until the patient is ready and has been treated. Sometimes the potential patient declines surgery once the psychological problems have been resolved and this is a financial risk the surgeon must be prepared to take. It is a greater risk to operate unwisely on a disturbed patient.

How to make a referral to a mental-health worker

Surgeons and other clinicians in the medical field may find it difficult to make this referral. They may feel that the potential patient would resist and be insulted. They may themselves be unsure of what they want from the referral and mistrust the psychologist or psychiatrist. Thus they may share the patient's scepticism, and this will inevitably be conveyed to the patient, ensuring resistance and non-attendance.

The most straightforward way to make such a referral is to encourage the patient to recognize that the desire for surgery is driven by emotions and a desire to feel better, and that it would be useful to have a session with someone who is able to address these issues. It is also helpful to encourage the patient to recognize that surgery can have a major impact on their lives and that they need to take time before surgery to consider what the effect will be and whether this is what they want.

It helps the clinician to build contacts with a counsellor, psychologist or psychiatrist. The mental-health worker can then gain information about surgical and other techniques, and the likely technical outcome; the surgeon can gain confidence in the psychological process. Thus mutual trust is developed, leading to future collaboration.

A word of caution! Sometimes clinicians want the psychologist to give them a reason *not* to operate when they have already made up their mind to refuse surgery: they use the referral as a way of saying 'no' to the patient. However, this should be clearly stated in the referral letter. If not, the psychologist may write back to say that there are no reasons to refuse on psychological grounds. This leaves the surgeon in the difficult position of having to operate against his or her better judgement. It also sours relationships between the surgeon and the mental-health worker, impeding further collaboration.

ASSESSING SATISFACTION WITH OUTCOME

Elsewhere in this book there will be measurements of good technical outcome. However, people seek facial rejuvenation treatment to improve their psychological and social well-being and not for technical reasons. Obviously, a poor technical result will not benefit them, but patients are remarkably tolerant of the result and the surgeon is often more critical of his or her work than the patient. If patients feel happier, more confident and less self-conscious, they tend to rate the operation as a success, even if the technical result is less than optimal.

The surgeon may be misled by the responses of the patient who feels grateful for the care and attention shown and who may not want to say anything to upset the surgeon. Measures of satisfaction which ask the question 'Are you satisfied?' tend to achieve the same bell-shaped distribution: 85%, very satisfied; 10%, satisfied; 5%, dissatisfied. This is because the patient is answering a different question, i.e. 'Have you been treated well?' If the surgeon is serious about measuring satisfaction he or she will need to separate process from outcome. This requires the clinician to ask two separate and distinct questions: (1) how does the patient feel about the process of treatment, the consultation, the preoperative care, the operation itself, the postoperative care; (2) how does the patient feel about the way the face looks now, the details of appearance, the physical sensations? Given the need patients often have to be polite and be grateful, such questions are best asked and answered anonymously, using unsigned questionnaires.

CONCLUSIONS

Those involved in facial rejuvenation treatment are dealing with psychological and social need. The best technical outcome may not result in the most successful procedure. In order to be effective, clinicians must be aware of their patients' relevant history, understand the aims and motivation of their patients, and make a good preoperative assessment based on this understanding.

References

1. Langlois JH, Kalakanis L, Rubenstein AJ, Larson A, Hallam M, Smoot M. Maxims or myths of beauty? A meta-analytic and theoretical review. Psychol Bull 2000;126(3):390–423.

2. Zebrowitz LA, Olson K, Hoffman K. Stability of babyfaceness and attractiveness across the life span. J Pers Social Psychol 1993;64(3):453–66.

3. Mealey L, Bridgstock R, Townsend GC. Symmetry and perceived facial attractiveness: a monozygomatic co-twin comparison. J Pers Social Psychol 1999;76(1):151–8.

4. Kowner R. Facial asymmetry and attractiveness judgement in developmental perspective. J Exp Psychol Human Percep Perform 1996;22(3): 662–75.

5. Maisey DS, Vale EL, Cornelissen PL, Tovee MJ. Characteristics of male attractiveness for women. Lancet 1999;353(9163):1500.

6. Cunningham MR, Narbee AP, Pike CL. What do women want? Facialmetric assessment of multiple motives in the perception of male facial physical attractiveness. J Pers Social Psychol 1990;59(1): 61–72.

7. Deffenbacher KA, Vetter T, Johanson J, O'Toole AJ. Facial aging, attractiveness and distinctiveness. Perception 1998;27(10):1233–43.

8. Rubenstein AJ, Kalakanis L, Langlois JH. Infant preferences for attractive faces: a cognitive explanation. Dev Psychol 1999;35(3): 848–55.

9. Patzer GL. Improving self-esteem by improving physical attractiveness. J Esthetic Dentist 1997;9(1):44–6.

10. Davis C, Claridge G, Fox J. Not just a pretty face: physical attractiveness and perfectionism in the risk for eating disorders. Int J Eating Disord 2000;27(1):67–73.

11. Perlini AH, Bertolissi S, Lind DL. The effects of women's age and physical appearance on evaluations of attractiveness and social desirability. J Social Psychol 1999;139(3): 343–54.

12. Rudd NA. Appearance and self-presentation research in gay consumer cultures: issues and impact. J Homosex 1996;31(1–2):109–34.

13. Silverthorne ZA, Quinsey VL. Sexual partner age preferences of homosexual and hetrosexual men and women. Arch Sex Behav 2000;29(1): 67–76.

14. Bradbury ET. The psychology of aesthetic plastic surgery. Aesthetic Plastic Surg 1994;18:301–5.

15. Phillips KA, McElroy SL, Keck PE, Pope HG, Hudson JI. Body dysmorphic disorder: 30 cases of imagined ugliness. Am J Psychol 1993;150(2): 302–8.

16. Munro A. Monosymptomatic hypochondriacal psychosis. Br J Psychiatry 1998;153(2):37–40.

6. Glycolic acid and other superficial peels

Zoe Diana Draelos

INTRODUCTION

Dermatologists and consumers alike have become fascinated by an interesting group of substances known as hydroxy acids, which provide antiaging and skin-smoothing effects. Hydroxy acids, which are incorporated into a seemingly infinite array of skin and hair products, have been used as part of the cosmetic armamentarium for thousands of years. The Egyptians were the first people known to rub fermented grape skins from the bottom of wine barrels over their skin to enhance beauty. The grape skins were rich in the hydroxy acid known as tartaric acid. The hydroxy acids form a family of chemicals intended to induce exfoliation, or removal of desquamating corneocytes from the skin surface. It is the removal of these dead skin cells that improves skin-surface smoothness and skin color. The benefits of cutaneous exfoliation are easily perceived by patients in a relatively short period of time, accounting for the continued research and development in this area. As opposed to photoprotection, where the benefits are delayed, exfoliation offers smoother skin with better color within one week.

The hydroxy acids can be subdivided into the following categories based on chemical composition: alpha-hydroxy acids, triple hydroxy acids, beta-hydroxy acids, combination hydroxy acids, and polyhydroxy acids. The most important issues regarding hydroxy acid performance can be evaluated in terms of type, concentration, and pH of the hydroxy acid, combined with the vehicle effects. The hydroxy acids can be applied to the skin in several different forms: lower concentration prolonged-contact hydroxy acid moisturizers or higher concentration short-contact skin peels. This chapter reviews the chemistry regarding hydroxy acids and their cutaneous effects, followed by a discussion of their use and formulation as topical peeling agents.

HYDROXY ACID CHEMISTRY AND MECHANISM OF ACTION

Alpha-hydroxy acids (AHA)

Alpha-hydroxy acids (AHA) are a group of organic carboxylic acids distinguished by a substituted hydroxy group (−OH) covalently bonded to the alpha carbon of a carboxylic acid. The linear, aliphatic nature of the AHA structure accounts for its water-soluble (hydrophilic) properties. The three subcategories of AHA consist of monocarboxylic acids [glycolic (2-hydroxyethanoic acid), lactic acid (2-hydroxy-propanoic acid), mandelic acid (2-hydroxy-2-phenylethanoic acid)], dicarboxylic acids [malic acid (2-hydroxy-1,4-butanedioic acid), tartaric acid (2,3-dihydroxy-1,4-butanedioic acid)], and tricarboxylic acids [citric acid (2-hydroxy-1,2,3-propanetricar-boylic acid)]. The intricacies of the formulation are more important than the nature of the AHA in terms of efficacy.[1]

AHA induce immediate epidermal effects through corneocyte disadhesion, which is thought to be operative by disruption of ionic bonding.[2] Several mechanisms have been proposed for this ionic

Table 6.1. *Alpha-hydroxy acid proposed mechanisms for corneocyte disadhesion from disruption of ionic bonding*

Mechanism 1	Increased distance between corneocytes due to hydration reducing cell cohesion
Mechanism 2	Enzymatic inhibition of transferases and kinases resulting in decreased electronegative sulfate and phosphate groups on the outer walls of the corneocytes reducing cell cohesion
Mechanism 3	Decreased pH leading to dissolution of desmosomes and reduced corneocyte adhesion

bonding alteration, summarized in Table 6.1.[3] This corneocyte disadhesion occurs histologically in the stratum corneum at the level of the stratum granulosum, until the cutaneous barrier has been disrupted, followed by dermal penetration.[4] The epidermal effects of AHA are a thinned stratum corneum with epidermal acanthosis.

The dermal effects of AHA are delayed and include decreased melanogenesis, unaltered angiogenesis, increased synthesis of glycosaminoglycans, prevention of topical corticosteroid atrophy, and increased dermal thickness, possibly due to the production of collagen through fibroblast proliferation, in a dose-dependent manner.[5,6] AHA have also been shown by Griffin et al. to induce factor XIIIa transglutaminase expression in dermal dendrocytes, which may account for some of the dermal changes seen in photoaged skin.[7] This proliferative effect is more pronounced with glycolic acid than with lactic or malic acid.[8] Penetration of the AHA into the deeper dermis can cause burning and stinging, as well as inflammation. It is currently unknown whether the antiaging dermal effects observed are due to this inflammation or a direct effect on cellular metabolism through actively or passively changing the ionic structure of various molecules in various pathways.

Triple hydroxy acids (THA)

Triple hydroxy acids are a variant of AHA. Usually, THA contain three complementary hydroxy acids, such as glycolic acid, lactic acid, and malic acid. The ultimate effect on the epidermis and dermis is the same as discussed previously, since in final formulation it is impossible to separate out the distinct contribution of the three distinct AHA entities.

Neutralized, esterified, and buffered alpha-hydroxy acids (AHA)

AHA are acidic substances, as discussed previously, that function to induce exfoliation through disruption in ionic bonding, which is in part due to the acidic pH of the hydroxy acids. Low-pH substances can be irritating to the skin, causing itching, stinging, and burning. Thus, formulating hydroxy acid preparations requires balancing efficacy with skin compatibility. In order to accomplish this end, several methods are used to alter the pH of AHA preparations: neutralization, esterification, and buffering.[9]

Hydroxy acids are frequently neutralized with an inorganic alkali or organic base to raise the product pH; this minimizes skin irritation but also decreases peeling efficacy, a topic of later discussion. For example, glycolic acid preparations are frequently neutralized with sodium hydroxide. However, completely neutralized glycolic acid, with a pH > 4.8, contains largely sodium glycolate, which has no cutaneous exfoliation properties. Thus, hydroxy acid preparations designed to induce peeling are only partially neutralized.

Hydroxy acid preparations can also be esterified. The process of esterification also raises the pH of the peeling preparation, which miminizes stinging and burning upon application. However, the degree of cutaneous exfoliation induced may also be decreased.

Hydroxy acid preparations can also be buffered to create a solution that resists pH change when an acid or alkali is added. This is important because the pH of the product may change when it encounters eccrine and sebaceous secretions or the intercellular compartments of the skin. Buffered formulations are not necessarily less irritating than their unbuffered counterparts. Buffering is strictly a method of insuring that some free acid is available once the peeling agent reaches the skin to induce exfoliation.

Lastly, it is worth mentioning that some AHA peeling solutions contain agents designed to minimize skin irritation by functioning as an anti-inflammatory. For example, strontium has been added to some glycolic acid peels to reduce stinging and burning, thus allowing prolonged skin contact and minimal post-peel erythema. Unfortunately, peels that reduce irritation also seem to demonstrate reduced efficacy in terms of the amount of induced exfoliation. Further research is needed on the relationship between irritation, pH, and exfoliation for AHA peeling preparations.

Beta-hydroxy acid (BHA)

The previously discussed AHA form only one component of the hydroxy acid family, which have been demonstrated to induce cutaneous exfoliation. A similar but chemically different hydroxy acid is salicylic acid (orthohydrobenzoic acid), the only beta-hydroxy acid (BHA). Salicylic acid is an organic aromatic carboxylic acid with a hydroxy group in the beta position. This phenolic, hydrophobic, lipophilic compound is a white crystalline powder, chemically unrelated to the AHA. Perhaps even labeling it as a hydroxy acid is somewhat of a marketing misnomer.

Salicylic acid is unique among the hydroxy acids as it can enter the milieu of the sebaceous unit, inducing exfoliation in the oily areas of the face and scalp.[10] For this reason, it has been used for years by dermatologists as a peeling agent to treat comedonal acne.[11,12] Salicylic acid, approved under monograph by the Food and Drugs Administration at a level of $\leq$ 2%, is incorporated into many shampoos designed to induce scalp exfoliation in patients with seborrheic dermatitis or psoriasis.[13]

Salicylic acid is thought to function through solubilization of intercellular cement, thereby reducing corneocyte adhesion. It appears to eliminate the stratum corneum layer by layer from the outermost level downwards.[14] This is in contrast to the AHA that appear to diminish cellular cohesion between the corneocytes at the lowest levels of the stratum corneum. This is probably due in part to the water-soluble characteristics of the AHA, which readily penetrate into the stratum corneum and the oil-soluble characteristics of salicylic acid, which remains on the stratum corneum. Differences in penetration also explain the decreased stinging and burning experienced with topical salicylic acid over glycolic acid peels, since the salicylic acid does not readily penetrate to the dermis.

Combination hydroxy acids (CHA)

CHA formulations combine an AHA and the BHA salicylic acid, with the intention of retaining the cutaneous benefits of both exfoliants (as discussed above). Thus, CHA are not new chemical entities but rather combination products that are difficult, if not impossible, to optimally formulate. This is due to the fact that only the free-acid component of the hydroxy acid can provide antiaging benefit to the skin, an important clinically relevant concept. The hydroxy acid that exists in the acid form is biologically active, whilst the one that exists in the salt form is not. Most hydroxy acid formulations contain both free acid and salt forms, since the products have been partially neutralized to prevent a low-pH product from inducing a chemical burn. The amount of free acid and salt can be readily determined by considering the pK_a of AHA and BHA.

The pK_a for the AHA is 3.83, whilst that for the BHA is 2.98. Products must be formulated at a pH close to the pK_a for optimal free-acid concentration and optimal efficacy. Thus, when a CHA prolonged-contact antiaging moisturizer is formulated it must be either AHA or BHA dominant, due to the inherently different pK_a of the hydroxy acids. At this time, CHA moisturizers designed for antiaging benefits are more of a marketing success than a clinical success; however, CHA peels offer added exfoliation benefits (discussed later).

Polyhydroxy acids (PHA)

The stinging and burning induced by the rapid penetration of AHA preparations into the dermis has led to the search for equally effective peeling agents with less dermal irritation. It is chemically known that high-molecular-weight substances traverse the epidermis more slowly than low-molecular-weight substances. This has resulted in the development of PHA exfoliant preparations which are chemically similar to AHA, but their higher molecular weights limit dermal penetration. The decreased dermal penetration theoretically means that there will be less stinging, burning, and irritation upon application, possibly allowing sensitive skin patients with rosacea or atopic dermatitis to find the products acceptable. PHA, such as gluconolactone, are water soluble like the AHA, exfoliating on the skin surface and not within the sebaceous unit. Their benefit depends solely on the formulation selected, and the decrease in dermal penetration may be only 1–2%.[15]

HYDROXY ACID FORMULATION

The preceding discussion focused on the various types of hydroxy acids that could be formulated into peeling preparations. It is important to remember that the degree of cutaneous injury and exfoliation achieved is directly related to the details of formulation. Hydroxy acids can only induce exfoliation at an acidic pH and at a sufficient concentration to induce a biological effect. The hydroxy acid must also be applied to the skin in a vehicle that delivers the desired clinical benefit with minimal irritation.

All hydroxy acids induce more exfoliation at low pH, but the optimal pH for formulation is determined by the pK_a of the active ingredient. One method of controlling pH is by altering the concentration of the hydroxy acid.[16] For example, 10% glycolic acid is four times more acidic than 1% glycolic acid. The acidity is chemically determined by electrostatic, inductive, and steric effects. In general, higher hydroxy acid concentration yields a lower pH and a greater biological effect; however, there is a limit to the acidity of a chemical that can be safely placed on the skin without inducing an uncontrolled chemical burn.

Safe properly formulated hydroxy acid products have a profound effect on the skin, with pH changes persisting for up to 2 hours. The extent of these pH changes depends on concentration: low 1% hydroxy acid concentrations can alter the pH of the outer three layers of the stratum corneum, while higher 10% hydroxy acid concentrations can affect the stratum corneum pH 10–20 layers deep. Thus, higher concentration hydroxy acids yield greater dermal penetration. For example, following glycolic acid application to the skin, 2.4% remains on the stratum corneum, 11.6% reaches the epidermis, and 8.6% resides in the dermis.[17] It is possible to enhance this dermal penetration through the use of substances that increase epidermal permeability, such as propylene glycol.[18]

HYDROXY ACID PEELS

Glycolic acid peels

Glycolic acid is the most frequently used AHA for skin peeling. It is formulated in concentrations varying from 10% to a fully saturated solution of 70%. Peel concentrations up to, but not including, 20% can be performed by an unsupervised esthetician, but > 20% concentration glycolic acid peels must be performed under the supervision of a physician. The danger from the use of glycolic acid peels arises from the fact that the material must be neutralized or removed from the skin surface to prevent further cutaneous effects. Chemical burns can result from prolonged exposure to high concentrations of glycolic acid. Moy et al. demonstrated the antiaging benefit of 50–70% glycolic acid solutions left on the skin for 3–7 minutes at 4-week intervals in patients with wrinkles and photoaging.[19] Table 6.2 lists the aesthetic benefits attributed to the use of glycolic acid peels.

Glycolic acid peels are also valuable in a large variety of dermatologic conditions.[20] For example, AHA can be incorporated into an acne treatment regimen for their ability to induce epidermolysis and dislodge comedones.[21] Briden et al. have used monthly glycolic acid peels in the treatment of rosacea.[22] Glycolic acid peels appear to be appropriate for individuals of both fair and dark complexions.[23]

Glycolic acid is readily available in a 70% aqueous stock solution and can be easily diluted with water to the desired strength for the physician who likes to self-formulate peels in strengths of 20%, 30%, 40%,

Table 6.2. *Aesthetic benefits of glycolic acid peels*

1. Improved skin color
2. Enhanced skin brightness
3. Smoother surface texture
4. Better skin tone
5. Increased skin firmness
6. Decreased wrinkling
7. Decreased dyspigmentation
8. More even facial cosmetic application
9. Enhanced benefits from the use of topical retinoids

Table 6.3. *Glycolic acid peel solution*

Glycolic acid peel (%)	Volume of 70% glycolic acid stock liquid (cm³)	Volume of water (cm³)
20	29	71
30	43	57
40	57	43
50	71	29
60	86	14
70	100	0

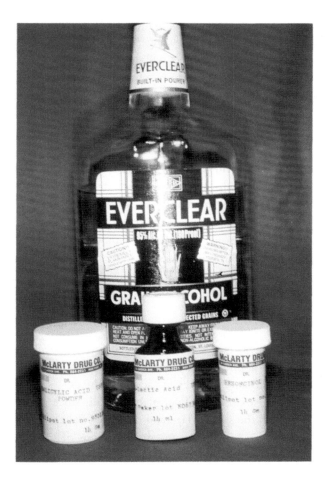

Figure 6.1 *Patented glycolic and salicylic acid peel solutions can be purchased for use in the office or self formulated as demonstrated.*

50%, 60%, and 70% (Table 6.3). These are unneutralized and unbuffered peels, which induce noticeable exfoliation. The different strengths are necessary to tailor the peel results to the patient's skin type and desired degree of exfoliation. The guidelines the author uses for peel selection are listed in Table 6.4. Many patented glycolic acid peels are also available for purchase (Figure 6.1).

The equipment used in performing a glycolic acid peel is shown in Figure 6.2. A basin filled with ice-water, ice cubes, and disposable towels is placed on the Mayo stand, along with a large rayon-tipped applicator. A stack of gauze and a small rayon-tipped applicator are kept close by in case the glycolic acid solution is inadvertently dripped. The desired concentration of glycolic acid is poured into a small crucible. Approximately 3 cm³ are used to peel an entire adult face. A fan is placed on the counter nearby and turned to a medium speed to move cool air over the face of the patient. The rayon-tipped applicator is inserted into the crucible and gently stroked over the face of the patient. Care is taken to avoid applying the glycolic acid peel to the nasal groove and to the corners of the mouth. The patient is asked to rate the degree of stinging and burning on a scale of 0–10, with 10 indicating a severe amount of discomfort. When the patient states that the discomfort has reached a level of 5, the peel is neutralized with copious amounts of ice-water to completely remove the acid from the skin. The face is rinsed with the disposable towels and ice-water at least five times, paying special attention to all the folds of the face. Following drying with a tissue, the face is coated with a layer of bland moisturizing cream.

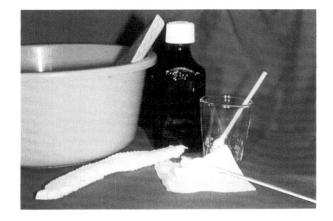

Figure 6.2 *Equipment used to perform a glycolic or salicylic acid peel: basin filled with ice cubes and ice-water, several disposable towels, disposable hairnet, peel solution, short rayon-tipped applicator, small glass, and bland cream moisturizer.*

It is important to remember that glycolic acid peels are not self-neutralizing. Any acid inadvertently left on the skin surface will be absorbed into the dermis and produce continued stinging and burning. Whether this dermal absorption is valuable remains controversial. The exfoliant effect of the peel is epidermal; however, some dermatologists feel that the dermal penetration leads to wrinkle reduction through the synthesis of glycosaminoglycans, such as hyaluronic acid. At present, no PHA peels with reduced dermal penetration are available. Further research should focus on methods of obtaining the desired post-peel exfoliation without the dermal stinging and burning.

BHA peels

Salicylic acid is the only BHA used for skin peeling. It can be applied to the skin in concentrations in the 10–50% range. Salicylic acid produces a more complete exfoliation than glycolic acid, since it can peel both the skin surface and the pores. Salicylic acid will remain in solution in concentrations of ≤ 20% or < 95% ethyl alcohol; however, at concentrations of ≥ 30% shaking of the peels is required prior to use. In contrast to glycolic acid peels, salicylic acid is a self-neutralizing peel that ends with the formation of white salicylic acid crystals on the skin.[24] The crystals are easily rinsed off the skin surface with water, but they do remain in the follicular ostia providing a prolonged keratolytic effect. Thus, salicylic acid peels are useful for general exfoliation in patients with photoaging, comedolysis in acne patients, and sensitive-skin patients, such as rosacea patients, in the author's experience, where dermal penetration should be minimized.

BHA peels are formulated from salicylic acid powder and 95% ethyl alcohol (Everclear). The author prefers to mix these peels in strengths of 10%, 20%, 30%, 40%, and 50%, as demonstrated in Table 6.5. As mentioned previously, salicylic acid peels of ≥ 30% are suspensions, which require shaking immediately prior to application to ensure an accurate concentration and even distribution of the salicylic acid (Figure 6.3). The application technique is identical to that described for glycolic acid peels, except that fewer coats of the peel solution are

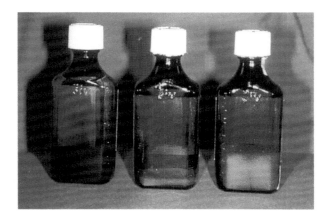

Figure 6.3 These bottles contain salicylic acid peels in concentrations of 20%, 30%, and 40% (from left to right). Salicylic acid peels in strengths of ≥ 30% are suspensions and require shaking immediately prior to application.

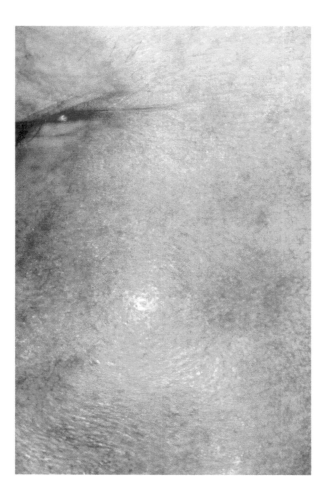

Figure 6.4 Whitish salicylic acid crystals and mild frosting can be seen on the lower cheek of this patient who underwent a 40% salicylic acid peel for dermatoheliosis.

Table 6.4. *Hydroxy acid peel selection criteria*

Type and concentration of peel solution	Expected results
20%, 30% glycolic acid	Produces minimal exfoliation, 20–30 minutes of erythema, resembles an aggressive facial, good in heavily retinized patients
40%, 50% glycolic acid	Produces mild exfoliation, 4 hours of erythema, good maintenance peel for most patients repeated every 10–12 weeks
60%, 70% glycolic acid	Produces moderate exfoliation, 8 hours of erythema, good lightening of epidermal pigmentation when repeated every 3 weeks for six treatments
10% salicylic acid	Produces minimal exfoliation, 20–30 minutes of erythema, good in younger patients with comedonal acne to initiate comedolysis, peel for rosacea and sensitive-skin patients
20%, 30% salicylic acid	Produces mild to moderate exfoliation, 1 hour of erythema, good peel for patients with acne and dyspigmentation repeated every 10–12 weeks
40%, 50% salicylic acid	Produces moderate exfoliation, 2 hours of erythema, good peel for patients with more pronounced photoaging repeated every 3 weeks for five treatments
Jessner's solution (combination hydroxy acid)	Produces moderate to dramatic exfoliation in the retinized patient, 12 hours of erythema, best peel to lighten epidermal pigmentation without the need for frequent repetition

applied to the face since the salicylic acid crystals form almost immediately upon application. Salicylic acid is a versatile peeling solution that can be safely used in all skin types, since it rarely produces hyperpigmentation. Additionally, salicylic acid is the author's preferred peel for the neck, upper chest, and back of the hands. The guidelines used for selection of the peel strength are presented in Table 6.4; the appearance of the face immediately following a salicylic acid peel is demonstrated in Figure 6.4. All equipment used in the peeling process must be washed with detergent and water since the salicylic acid peel solution also crystallizes on everything it makes contact with (Figure 6.5).

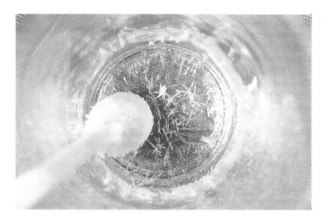

Figure 6.5 *Salicylic acid crystallizes on all of the equipment used during the peel, requiring detergent and water removal.*

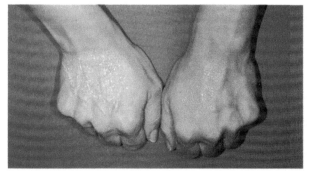

Figure 6.6 *Glycolic acid has been applied to the hand on the left while salicylic acid has been applied to the hand on the right. Glycolic acid requires water rinsing to remove the excess peel solution from the skin, while salicylic acid crystallizes on the skin surface and self-neutralizes.*

BHA peels differ from glycolic acid peels in that the salicylic acid crystallizes on the skin surface, leaving a white film (Figure 6.6) (not to be confused with the acetowhitening achieved with trichloroacetic acid peels).

Combination hydroxy acid peels (Jessner's solution peels)

Glycolic and salicylic acid peels produce mild exfoliation with short-lived erythema. They are most appropriately used in the patient who desires mild treatment with minimal recovery time, but has also been counseled as to the desired outcome – realistic expectations are important. Glycolic and salicylic acid peels do not remove facial wrinkles or dyspigmentation after one treatment. They are best used in patients who are looking for a smoother skin surface over which cosmetics can be more attractively applied. Salicylic acid peels can also be valuable in the patient who requires comedolysis for the treatment of comedonal acne. Yet, in patients with more advanced photoaging, there is the need for a deeper peel that produces greater benefit, but with a longer recovery period.

Combination hydroxy acid peels form an intermediate peel category that is useful in many patients (Table 6.4). The most popular combination hydroxy acid peel is known as Jessner's peel and is composed of lactic acid (an AHA) and salicylic acid (a BHA) combined with resorcinol and ethyl alcohol (Table 6.6). The author applies the peel in the same manner as a pure salicylic acid peel, but more intense whitening, or frosting, is achieved. Some of this whitening is due to crystallization of the salicylic acid on the skin surface; however, there is also immediate whitening of the upper layers of the stratum corneum, giving the face a white appearance even after water rinsing of the crystallized salicylic acid. This peel is the author's preferred choice in men wishing to improve skin texture. The increased sebum production of the male face along with the coarser skin texture responds well to a Jessner's peel, as only minimal peeling occurs with a glycolic acid peel alone.

Table 6.5. *Salicylic acid peel recipe*

Salicylic acid peel (%)	Weight of salicylic acid powder (g)	Volume of ethyl alcohol 95% (cm³)
10	10	100
20	20	100
30	30	100
40	40	100
50	50	100

Table 6.6. *Combination hydroxy acid peel or Jessner's peel solution*

Ingredient	Amount
Lactic acid liquid	14 ml
Salicylic acid powder	14 g
Resorcinol powder	14 g
Ethyl alcohol 95%	Enough to make 100 cm³ total volume

Jessner's solution is also an excellent prepeel treatment for the medium depth 25–30% trichloroacetic acid (TCA) peels. It serves to enhance penetration of the TCA yielding a more even, deeper peel.

SUMMARY

This chapter has detailed the chemistry and physiology of the hydroxy acids and their utility in achieving cutaneous exfoliation. Formulation issues and their relevance to the desired cutaneous effect have also been discussed. Methods of making peel solutions and their use in appropriate patient populations have been described for the physician who wishes to administer these peels to patients. In summary, the hydroxy acids are a valuable part of the physician's antiaging armamentarium.

References

1. Stiller MJ, Bartolone J, Stern R, et al. Topical 8% glycolic acid and 8% l-lactic acid creams for the treatment of photodamaged skin. Arch Dermatol 1996;132:631–6.

2. Dietre CM, Griffin TD, Murphy GF, et al. Effects of alpha-hydroxy acids on photoaged skin. J Am Acad Dermatol 1996;34:187–95.

3. Berardesca E, Maibach H. AHA mechanism of action. Cosmet Toilet 1995;110:30–1.

4. Van Scott EJ, Yu RJ. Hyperkeratinization, corneocyte cohesion and alpha hydroxy acids. J Am Acad Dermatol 1984;11:867–79.

5. Bernstein EF, Uitto J: Connective tissue alterations in photoaged skin and the effects of alpha hydroxy acids. J Geriatr Dermatol 1995;3 Suppl:7A–18A.

6. Lavker RM, Kaidbey K, Leyden JJ. Effects of topical ammonium lactate on cutaneous atrophy from a potent topical corticosteroid. J Am Acad Dermatol 1992;26:535–44.

7. Griffin TD, Murphy GF, Sueki H, et al. Increased factor XIIIa transglutaminase epxression in dermal dendrocytes after treatment with alpha-hydroxy acids: potential physiologic significance. J Am Acad Dermatol 1996;34:196–203.

8. Kim SJ, Park JH, Kim DH, Won YH, Maibach HI. Increased in vivo collagen synthesis and in vitro cell proliferative effect of glycolic acid. Am J Dermatol Surg 1998;24:1054–8.

9. Yu RJ, Van Scott EJ. Bioavailability of alpha-hydroxy acids in topical formulations. Cosmet Dermatol 1996;9:54–62.

10. Davies M, Marks R. Studies on the effect of salicylic acid on the normal stratum corneum. Br J Dermatol 1980;103:191–6.

11. DiNardo JC. A comparison of salicylic acid, salicylic acid with glycolic acid and benzoyl peroxide in the treatment of acne. Cosmet Dermatol 1995;8.

12. Kligman A, Kligman AM. Salicylic acid as a peeling agent for the treatment of acne. Cosmet Dermatol 1997;10:44–7.

13. Draelos ZD. Salicylic acid in the dermatologic armamentarium. Cosmet Dermatol 1997;10 Suppl:7–8.

14. Roberts DL, Marshall R, Marks R. Detection of the action of salicylic acid on the normal stratum corneum. Br J Dermatol 1980;103:191–6.

15. Kraeling ME, Bronaugh RL. In vitro percutaneous absorption of alpha hydroxy acids in human skin. J Soc Cosmet Chem 1997;48:187–97.

16. DiNardo JC, Grove GL, Moy L. Clinical and histological effects of glycolic acid at different concentrations and pH levels. Dermatol Surg 1996;22:421–4.

17. Smith WP. Hydroxy acids and skin aging. Cosmet Toilet 1994;109:41–8.

18. Sah A, Mukherjee S, Wickett RR. An in vitro study of the effects of formulation variables and product structure on percutaneous absorption of lactic acid. J Cosmet Sci 1998;49:257–73.

19. Moy LS, Murad H, Moy RL. Glycolic acid peels for the treatment of wrinkles and photoaging. J Dermatol Surg Oncol 1993;19:243–6.

20. Van Scott EJ, Yu RJ. Alpha hydroxy acids: procedures for use in clinical practice. Cutis 1989;43:222–8.

21. Van Scott EJ, Yu RJ. Alpha hydroxy acids: therapeutic potentials. Can J Dermatol 1989;1:108–12.

22. Briden ME, Rendon-Pellerano MI. Treatment of rosacea with glycolic acid. J Geriatr Dermatol 1996;4(SB):17B–21B.

23. Kakita LS, Petratos MA. The use of glycolic acid in asian and darker skin types. J Geriatr Dermatol 1996;4(SB):8B-11B.

24. Kligman D, Kligman AM. Salicylic acid peels for the treatment of photoaging. Dermatol Surg 1998;24:325–8.

COMBINATION TREATMENT

Nicholas J Lowe

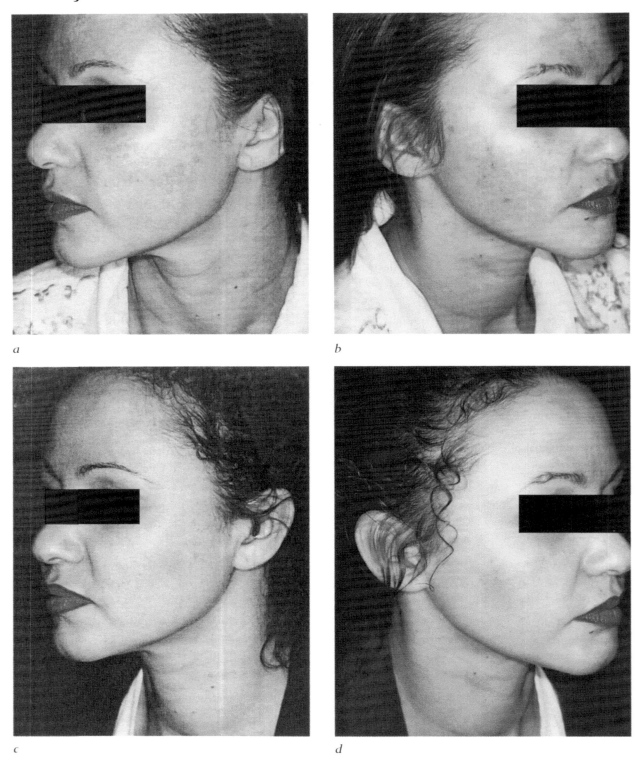

a

b

c

d

Figure 6.7 *A good example of combination topical therapy. A 39-year-old female with mild acne and facial pigmentation (melasma) (A,B) before and (C,D) after using lightening cream (tretinoin, hydroquinone, desuride cream) and 4-glycolic acid peels. She will use 'maintenance' creams twice daily and broad spectrum sunscreens each morning.*

7. Combination chemical peels

Gary D Monheit

BACKGROUND

The explosion of interest in chemical peeling and laser resurfacing on the part of cosmetic surgeons has paralleled the general public's interest in acquiring a youthful appearance by rehabilitating the photoaged skin. The public's interest has been further heightened by advertising for cosmetic agents, over-the-counter chemicals and treatment programs that have entered the general market of products meant to rejuvenate skin, and erase the marks of sun damage and age. Most of these over-the-counter, do-it-yourself programs have been tried by patients and by the time they consult their cosmetic surgeon or dermatologist they are ready for a more definitive procedure, performed either by chemical peeling or laser resurfacing. It is the obligation of the physician to analyze the patient's skin type and the degree of photoaging skin, and thus prescribe the correct facial rejuvenation procedure that will give the greatest benefit with the fewest risk factors and the lowest morbidity. The cosmetic surgeon should have available for his/her consumer the options of medical or cosmeceutical topical therapy, dermabrasion, chemical peeling and lasers available for selective skin destruction and resurfacing. Each of these techniques maintains a place in the armamenteria of the cosmetic surgeon to provide the appropriate treatment for each individual patient and their specific problem. In particular instances, a combination of these approaches is the correct procedure.

With an aging baby-boomer population expressing an interest in rehabilitating weathered and photoaging skin, the patient has become a major consumer for the cosmetic surgeon. The approach to photoaging skin has expanded beyond a one-stage procedure to now include preparatory medical therapy and post-treatment cosmeceutical topical therapy to maintain results and prevent further photodamage. Thus, the cosmetic surgeon's office has become not only the setting for surgical treatment but also an educational setting for skin, protection and care, and a marketplace for the patient to obtain the necessary topical treatments for skin protection.[1] It is up to the dermatologist, cosmetic surgeon, or plastic surgeon to fully understand the nature of skin and sun damage, the protective techniques available, and the active agents that work as cosmeceutical preparations. Having available multiple procedures to solve these problems will make the patients better candidates for the right procedure to restore and rehabilitate their skin.

Chemical peeling involves the application of a chemical exfoliant to wound the epidermis and/or dermis for the removal of superficial lesions and improve the texture of the skin. Various acidic and basic chemical agents are used to produce the varying effects of light to medium to deep chemical peels through differences in their ability to destroy skin. The level of penetration, destruction and inflammation determines the level of peeling. The histologic studies of Stegman,[2] over 10 years, ago have provided the scientific basis for peeling by linking the strength of an agent to the depth level of destruction.[2] Using trichloracetic (TCA) acid as the benchmark, the percentage concentration of acid has been correlated to a superficial, medium or deep procedure. This has been confirmed by the histologic studies that document the following levels of destruction with concentration: (1) superficial chemical peel, 10–30%; (2) medium-depth chemical peel, 30–45%; (3) deep chemical peel, > 45%. Thus, this classification was able to simplify chemical peeling in that the agent itself, or the generic name, is not the important component but rather the level of destruction, which in fact determined the efficacy and extent of the resurfacing procedure.[3]

Similarly, laser resurfacing has been documented to destroy tissue as a superficial, medium or deep procedure. The Er:YAG laser has been used for most superficial procedures while the pulsed CO_2 laser has been used for medium-depth and deep resurfacing. Biopsies directly after surgery, as well as in healing phases, have confirmed these levels to be similar to those using chemical peeling. In addition, dermabrasion has been documented as a superficial, medium and deep resurfacing procedure, depending on the depth of mechanical removal and destruction. Most recently, microdermabrasion has been added as an adjunct procedure, which can be classified as a very superficial or superficial resurfacing procedure. It is the equivalent 'lunchtime' procedure in mechanical abrasives, used to remove the stratum cornea and portions of the outer epidermis. The procedure is performed within a closed suction system through which aluminum oxide crystals are sprayed onto the skin surface to abrade the stratum corneum (Table 7.1).

The stimulation of epidermal growth through the removal of the stratum corneum without necrosis consists of a light superficial peel. Through exfoliation, it thickens the epidermis with qualitative regenerative changes. Destruction of the epidermis defines a full superficial chemical peel inducing the regeneration of the epidermis. Further destruction of the epidermis and induction of inflammation within the papillary dermis constitutes a medium-depth peel.[2] Then, further inflammatory response in the deep reticular dermis induces new collagen production and ground substances, constituting a deep chemical peel. These have now been well classified and usage has been categorized for various degenerative conditions associated with photoaging skin based on levels of penetration. Thus, the physician has the tools capable of solving problems that may be mild, moderate or severe with agents that are very superficial, superficial, medium-depth or deep peeling chemicals.[4]

The present author has devised a system of quantitating photodamage and has developed numerical scores that would fit into corresponding rejuvenation programs.[5] In analyzing photodamage, the major categories include epidermal color with skin lesions and dermal changes with textural changes. Dermal changes include wrinkles, cross-hatched lines, sallow color, leathery appearance, crinkly thin parchment skin and the pebblish white nodules of milia. Each of these is classified, giving the patient a point score of 1–4. In addition, the number and extent of lesions are categorized from freckles, lentigenes, telangiectasias, actinic and seborrheic keratoses, skin cancers and senile comedones. These also are added in a classification system of 1–4 and the final score results are tabulated. A total score of 1–4 would indicate very mild damage and the patient would respond adequately to a five-step skin-care program including sunscreen protection, retinoic acid, glycolic acid peels

Table 7.1. *Levels of resurfacing*

Level	Histology	Peel	Abrasion	Laser
Superficial	Destruction of epidermis alone	10–20% TCA Glycolic 50–70% Jessner's solution	Microdermabrasion	None
Medium	Destruction of epidermis plus papillary dermis	Combination: Jessner's solution + 35% TCA Glycolic acid + 35% TCA Solid CO_2 + 35% TCA	Manual dermasanding	Er
Deep	Destruction of upper reticular dermis	Baker's phenol	Mechanical dermabrasion	CO_2 Er, CO_2

Texture changes	Points				Score
Wrinkles – dynamic	1	2	3	4	
(% of potential lines)	< 25%	< 50%	< 75%	< 100%	
Wrinkles – photoaging	1	2	3	4	
(% of potential lines)	< 25%	< 50%	< 75%	< 100%	
Cross-hatched lines – fine lines	1	2	3	4	
(% of potential lines)	< 10%	< 20%	< 40%	< 60%	
Sallow color and dyschromia	1	2	3	4	
	Dull	Yellow	Brown	Black	
Leathery appearance	1	2	3	4	
Crinkly (thin and parchment)	1	2	3	4	
Pebbly (deep whitish nodules)	2	4	6	8	
(% of face)	< 25%	< 50%	< 75%	< 100%	
Pore number and size	2	4	6	8	
	< 25%	< 50%	< 75%	< 100%	

Lesions	Points				Score
Freckles – mottled skin	1	2	3	4	
(number present)	< 10	< 25	< 50	< 100	
Lentigenes (dark/irregular) and	2	4	6	8	
seborrheic keratoses (size)	< 5 mm	< 10 mm	< 15 mm	< 20 mm	
Telangiectasia – erythema flush	1	2	3	4	
(number present)	< 5	< 10	< 15	> 15	
Actinic and seborrheic keratoses	2	4	6	8	
(number present)	< 5	< 10	< 15	> 15	
Skin cancers	2	4	6	8	
(number present – now or by history)	c. 1	c. 2	c. 3	c. > 4	
Senile comedones	1	2	3	4	
(in cheekbone area)	< 5	< 10	< 20	> 20	

Total score

Corresponding rejuvenation program

Score	Needs
1–6	Skin-care program with tretinoin and glycolic acid peels
7–11	As for 1–6 plus Jessner's solution peel, pigmented lesion laser and/or vascular laser
12–16	As for 7–11 plus medium peels (Jessner's solution + TCA peels), skin fillers and/or Botox
17 or more	As for 12–16 plus laser resurfacing

Staff signature   Date   Patient signature   Date

Figure 7.1 Index of photoaging (courtesy of Monheit Dermatology Associates).

and selective lesional removal. A score of 5–9 would include all of the above plus a repetitive superficial peeling agents program, such as glycolic acid, Jessner's solution or lactic acid peels. A score of 10–14 would include medium-depth chemical peeling and a score of 15 or above would include deep chemical peeling or laser resurfacing. Thus, during the consultation, the patient could understand their degree of photodamage and the necessity for an individual peeling program (see Figure 7.1).

In addition to resurfacing procedures, other procedures to correct photoaging skin include:

(1) chemodenervation with botulinum toxin;
(2) skin and soft-tissue implants with collagen, e.g. Zyderm®, Zyplast® (both McGhan Medical Corporation, Santa Barbara, CA), Dermalogen® (Collagenesis, Beverly, MA), fat;
(3) cosmeceutical agents.

These tools can be combined with resurfacing techniques to produce the most efficacious benefits with reduced risks and down time.

The peeling agent is a chemical escharotic that damages the skin in a therapeutic manner. It is important that the physician understands the patient's skin and its ability to withstand this damage. Certain skin types withstand the damage to a greater degree than others, and particular skin disorders have a greater tendency to produce side-effects and complications from chemical peels. Patients with extensive photodamage may require stronger peeling agents and repeated applications of medium-depth peeling solutions to obtain therapeutic results. Patients with skin disorders such as atopic dermatitis, seborrheic dermatitis, psoriasis or contact dermatitis may find their disease exacerbated in the postoperative period, and they may even develop problems with postoperative healing such as prolonged healing, post-erythema syndrome or contact sensitivity. Rosacea is a disorder of vasomotor instability in the skin and may develop an exaggerated inflammatory response to the peeling agents. Other important factors include a history of radiation therapy to the proposed facial skin, as chronic radiation dermatitis decreases the body's ability to heal properly (Table 7.2).[6]

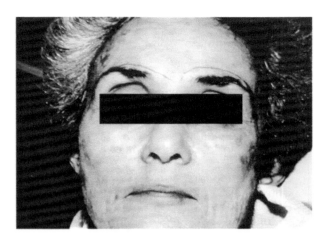

Figure 7.2 *Preoperative appearance of Glogau level II photoaging facial skin.*

Herpes simplex fascial can be a postoperative problem with significant morbidity. Susceptible patients should be pretreated with antiherpetic agents such as acyclovir or valcyclovir to prevent herpetic activation. These patients can be identified in the preoperative consultation and placed on appropriate therapy at the time of the chemical peel. All antiherpetic agents act by inhibiting viral replication in the intact epidermal cell. The significance of this in chemical peeling is that the skin must be re-epithelialized before the agent has its full effect. Thus, the antiviral agent must be continued in deep chemical peeling for the entire 2 weeks, or in medium-depth peeling for at least 10 days.[7] The present author rarely uses antiviral agents in light or superficial chemical peeling, as the injury pattern is usually not enough to activate the herpes simplex virus.

The chief indications for chemical peeling are associated with the reversal of actinic changes such as photodamage, rhytides, actinic growths, pigmentary dyschromias and acne scars (Figure 7.2). The physician thus can use his/her classification systems to quantitate and qualitate the level of photodamage and prescribe the appropriate chemical peeling combination.

Table 7.2. *Fitzpatrick's classification of skin types*

Skin type	Color	Reaction to sun
I	Very white or freckled	Always burns
II	White	Usually burns
III	White to olive	Sometimes burns
IV	Brown	Rarely burns
V	Dark brown	Very rarely burns
VI	Black	Never burns

COMBINATION MEDIUM-DEPTH CHEMICAL PEELING

Medium-depth chemical peeling is defined as controlled damage from a chemical agent to the

Table 7.3. *Agents for medium-depth chemical peels*

Agent	Comment
1. TCA – 50%	Not recommended because of risk of scarring
2. Combination – 35% TCA + solid CO_2 (Brody 1995[9])	The most potent combination
3. Combination – 35% TCA + Jessner's solution (Monheit 1989[10])	The most popular combination
4. Combination – 35% TCA + 70% glycolic acid (Coleman and Futrell 1994[11])	An effective combination
5. 89% Phenol	Rarely used

papillary dermis resulting in specific changes that can be performed in a single setting. Agents currently used include combination products such as Jessner's solution, 70% glycolic acid and solid CO_2 alloy with 35% TCA. The benchmark for this level peel was 50% TCA, which traditionally achieved acceptable results in ameliorating fine wrinkles, actinic changes and pre-neoplasia. However, since high quantitative TCA is an agent more likely to be fraught with complications, especially scarring, in strengths of 50% or higher, it has fallen out of favor as a single-agent chemical peel.[8] It is for this reason that the combination products, along with a 35% TCA formula, have been found equally effective in producing this level of control damage without the risk of side-effects (Table 7.3).

Brody[9] first developed the use of solid CO_2 applied with acetone to the skin as a freezing technique prior to the application of 35% TCA, which appears to break the epidermal barrier for a more even and complete penetration of the 35% TCA. Monheit[10] then demonstrated the use of Jessner's solution prior to the application of 35% TCA (Table 7.4). The Jessner's solution was found to be effective in destroying the epidermal barrier by breaking up individual keratinocytes, thus allowing deeper penetration of the 35% TCA and a more even application of the peeling solution.[11] Similarly, Coleman and Futrell[11] demonstrated the use of 70%

Table 7.4. *The Jessner's solution formula*

Resorcinol	14 g
Salicylic acid	14 g
Lactic acid	14 ml
Ethanol (qs)	100 ml

glycolic acid prior to the application of 35% TCA, the effect of which is very similar to that of Jessner's solution (see Table 7.3).

All three combinations have been proven more effective and safer than the use of 50% TCA. Both acid application and frosting are better controlled with the combination procedures such that the hot spots caused by higher concentrations of TCA, which can produce dyschromias and scarring, are not a significant problem with these medium-depth peels. The Monheit version of the Jessner's solution +35% TCA peel is a relatively simple and safe combination. The technique is used for mild to moderate photoaging, including pigmentary changes, lentigines, epidermal growths, dyschromias and rhytides. It is a single procedure with a healing time of 7–10 days. It is also useful for the removal of diffuse actinic keratoses, providing an alternative to chemical exfoliation with topical 5-fluorouracil (5-FLL) chemotherapy. It reduces the morbidity of a 3-week course for topical 5-FU and gives the cosmetic benefits of improved photoaging skin.[12]

The procedure is usually performed with mild preoperative sedation and non-steroidal anti-inflammatory agents. The patient is told that the peeling agent will sting and burn temporarily and a non-steroidal anti-inflammatory agent, such as aspirin, is given before the peel and continued for the first 24 hours if the patient can tolerate the medication. Its anti-inflammatory effect is especially helpful in reducing swelling and relieving pain. If given before surgery, it may be all the patient requires during the postoperative phase. However, for full-face peels, it is useful to give preoperative sedation (diazepam, 5–10 mg orally) and mild analgesia [meperidine 25 mg (Demerol®; Sanofi Winthrop, New York)], and hydroxyzine hydrochloride [25 mg intramuscularly

(Vistaril®; Lorec, New York)]. The discomfort from this peel is not long lasting so short-acting sedatives and analgesics are all that are necessary.[13]

Vigorous cleansing and degreasing is necessary for even penetration of the solution. The face is scrubbed gently with Irgasam (Septisol; Calgon Vestal Laboratories, St Louis, MO) and 4 inch × 4 inch gauze pads and water, then rinsed and dried. Next, an acetone preparation is applied to remove residual oils and debris. The skin is essentially debrided of stratum corneum and excessive scale. The necessity for thorough degreasing for an even fully penetrant peel cannot be overemphasized. The physician should feel the dry, clean skin to check the thoroughness of

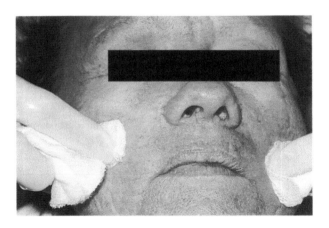

Figure 7.4 *Appearance of skin after application of Jessner's solution.*

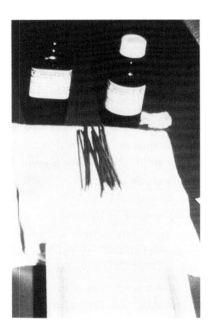

Figure 7.3 *Peel solutions with cotton tips, 2 inch × 2 inch; gauze and saline. .*

degreasing. If oil is felt, degreasing should be repeated. A splotchy peel is usually the result of uneven penetration of peel solution due to residual oil or stratum corneum from inadequate degreasing.

The Jessner's solution is then applied with either cotton-tipped applicators or 2 inch × 2 inch gauze (Figures 7.3 and 7.5). The Jessner's solution is applied evenly, usually only one coat, to achieve a light but even frosting. The frosting achieved with Jessner's solution is much lighter than that produced by TCA and there is usually little discomfort. A mild erythema appears with a faint tinge of frost dispersed over the face (Figure 7.4). Even strokes are used to apply the solution to the unit area covering the forehead to the cheeks to the nose and chin. The eyelids are treated last, creating the same erythema with blotchy frosting.

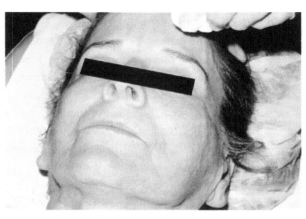

a

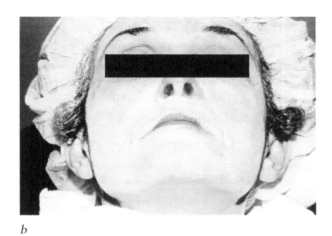

b

Figure 7.5 *(A) Full application of 35% TCA with frosting. (B) Jessner's solution applied with 2 inch × 2 inch gauze pads*

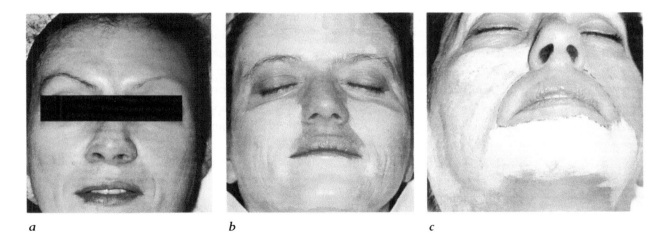

a   *b*   *c*

Figure 7.6 *Levels of frosting: (A) level I — erythema with streaky frosting; (B) level II — even white frosting with erythema showing through; (C) level III — solid white enamel frosting.*

The TCA is then applied evenly with one to four cotton-tipped applicators that can be applied over different areas with lighter or heavier doses of the acid. Four cotton-tipped applicators are applied in broad strokes over the forehead and also on the medial cheeks. Two mildly soaked cotton-tipped applicators can be used across the lips and chin, and one damp cotton-tipped applicator on the eyelids. Thus, the dosage of application is technique dependent, varying with the amount of acid used and the number of cotton-tipped applicators applied. The cotton-tipped applicator is useful in quantitating the amount of peel solution to be applied.

The white frost from the TCA application appears on the treated area within 30 seconds to 2 minutes (Figure 7.5). Even application should eliminate the need to go over areas a second or a third time, but if frosting is incomplete or uneven, the solution should be reapplied. TCA takes longer to frost than Baker's formula or straight phenol, but a shorter period of time than the superficial peeling agents do. The surgeon should observe the frosting at least 3–4 minutes after the application of TCA to ensure that frosting has reached its peak; the completeness of a frosted cosmetic unit can then be determined and the area touched-up as needed. Areas of poor frosting should be retreated carefully with a thin application of TCA. The physician should achieve a level II–III frosting (Figure 7.6a–c). Level II frosting is defined as a white-coated frosting with a background of erythema.[14] A level III frosting, which is associated with a deeper penetration in the dermis, is a solid white enamel frosting with no background of erythema (Figure 7.7). A deeper level III frosting should be restricted only to areas of heavy actinic damage and thicker skin. Most medium-depth chemical peels use a level II frosting, and this is especially true over the eyelids and other areas of sensitive skin. Those areas with a greater tendency to scar formation, such as the zygomatic arch, the bony prominences of the jawline and the chin, should receive only up to a level II frosting. Overcoating TCA will increase its penetration, so a second or third application will increase the risk of further damage. One must be careful to overcoat only in areas where the take-up or frosting was not adequate.

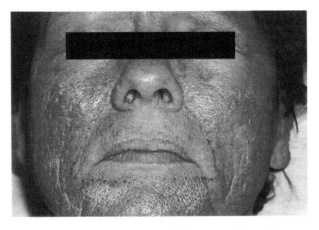

Figure 7.7 *The appearance of frosting with erythema and blotches after use of Jessner's solution.*

Anatomic areas of the face are peeled sequentially from forehead to temple to cheeks and finally to the lips and eyelids. The white frosting indicates kerato-coagulation and at that point the reaction is complete. Careful feathering of the solution into the hairline and around the rim of the jaw and brow conceals the line of demarcation between peeled and non-peeled areas. The perioral area has rhytides that require a complete and even application of solution over the lip skin to the vermilion. This is best accomplished with the help of an assistant who stretches and fixates the upper and lower lips while the peel solution is applied.

Certain facial areas and particular skin lesions require special attention. Wrinkled skin should be stretched to allow an even coating of solution into the folds and troughs. Oral rhytides require peel solution to be applied with the wood portion of a cotton-tipped applicator and extended into the vermilion of the lip. Deeper furrows such as expression lines will not be eradicated by peel solution and thus should be treated like the remaining skin. Thicker keratoses do not frost evenly and thus do not pick up peel solution. Additional applications rubbed vigorously into the lesion may be needed for peel solution penetration. Other adjunctive procedures may be needed to remove thick keratotic lesions that may not respond fully to the medium peel alone. These include cryosurgery, spot CO_2 laser and/or dermasanding. The present author's preference is dermasanding, performed regularly in combination with medium-depth peeling.

Eyelid skin must be treated delicately and carefully. A semi-dry applicator should be used to carry the solution to within 2–3 mm of the lid margin. The patient should be positioned with the head elevated at 30° and the eyelids closed. Excess peel solution on the cotton tip should be drained gently on the bottom before application. The applicator is then rolled gently on the lids and periorbital skin. Excess peel solution should never be left on the lids because the solution can roll into the eyes. Tears must be dried with a cotton-tipped applicator during peeling because they may pull peel solution to the puncta and eye by capillary attraction. The solution is diluted immediately with cool saline compresses at the conclusion of the peel. The Jessner's–TCA peel procedure is as follows:

(1) the skin should be cleaned thoroughly with Septisol to remove oils;
(2) acetone or acetone alcohol is used to further debride oil and scale from the surface of the skin;
(3) Jessner's solution is applied;
(4) 35% TCA is applied until frost appears;
(5) cool saline compresses are applied to neutralize the solution;
(6) the peel will heal with 0.25% acetic acid soaks and a mild emollient cream.

There is an immediate burning sensation as the peel solution is applied but this subsides as frosting is completed. Cool saline compresses offer symptomatic relief for a peeled area as the solution is applied to other areas. The compresses are placed over the face for 5–6 minutes after the peel until the patient is comfortable. The burning subsides fully by the time the patient is ready to be discharged. At that time, most of the frosting has faded and a brawny desquamation is evident.

At the conclusion of the peel, when maximal frosting is obtained, the clinician can assess the need for further treatment with dermasanding. The indications include:

(1) deeper rhytides beyond the reach of medium-depth peeling, including perioral lip rhagads, crow's-feet, forehead lines or creases;
(2) keratotic growths that do not respond to peel alone such as seborrheic keratoses, actinic keratoses, verrucae and lentigenes;
(3) removal of other growths such as syringomas, sebaceous hyperplasia and rhinophymatic changes;
(4) blending borders such as hairline and jawline, and blending cosmetic units around laser-treated areas.

The advantages of dermasanding include:

(1) simplicity of the technique when compared to lasers and motorized dermabrasion;
(2) safety and control of manual dermasanding over the other techniques, especially when treating rhytides on the lips, orbital rims and cheeks;
(3) blending of cosmetic areas that is hard to obtain with laser or dermabrasion;
(4) cost and simplicity of instrumentation;

(5) quick healing with less postoperative erythema than laser resurfacing;

(6) decreased incidence of hypopigmentation as compared to laser resurfacing or deep chemical peeling;

(7) simple touch-up procedures can be planned as adjuncts to the primary procedure.[15]

Indications

(1) Removal of skin lesions: epidermal growths;

(2) treatment of acne scars;

(3) treatment of localized photoaging skin;

(4) adjunct to superficial and medium-depth chemical peels;
  • full-face peel with perioral dermasanding;
  • full-face medium peel with dermasanding for skin growths;

(5) adjunct to Er and CO_2 laser resurfacing.

Dermasanding is performed after full-face CO_2 laser resurfacing over areas where it is needed, e.g. perioral rhytides needing deeper treatment; areas not treated with laser for blending, such as eyebrows, hairline, jawline and upper neck; removal of necrotic debris after full-face laser resurfacing.[16]

The silicone carbide sandpaper can be obtained in three grades: (1) fine, 400 grit; (2) medium, 220–320 grit; (3) coarse, 180 grit. The paper is cut into strips and wrapped around 4 inch × 4 inch gauze or a syringe for even dermal sanding. The area to be treated is first anesthetized with a local ring block or regional nerve block. The epidermis will come off first, revealing fine bleeding points. The end-point is the eradication of the lesion for the appearance of superficial dermal structures. It is best to treat an entire cosmetic unit, though individual unit areas can be blended with surrounding facial skin.

The resultant wound is healed like a dermabrasion with either the open occlusive technique (1/4% acetic acid soaks with Vaseline®, Lever Fabergé or Eucerin®, BDF, Morristown, NJ) or coverage with a bio-occlusive membrane (Vigilon®, Bard Medical, Covington, GA or 2nd Skin®, Spenco). The wound is usually re-epithelialized in 7–10 days. Dermasanding is thus another modality to be used in concert with peeling and CO_2 laser surgery for the treatment of photoaging skin.[17]

Postoperatively, edema, erythema and desquamation are expected. With periorbital peels, and even forehead peels, eyelid edema can be severe enough to close the lids. For the first 24 hours, the patient is instructed to soak the area four times a day with a 0.25% acetic acid compress made of 1 tablespoon of white vinegar in 1 pint of warm water. A bland emollient is applied to the desquamating areas after soaks. After 24 hours, the patient can shower and

Figure 7.8 *Appearance (A) 4 days postoperatively and (B) 6 months postoperatively.*

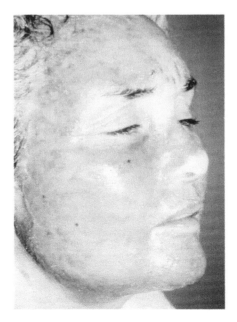
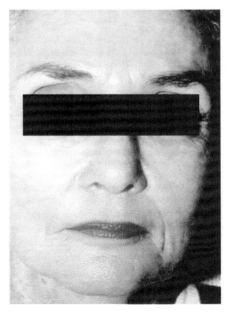

a *b*

clean gently with a mild non-detergent cleanser. The erythema intensifies as desquamation becomes complete within 4–5 days (Figure 7.8a). Thus, healing is completed within 1 week to 10 days. At the end of one week the bright red color has faded to pink and has the appearance of a sunburn; this can be covered by cosmetics and will fade fully within 2–3 weeks (Figure 7.8b).

The medium-depth peel is dependent on three components for its therapeutic effect: (1) degreasing; (2) Jessner's solution; (3) 35% TCA. The amount of each agent applied creates the intensity and thus the effectiveness of this peel. The variables can be adjusted according to the patient's skin type and the areas of the face being treated. In the present author's practice it is the workhorse of peeling and resurfac-

ing, as it can be individualized for most patients seen. By combining the agents, a more effective and safer medium-depth peel can be obtained.[18]

The medium-depth chemical peel thus has five major indications: (1) destruction of epidermal lesions, e.g. actinic keratoses; (2) resurfacing the level II moderate photoaging skin; (3) pigmentary dyschromias; (4) mild acne scars; (5) blending photoaging skin with laser resurfacing and deep chemical peeling.

Actinic keratoses

This procedure is well suited for epidermal lesions, such as diffuse, thin actinic keratoses, that have required repeated removal with either cryosurgery or chemoexfoliation (5-FU) (Figure 7.9a). The entire face can be treated as a unit or as subfacial cosmetic

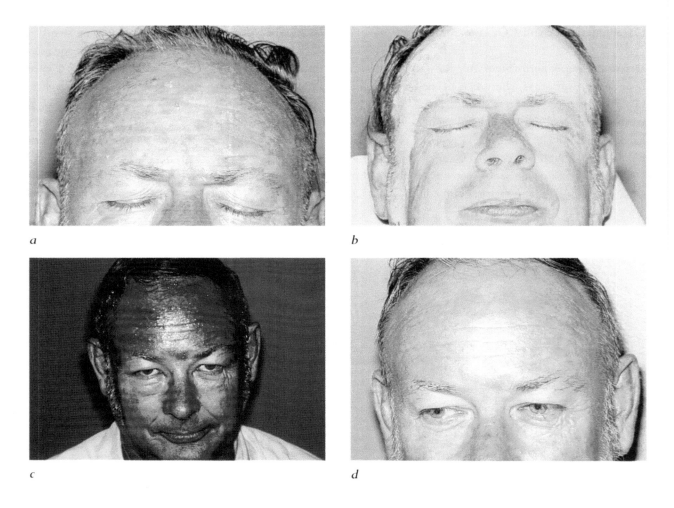

a   *b*

c   *d*

Figure 7.9 *Treatment of actinic keratoses with Jessner's solution + 35% TCA peel. (A) preoperative appearance; (B) application of Jessner's solution + 35% TCA; (C) appearance 4 days postoperatively showing inflammation and desquamation; (D) appearance 3 months postoperatively.*

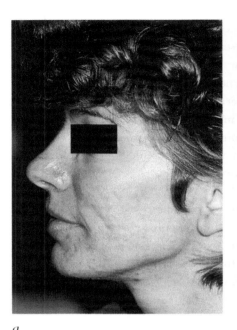

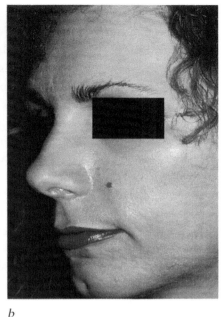

a

b

Figure 7.10 Jessner's solution + TCA peel for moderately photoaging skin: (A) preoperative appearance; (B) appearance 6 months postoperatively.

units such as forehead, temples and cheeks. Active lesions can be removed, and incipient growths as yet undetected will also be removed as the epidermis is sloughed (Figure 7.9b and d). Advantages include a short recovery period (7–10 days) with little postoperative erythema after healing. There is little risk of pigmentary changes, either hypo- or hyperpigmentation, so the patient can return to work after the skin has healed (Figure 7.9c). For thicker lesions, the addition of dermasanding will suffice.

Moderately photoaging skin
Glogau level II damage responds well to this peeling combination, with removal of the epidermal lesions and dermal changes that will freshen sallow, atrophic skin and soften other rhytides. It will heal in 10 days with minimal risk of textural or color complications. Deeper rhytides will require combinations with CO_2 laser resurfacing or dermasanding (Figure 7.10a and b).

Pigmentary dyschromias
Though color change can be treated with repetitive superficial chemical peeling, the medium-depth peel is a single treatment preceded and followed by the use of bleaching agents and retinoic acid.[19] In most cases, the pigmentary problems are resolved with this single-treatment program. The least inflammatory resurfacing procedure will give the greatest chance of success

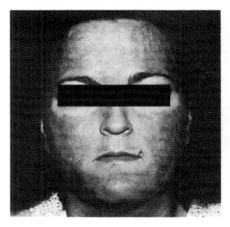

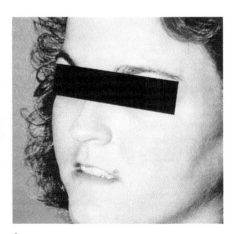

a

b

Figure 7.11 Treatment of pigmentary dyschromias with a medium-depth chemical peel and cosmeceutical treatment with tretinoin and hydroquinone (4%): (A) preoperative appearance; (B) appearance 6 months postoperatively.

without recurrent postinflammatory hyperpigmentation. Thus, the medium-depth peel is recommended over CO_2 laser resurfacing (Figure 7.11 and b).

Blending other resurfacing procedures

In a patient in whom there are advanced photoaging changes, such as crow's-feet and rhytides in the periorbital area with medium-depth changes on the remaining face, a medium-depth peel can be used to integrate deeper resurfacing procedures in selective cosmetic units. That is, laser resurfacing, deep chemical peeling, dermabrasion or dermasanding can be performed over the periorbital and perioral areas which may have more advanced photoaging changes while the medium-depth chemical peel is used for the rest of the face (Figure 7.12a–c).[16] Patients requiring laser resurfacing in a localized cosmetic unit will have the remaining areas of their face blended with this medium-depth chemical peel. Patients having laser resurfacing or deep peeling to the perioral or periorbital areas alone may develop a pseudohypopigmentation that is a noticeable deformity. The patient requiring laser resurfacing at a localized cosmetic unit will have the remaining areas of their face blended with this medium-depth peel. The alternatives, i.e. a full-face deep peel or laser resurfac-

ing, have an increased morbidity, longer healing times, and risk of scarring over areas such as the lateral jawline, malar eminences and the forehead. If deep resurfacing is needed only over localized areas, such as perioral or periorbital face, a blending medium-depth peel reduces morbidity and healing time. The present author has found that most patients requiring laser resurfacing in a localized cosmetic unit will have the remaining areas of their face blended with this medium-depth chemical peel.[18]

Postoperative complications most commonly result from local infection or contact dermatitis. The best deterrent for local infection is the continuous use of soaks to debride crusting and necrotic material. Streptoccal and staphylococcal infections can occur under biosynthetic membranes or thick occlusive ointments. The use of 0.25% acetic acid soaks seems to deter this, as well as the judicious removal of the ointment with each soak. *Staphylococcus, E. coli* and even *Pseudomonas* infection may result from improper care during healing and should be treated promptly with the appropriate oral antibiotic.

Frequent postoperative visits are necessary to recognize the early onset of a bacterial infection. It may present itself as delayed wound healing, ulcera-

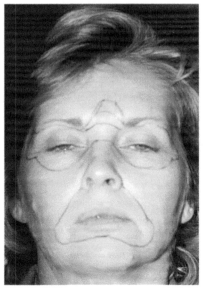 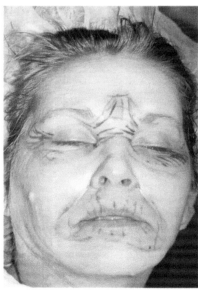 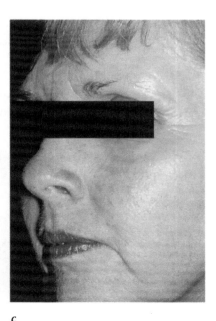

a   *b*   *c*

Figure 7.12 Combination deep chemical peel in the perioral area with a medium-depth peel over the remaining face: (A) preoperative appearance; (B) application of peel solution; (C) postoperative appearance.

tions, or the build-up of necrotic material with excessive scabbing, crusting, purulent drainage and odor. Early recognition will peel the skin and prevent the spread of infection and scarring.

Herpes simplex infection is the result of reactivation of the herpes simplex virus on the face and most commonly on the perioral area. A history of a previous herpes simplex virus infection should necessitate the use of prophylactic oral antiviral medications. Patients with a positive history can be treated with 400 mg of acyclovir three times a day, beginning on the day of the peel and continuing for 7–14 days depending on whether they have a medium-depth or a deep chemical peel. The mechanism of action is to inhibit viral replication in the intact epidermal cell, which means that the drug would not have an inhibitory effect until the skin re-epithelialized, i.e. 7–10 days in medium-depth and deep chemical peels. In the past, these agents were discontinued at day five and clinical infection became apparent 7–10 days later.[20] Active herpetic infections can easily be treated with antiviral agents and, caught early, they usually do not scar.

Delayed wound healing and persistent erythema are signs that the peel is not healing normally. The cosmetic surgeon must know the normal timetable for each of the healing events to occur so that it can be recognized at what time healing is delayed or the erythema is not fading adequately. Delayed wound healing may respond to physician debridement if an infection is present, corticosteroids if due to contact allergic or contact irritant dermatitis, along with the change of the offending contact agent, or protection with a biosynthetic membrane such as Flexzan™ or Vigilon®. When this diagnosis is made, these patients must be followed daily, with dressing changes and a close watch on the healing skin.

Persistent erythema is a syndrome where the skin remains erythematous beyond what is normal for the individual peel. A superficial peel loses its erythema in 15–30 days, a medium-depth peel within 60 days, and a deep chemical peel within 90 days. Erythema and/or pruritus beyond this period of time is considered abnormal and fits this syndrome. It may be due to contact dermatitis, contact sensitization, re-exacerbation of prior skin disease, or a genetic susceptibility to erythema; it may also indicate a sign of potential scarring. Erythema is the result of the angiogenic factors stimulating vasodilation, which also includes the phase of fibroplasia being stimulated for a prolonged period of time.[21] For this reason, it can be accompanied by skin thickening and scarring. It should be treated promptly and appropriately with topical steroids, systemic steroids, intralesional steroids if thickening is occurring, and skin protection, which would eliminate the factors of irritancy and allergy. If thickening or scarring becomes evident, other measures that may be helpful include the daily use of silicone sheeting and the dye pulsed laser to treat the vascular factors. With prompt intervention, in many cases scarring can be averted.

CONCLUSION

The physician has the responsibility of choosing the correct modality to treat skin conditions such as photoaging skin, scars, dyschromias and the removal of skin growths. There are many resurfacing techniques available, including the three levels of peeling, lasers and abrasion. A combination approach may give the best results with minimal morbidity and risk. It is the responsibility of the physician to have a thorough knowledge of all of these tools to give each patient the correct treatment warranted by their condition.

References

1. Fitzpatrick TB. The validity and practicality of sun-reactive skin types I through VI. Arch Dermatol 1988;124:869–71.

2. Stegman SJ. A comparative histologic study of the effects of three peeling agents and dermabrasion on normal and sun-damaged skin. Aesthetic Plast Surg 1982;6:123–5.

3. Monheit GD. Medium and deep chemical peels. In: Cosmetic Surgery, New York: Marcel Dekker; 2001: 37–69.

4. Glogau RG. Chemical peeling and aging skin. J Geriatr Dermatol 1994;2:30–5.

5. Monheit GD. Presentation at the American Academy of Dermatology in New Orleans, March 1999.

6. Wolfe SA. Chemical face peeling following therapeutic irradiation. Plast Reconstr Surg 1982; 69:859.

7. Monheit GD. Facial resurfacing may trigger the herpes simplex virus. Cosmet Dermatol 1995; 8:9–16.

8. Brody HJ. Variations and comparisons in medium-depth chemical peeling. J Dermatol Surg Oncol 1989;15:953–63.

9. Brody HJ. Trichloracetic acid application in chemical peeling, operative techniques. Plast Reconstr Surg 1995;2:127–8.

10. Monheit GD. The Jessner's + TCA peel: a medium depth chemical peel. J Dermatol Surg Oncol 1989;15:945–50.

11. Coleman WP, Futrell JM. The glycol acid/trichloracetic acid peel. J Dermatol Surg Oncol 1994;20:760–80.

12. Monheit GD. The Jessner's–TCA peel. Facial Plast Surg Clin North Am 1994;2:21–2.

13. Monheit GD. Skin preparation: an essential step before chemical peeling or laser resurfacing. Cosmet Dermatol 1996;9:13–14.

14. Rubin M. Manual of chemical peels. Philadelphia: Lippincott; 1995:50–67.

15. Harris DR, Noodleman FR. Combining manual derm sanding with low strength trichloracetic acid to improve actinically injured skin. J Dermatol Surg Oncol 1994;20:436–42.

16. Monheit GD, Zeitouni NC. Skin resurfacing for photoaging: laser resurfacing versus chemical peeling. Cosmet Dermatol 1997;10:11–22.

17. Chiarello SC. Tumescent dermasanding with cryospraying: a new wrinkle in the treatment of rhytids. Dermatol Surg 1996;22:601–10.

18. Monheit GD. The Jessner's–trichloracetic acid peel. Dermatol Clin 1995;13:277–83.

19. Monheit GD. Chemical peeling for pigmentary dyschromias. Cosmet Dermatol 1995;8:10–15.

20. Monheit GD. Facial resurfacing may trigger the herpes simplex virus. Cosmet Dermatol 1995; 8:9–16.

21. Goslen JB. Wound healing after cosmetic surgery. In: Coleman WP, Hanke CW, Alt TH, et al, editors. Cosmetic surgery of the skin. Philadelphia: Decker; 1991:47–63.

COMBINATION TREATMENT (Nicholas J Lowe)

Indications	Potential combination treatments	Chapter reference
Facial aging	Photoprotection	2
Dyspigmentation	Topical agents	3,4
Actinic keratoses	Glycolic acid peels	6
Post-acne scarring	Treatment for dyspigmentation, e.g. skin lightening agents	8
	Non-ablative laser	12
	Botox	13–15
	Fillers	16,17,19
	Liposuction	18
	Ocular plastic	23
	Surgical approaches	24
	Neck rejuvenation	25

8. Pigmentation of the ageing face – evaluation and treatment

Nicholas J Lowe and Suzanne Kafaja

INTRODUCTION

The face ages in a variety of ways. In addition to rhytides and sagging many patients complain that pigmented skin lesions give their faces an older appearance than they desire. One of the lay terms for solar lentigo – age spots – reveals patients' sentiments about this type of pigmentation.

There are numerous benign pigmentation disorders that can lead to the appearance of increased facial ageing. These include solar lentigo, pigmented seborrhoeic keratoses, melasma and facial melanosis from other causes, e.g. postinflammatory hyperpigmentation.[1] These problems usually require a combination of therapeutic approaches to ensure maximum improvement, including the following:

- photoprotection;
- topical skin lightening treatments;
- combination of lightening agents with topical retinoids;
- chemical peels with or without microdermabrasion;
- laser therapy may be used to treat some causes of facial pigmentation, but may be disappointing for diseases such as melasma;
- options for laser treatment include pigment-specific lasers (e.g. ruby or alexandrite lasers) or non-specific lasers (e.g. Er:YAG or CO_2 lasers).

EVALUATION OF FACIAL PIGMENTATION

Clinical assessment of dyspigmentation is the most important part of treatment selection.[1] Careful clinical evaluation is essential but a variety of other techniques, including chromometer and filtered photography, are also useful.[2]

Ultraviolet A (UVA) light has been known for many years to reveal pigmented areas in the skin.[3] It has been used previously to assess the skin level of pigmentation present in café au lait lesions, melasma and other pigmented lesions such as solar lentigo.[2–4]

Filtered UVA phototherapy is used to assess the extent and depth of facial pigmentation. It can also be successfully used to evaluate effective application of some sunscreens.

In general, superficial epidermal pigmentation will be accentuated by UVA photography, whereas dermal pigmentation becomes less obvious.

Ultraviolet filtered photography

Equipment: See Figure 8.1
Film: Kodak TMY 400 Black and White (24 exposure)
Camera: Nikon N-600
Lens: Nikkor 60 mm with a reproduction ratio of 1:6 and an aperture of f16
Flashes: CSI UV System 100 consisting of two Norman flashheads with filters passing UV at 365 nm

For the purposes of recording depigmentation or hyperpigmentation in dermatology, UVA works extremely well. Pigment in the skin strongly absorbs long-wave UV light, providing an excellent record of the pigmented areas on film.

ULTRAVIOLET PHOTOGRAPHY

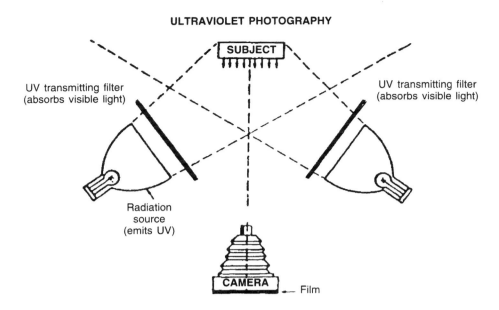

Figure 8.1 Equipment for reflected ultraviolet photography.

UVA photography acts on the premise that some materials will absorb UV light, others will reflect it and yet others will partially absorb or reflect it. When a strong light source (filtered so as to pass only UVA) is fired onto the object being photographed, the film is actually able to record this event. UVA (320–400 nm) is the most practical type of UV light since it passes through most optical glass very easily. This is the range that is being passed from the filtered light source to the film plane inside the camera.

UVA filtered photography is a very useful additional means of evaluating the severity of dyspigmentation in photodamaged facial skin. The technique, particularly when used with computer image analysis of the standardized photography, allows an objective measurement of the severity of dyspigmentation and its response to therapy to be made. Figure 8.2 shows a patient recorded by conventional and UVA filtered photography.

This method can also be used to examine uniformity of application of sunscreens, and thus allowing

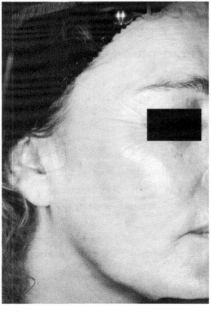

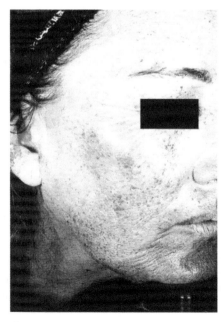

a   *b*

Figure 8.2 Conventional (A) and filtered UVA photography (B) of the face. (B) shows much more significant pigmentation than is evident in conventional photograph (A). The pigment is mainly superficial (epidermal) in location.

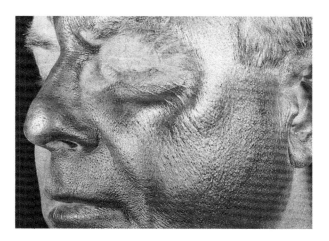

Figure 8.3 *Unfiltered photography. A sunscreen (containing UVA sunscreens) has been applied to the left side of the face and the areas where sunscreen application is missing are visible.*

instruction of the patient on uniform sunscreen application. Figure 8.3 shows application of a sunscreen containing a UVA filter ingredient.

The use of UVA filtered photography has been previously described by several investigators.[2–4]

TOPICAL THERAPY OF FACIAL PIGMENTATION

Numerous non-invasive treatment modalities exist for the treatment of hyperpigmented skin lesions. These treatments centre on the prevention of the synthesis of melanin, increasing its degradation or removal, and reduced proliferation of melanocytes.

Daily broad-spectrum sunscreen use represents a major first step in the management of hyperpigmented skin lesions. In fact, the use of sunscreen against UVA, UVB and visible light, which have been shown to play a critical role in the formation of melanin, should be strongly stressed to all patients. Other topical treatments include hydroquinones, kojic acid, tretinoins, other retinoids and glycolic acid, as well as chemical peels and combinations of all of these treatments.

Hydroquinones

Hydroquinones are hydroxyphenolic compounds that inhibit the formation of melanin by inhibiting the action of the enzyme tyrosinase, thus preventing the conversion of dopa to melanin. Hydroquinone may be formulated in multiple strengths, varying from 2% to 10%. The higher strengths are usually reserved for use in the treatment of severe cases of hyperpigmentation. While hydroquinones have been used as a single mode of treatment of hyperpigmentation, the current recommendations favour the use of combination treatment of hydroquinones, tretinoin and low-potency corticosteroid (e.g. hydrocortisone 1%), which have been shown to potentiate the efficacy of hydroquinone treatment (Figures 8.4 and 8.5).[5]

Common side-effects seen with hydroquinones include irritant contact dermatitis, depigmentation of the surrounding skin, postinflammatory hyperpigmentation and ochronosis, a rare side-effect more commonly seen in black patients.[6] Despite the fact that it was initially believed that ochronosis resulted from the use of higher-concentration hydroquinones, recent studies suggest that the culprit appears to be the overuse of these compounds rather than the strength. Multiple modalities of treatment of ochronosis are currently in use but appear to have minimal benefits. These treatments range from tretinoin creams to trichloroacetic acids. It may be worth trying pigment-specific lasers on ochronosis.

Azelaic acid

This medium chain length saturated nine carbon dicarboxylic acid non-phenol compound is approved for the treatment of acne. It has since been recognized as a treatment for hyperpigmentation by inhibiting tyrosine. This dicarboxylic acid, at 20% strength, has been shown to be as effective as 5% hydroquinone cream in the treatment of melasma. Other non-phenol agents that are currently in use for the treatment of hypermelanosis include kojic acid and alpha-hydroxy acids; 5-hydroxy-anisole is used in some countries and is awaiting the Food and Drug Administration's approval in the USA as a combined treatment with tretinoin.

Topical retinoids

The use of tretinoin creams alone or in combination with hydroquinones has also been shown to significantly improve melasma and postinflammatory hyperpigmentation.[7,8] Common side-effects seen

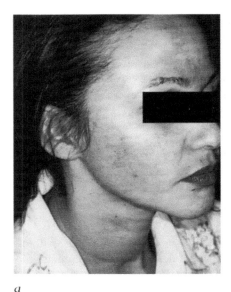
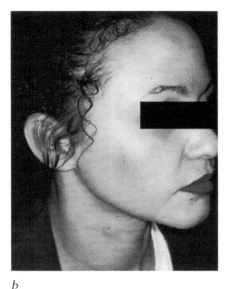

a   *b*

Figure 8.4 *Melasma plus postinflammatory hyperpigmentation before (A) and after (B) hydroquinone 5% and tretinoin 0.05% plus low-potency cortisone at night, broad-spectrum sunscreen each morning and four glycolic acid peels.*

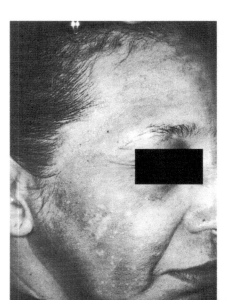
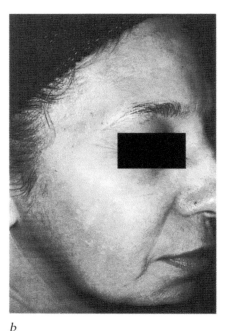

a   *b*

Figure 8.5 *(A) Severe melasma (facial pigmentation) before treatment. Reprinted with permission from Retinoids: A Clinicians' Guide. Lowe NJ and Marks R, 2nd edition, Martin Dunitz, London, 1998. (B) Melasma following 3 months of combined hydroquinone, tretinoin, Desonide cream nightly and broad-spectrum sunscreen each morning (4 months' therapy).*

with the use of tretinoin include erythema and peeling, and possible inflammatory hyperpigmentation.[7,8]

Newer retinoids such as tazarotene gel and cream may also be effective in improving facial hypermelanosis.

Chemical peels

Superficial and medium-depth chemical peels are recognized as decreasing the hyperpigmentation of melasma, particularly in patients with different skin tones.[9–11] These peels are less effective in patients with darker coloured skins, as peels then are more likely to cause postinflammatory hyperpigmentation. Despite the fact that these chemical peels may offer long-term benefits for the treatment of hypermelanosis, patients must be advised of the side-effects seen with this mode of treatment, e.g. skin irritation with erythema and exudation in some patients. Recent studies also suggest that the combination of pretreatment with tretinoin cream followed by chemical peels may offer a more notable decrease in the hypermelanosis, as with solar lentigines.

While these multiple topical modalities seem to have significant effects on melasma and postinflammatory hyperpigmentation, they tend to have minimal or no effect on pigmented lesions such as Becker's naevus. The current management of these lesions tends to centre mainly on laser treatment. In considering the optimal treatment of hypermelanosis it is crucial to consider the advantages as well as the side-effects of each treatment. Some of the advantages of topical treatments of hypermelanosis include the ease of application and the uniformity of results. Laser and chemical peels, on the other hand, may provide faster results of depigmentation. However, it is important to consider that some of their effects may not be reversible and hypopigmentation can result.

Microdermabrasion

Other treatments combined to treat facial pigmentation are skin lightening topical agents together with alternating glycolic acid peels and microdermabrasion. Microdermabrasion is employed using a variety of skin vacuum machines that use different skin abrading powders, e.g. aluminium salts, sodium bicarbonate crystals or sodium chloride crystals. The use of this treatment has expanded widely in the USA recently.

The hypothesis is a partial removal of the pigmented stratum. It may also partially disrupt the epidermal barrier and lead to enhanced effects of topical depigmenting creams. Microdermabrasion has also been claimed to improve superficial scars, acne, postinflammatory hyperpigmentation and facial melanosis. Controlled comparison studies of the different microdermabrasion machines are needed. In the present authors' clinics microdermabrasion is used as an alternating treatment with glycolic acid peels. Initially, the patient is treated every 2 weeks with glycolic acid peel or microdermabrasion. Following improvement the patient receives monthly maintenance treatment plus continuation of their topical therapy routine.

LASERS FOR PIGMENTED SKIN LESIONS OF THE FACE

A variety of lasers are used to treat benign pigmented skin lesions as well as tattoos. The basic principle for the use of these lasers in the management of pigmented skin lesions concerns melanin absorption characteristics.[12–15] Melanin, the main target in the laser treatment of pigmented lesions, has a broad absorption spectrum ranging between 351 and 1064 nm. Hence lasers with corresponding wavelengths target pigmented lesions of varying depths, with longer wavelengths producing damage to pigmentation at greater depth.[15,16] These lasers include the pulsed dye laser (510 nm wavelength),[17] the frequency doubled Q-switched Nd:YAG laser (532 nm),[18] the Q-switched ruby laser (694 nm),[19] the Q-switched alexandrite laser (755 nm) and the Q-switched Nd:YAG laser (1064 nm). Several of these lasers have been widely used in hair removal in the longer pulsed mode. By taking into account the effect of these lasers on melanin, these devices have recently been recognized as a tool for the management of some hyperpigmented lesions of the skin.

Q-switched ruby laser

The main chromophore at this laser's wavelength (694 nm) is melanin. The major benefit of the long red wavelength provided by this laser is that it allows deeper penetration of the skin layers into the dermis, thus allowing for an ideal treatment modality of the deep dermal pigmented lesions. This laser is valuable for solar lentigo, postinflammatory hyperpigmentation, naevus of Ota, but less so for melasma (Figures 8.6).[20–25]

Q-switched Nd:YAG laser

This laser produces a near-infrared beam with a wavelength of 1064 nm, allowing for a penetration depth of 5–8 nm. The pulse width achievable with this laser varies between 5 and 10 ns, with high energy fluences of 8–12 J/cm². This laser has been especially useful in the management of black and blue tattoos.

When the laser beam is passed through a potassium titanyl phosphate (KTP) crystal it produces a green light as the wavelength is halved to 532 nm, while the frequency is doubled.[26] The achievable pulse width with this laser appears to vary between 10 and 40 ns. This green light of the frequency-doubled Q-switched Nd:YAG laser is able to

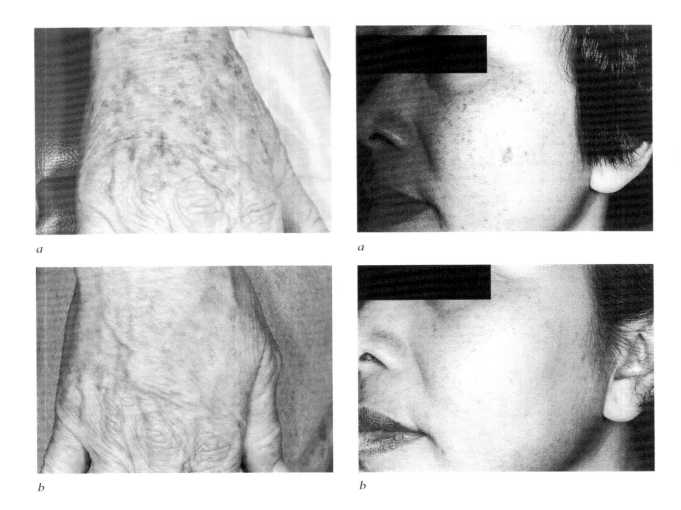

a

b

a

b

Figure 8.6 *Extensive solar lentigo lesions before (A) and after (B) 3 months of treatment with a Q-switched ruby laser. Note the improved skin texture as well as reduced pigmentalia.*

Figure 8.7 *A combination of solar lentigo plus upper facial melasma (A). The lentigo has cleared after Q-switched ruby laser and the melasma has improved (B).*

penetrate only into the epidermis and the upper dermis layer, thus providing an optimal means of treating superficial pigmented lesions, such as lentigines, café au lait spots, and red, orange and purple tattoos.[26]

Q-switched alexandrite laser

This laser provides a high intensity red beam with a wavelength of 755 nm. The achievable pulse width of this laser varies between 50 and 100 ns. The red beam wavelength allows this laser to penetrate not only the epidermis but also the dermis, as with the ruby laser, thus allowing for its use in the management of dermal

pigmented lesions. Despite the fact that the wavelength of this laser appears to match less selective melanin absorption, it has proven effective in removing dermal pigmentation such as that of postinflammatory hyperpigmentation.

Pulsed dye laser

The 510 nm wavelength of this laser lends itself to targeted epidermal lesions. The pulse width of this laser is 300 ns and the energy fluence is 2–4 J/cm^2. These properties make the pulsed dye laser particularly useful in treating benign epidermal lesions with minimal risks of injury and scarring.[17] However, there appear to be transient complications associated with the use of this laser, such as hyper- and hypopigmentation; other side-effects commonly seen with this laser include mild pain, ash white appearance to the skin immediately following treatment and purpura, which often lasts no longer than 2 weeks post-treatment. This laser is now rarely used, as the resulting hypopigmentation is more transient than that seen with the Q-switched lasers.

Long-pulsed ruby laser

This laser was used by the present authors as their initial hair removal laser. The laser beam produced is a red light at 694 nm with pulse duration of 3 μs. This system was originally introduced for laser-assisted hair removal. It targeted melanin within the hair follicle, causing thermal injury to the follicle and hair shaft. However, it has been recognized that these photoepilation systems also affect the melanocytes located in the superficial layers of the skin due to their longer pulse duration. When the system is used as a hair removing device, a cooling handpiece device is used to prevent thermal injury to superficial melanocytes as the energy is transmitted to the target region through a cooling-tip delivery system, which is composed of a sapphire lens. These properties lend themselves to the use of these systems in the management of hyperpigmented lesions of the skin. In fact,

the normal mode ruby laser (694 nm) has been shown to be superior to the Q-switched lasers in causing thermal damage to the superficial cells' naevus cell nests, with no evidence of malignant transformation of the treated region.[27] Despite clinical improvements of naevi, the complete destruction of the nevomelanocytes is thought to require multiple treatments.

Normal mode alexandrite laser

This laser uses a 755 nm wavelength with an average duration pulse of 10 ms. The energy fluence delivered ranges from 10 to 80 J/cm². The long-pulsed alexandrite laser system seems to affect follicular melanin in the same fashion as does the long-pulsed ruby system, and has also been in use primarily as a hair removal device. The alexandrite laser may offer an alternative to the multiple treatments required with long-pulsed ruby lasers, as the longer wavelength of the former provides deeper penetration of the skin layers. A recent study by Reda et al.[28] to evaluate the clinical and histological effects of a single treatment on benign pigmented naevi, using normal mode alexandrite lasers, showed either clearance or near clearance of the naevi.[28] The present authors have been evaluating this laser for a variety of benign pigmented lesions (Figure 8.8).

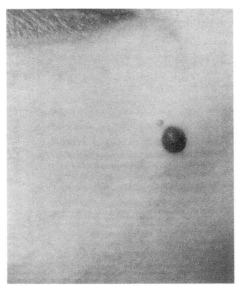 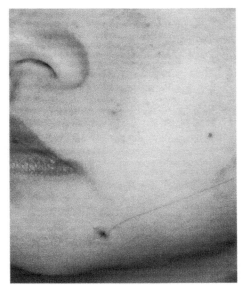

Figure 8.8 (A) Prominent pigmented naevus on the left hand side of the chin treated with shave biopsy to confirm a benign compound naevus. (B) Following one treatment with the long-pulsed alexandrite (755 nm). The patient may need a second treatment to clear the residual naevus.

a   *b*

SUMMARY OF COMBINED TREATMENT OF PIGMENTED SKIN LESIONS OF THE FACE

Topical therapy

Broad-spectrum sunscreens daily. Tretinoin, tazarotene, hydroquinone. Modified Kligmans Combination Formula. Azalaic acid, kojic acid, other topical agents: e.g. liquorice extracts, 5-hydroxyanisole.

Superficial procedures

Superficial peels, e.g.:
glycolic acid peels;

Jessner's solution;
microdermabrasion.

Lasers

Pigment-specific lasers
ruby;
alexandrite;
Nd:YAG.

(See Figures 8.9–8.13.)

Non-specific lasers
CO_2 laser;
Er:YAG laser.

(See Figure 7.12.)

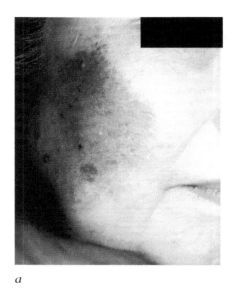
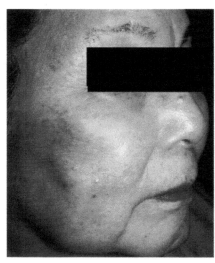

a   *b*

Figure 8.9 (A) Naevus of Ota. (B) After 3 treatments with Q-switched ruby laser 6 months apart. Photographs courtesy of Dr NJ Lowe.

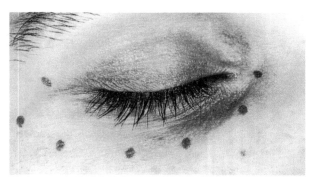
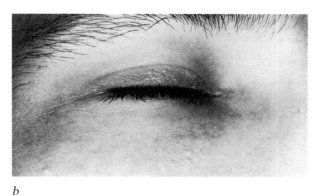

a   *b*

Figure 8.10 (A) Infraorbital skin pigmentation from a combination of dermal pigmentation plus shadows from fine infraorbital lines. (B) Following treatment with erbium YAG laser. In addition to reduced pigment there is good skin smoothing. See chapters 10 and 11.

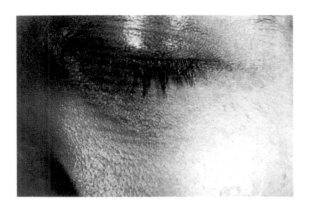
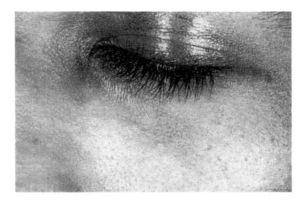

a   b

Figure 8.11 *Infraorbital dark circle (A) before and (B) after two treatments with the Q-switched ruby laser using 7.5 J/cm². Grade 2 improvement. Reprinted from Dermatol Surg 1995;21:769.*

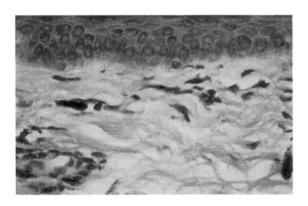
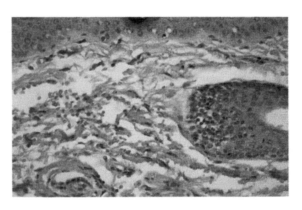

Figure 8.12 *Skin biopsy taken prior to treatment showing melanin pigment granules within mid and upper dermal macrophages (×200). Reprinted from Dermatol Surg 1995;21:769.*

Figure 8.13 *Twelve weeks post-laser treatment. There has been a marked reduction of dermal pigment. Occasional vacuolated basal epidermal cells are observed (×200). Reprinted from Dermatol Surg 1995;21:769.*

References

1. Ortonne JP. In: Parish LC, Lask GP, editors. Pigmentory changes in aesthetic dermatology. New York: McGraw-Hill, 1991:74–83.

2. Mustakallio KK, Korhonen P. Monochromatic ultraviolet photography in dermatology. J Investi Dermatol 1996;47:351–5.

3. Gilchrest BA, Fitzpatrick TB, Anderson RR, Parrish JA. Localization of melanin pigmentation in the skin with wood's lamp. Br J Dermatol 1997;96:245–9.

4. Arai J, et al. Ultraviolet photography. Int J Cosmet Sci 1989;1:103–10.

5. Kligman AM, Willis I. A new formula for depigmenting human skin. Arch Dermatol 1975;111:40–8.

6. Findlay GH, Morrison JGL, Sinson IW. Exogenous ochronosis and pigmented colloid milium from hydroquinone bleaching creams. Br J Dermatol 1975;93:613–22.

7. Griffiths CEM, Goldfarb MT, Finkel LJ, et al. Topical tretinoin (retinoic acid) treatment of hyperpigmented lesions associated with photo aging in Chinese and Japanese patients: a vehicle controlled clinical trial. J Am Acad Dermatol 1994;30:76–84.

8. Griffiths CEM, Finkel LJ, Ditre CM, et al. Topical tretinoin (retinoic acid) improves melasma. A

vehicle controlled clinical trial. Br J Dermatol 1993;129:415–21.

9. Burns RL, Prevost-Blank PL, Lawry MA, et al. Glycolic acid peels for postinflammatory hyperpigmentation in black patients. Dermatol Surg 1997;23:171–5.

10. Lim JTE, Tham SN. Gylcolic acid peels in the treatment of melasma among Asian women. *Dermatol Surg* 1997;23:177–9.

11. Garcia A, Fulton JE. The combination of glycolic acid and hydroquinone or kojic acid for the treatment of melasma and related conditions. Dermatol Surg 1996;22:443–7.

12. Apfelberg DB, Maser MR, Lash H, et al. The argon laser for cutaneous lesions. J Am Med Ass 1981;245:2073–5.

13. Trelles MA, Verkuysse W, Pickering JW, et al. Mono-line argon laser (514 nm) treatment of benign pigmented lesions with long pulse widths. J Photobiol 1992;16:357–65.

14. Ohishiro T, Maruyana Y. The ruby and argon lasers in the treatment of neavi. Ann Acad Med Singapore 1983;12:385–95.

15. Anderson RR, Parish JA. Selective photothermolysis: precise micro surgery by selective absorption of pulsed radiation. Science 1983;220:524–7.

16. Sherwood K, Murray S, Kurban K, et al. Effects of wavelength on cutaneous pigment using pulsed irradiation. J Invest Dermatol 1989;92:717–20.

17. Fitzpatirck RE, Goldman MP, Ruiz-Esparaza J. Laser treatment of benign pigmented epidermal lesions using a 300 ns pulse and 510 nm wavelength. J Dermatol Surg Oncol 1993;18:341–7.

18. Anderson RR, Margolis RJ, Watanabe S, et al. Selective photothermolysis of cutaneous pigment by Q-switched Nd:Yag laser pulsed at 1064, 532, and 535 nm. J Invest Dermatol 1989;93:28–32.

19. Nelson JS, Applebaum J. Treatment of superficial cutaneous pigmented lesions by melanin specific selective photomolysis using the Q-switched ruby laser. Ann Plast Surg 1992;29:231–7.

20. Levins PC, Anderson RR. Q-switched ruby laser for the treatment of pigmented lesions and tattoos. Clin Dermatol 1995;13:75–9.

21. Goldberg DJ. Benign pigmented lesions of the skin: treatment with the Q-switched ruby laser. J Dermatol Surg Oncol 1998;19:376–9.

22. Taylor CR, Anderson RR. Treatment of benign pigmented epidermis lesions by Q-switched ruby laser. Int J Dermatol 1993;32:908–12.

23. Lowe NJ, Wieder JM, Sawcer DE, et al. Nevus of Ota: treatment with high energy fluences of the Q-switched ruby laser. J Am Acad Dermatol 1993;29:997–1101.

24. Goldberg DJ, Nychay SG. Q-switched ruby laser treatment of nevus of Ota. J Dermatol Surg Oncol 1992;18:817–21.

25. Lowe NJ, Wieder JM, Shorr N, et al. Infraorbital pigmented skin Dermatol Surg 1995;21:767–70.

26. Lask GP, Glassberg E. Neodymium: yttrium–aluminium–garnet laser in the treatment of cutaneous lesions. Clin Dermatol 1995;13:81–6.

27. Ueda S, Imayana S. Normal mode ruby laser for treating congenital nevi. Arch Derm 1997;133:355–9.

28. Reda AM, Taha IR, Riad HA. Clinical and histological effect of a single treatment of normal mode alexandrite laser on small melanocytic nevi. J Cutan Laser Ther 1999;1:209–15.

COMBINATION TREATMENT (Nicholas J Lowe)

Indications	Potential combination treatments	Chapter reference
Facial pigmentation	Photoprotection	2
Lentigo	Topical agents	3
Melasma	Glycolic acid peels	6
Melanosis	Chemical peels	7
Congenital pigmentation	Botox	13–15
	Fillers	16–19
	Facial hair removal	22
	Photography very useful	26,27

9. Treating facial vascular lesions with lasers

Dina Yaghmai and Jerome M Garden

BACKGROUND

Facial vascular lesions comprise a large group of disorders commonly seen among patients. Such lesions exhibit considerable variation that include disfiguring congenital port-wine stains, hemangiomas, acquired telangiectasia, and diffuse erythema of rosacea.

The major causes for the development of vascular lesions on the face include: genetic or congenital predisposition, as in port-wine stains, hormonal factors seen in pregnancy and topical or systemic corticosteroid use, physical factors such as actinic-induced damage or ionized radiation, trauma, and post-surgical procedures such as rhinoplasty, collagen vascular disorders such as systemic lupus or dermatomyositis, and primary cutaneous disease of vascular disregulation such as rosacea or varicose veins.[1]

Facial telangiectases are visible superficial cutaneous vessels that measure 0.1–1 mm in diameter. Telangiectasias represent dilated venules, capillaries or arterioles.[2] Four classifications, based on clinical appearance, include: (1) simple or linear; (2) arborizing; (3) spider and; (4) papular.[3]

Multiple therapeutic modalities have been adopted for the treatment of vascular lesions. These include medical treatment with oral antibiotics or hormonal therapy, electrosurgery,[4] razor-blade surgery,[5] dermabrasion,[6] sclerotherapy,[7] and, most recently, laser surgery. Facial vascular lesions are asymptomatic and the main concern in treatment is good cosmesis with minimal adverse effects. The concept of selective photothermolysis, introduced by Anderson and Parrish,[8] help define the use of lasers in the treatment of vascular lesions with its concept of laser-induced thermal damage being limited only to the desired target.

Since the advent of lasers, a variety of different types of lasers have been used to treat vascular lesions. Several basic laser parameters must be evaluated in order to choose the best laser for treatment of different facial vascular lesions. The different lasers used for the treatment of vascular lesions include argon, CO_2, copper vapor, copper bromide, krypton, dye, and potassium titanyl phosphate (KTP) lasers. The main target chromophore in cutaneous blood vessel processes is hemoglobin and oxyhemoglobin. Oxyhemoglobin, with major absorption peaks at 418, 542, and 577 nm, has a high concentration in the blood vessels, making it an excellent target. The major lasers used in the treatment of vascular lesions have emission wavelengths that correspond to the absorption peaks of oxyhemoglobin. Although the 418 nm band is the strongest oxyhemoglobin absorption peak, it is also absorbed by the melanin chromophore in the epidermis. Therefore, the 577 nm band is more appropriate. This longer wavelength not only allows for deeper penetration into the dermis where blood vessels are found but also provides the least amount of absorption by the melanin chromophore in the epidermis.[9]

In order to effectively utilize the different lasers that are available today, it is imperative that the clinician is aware of certain basic laser parameters as well as the thermal properties of the lesions being treated. As mentioned above, for vascular lesions the target chromophore is oxyhemoglobin. While the site and depth of absorption are determined by the wavelength emitted by the laser, the tissue response is affected by the power density and the pulse duration of the exposed laser beam. The duration of exposure of the laser pulse, the pulse duration, determines the heat production within the target and its rate of dissipation to surrounding structures. In order to prevent damage to the surrounding tissue, high temperatures should be contained in the target, with gradual diffusion of cooler temperatures to the surrounding tissue. The temperature within the target tissue must be sufficient to cause selective destruction of the target while inflicting minimal damage on the surrounding structures.[8]

The thermal relaxation time is the time required for the target tissue to decrease the maximum central temperature obtained through heating by half. This value is dependent on the size of the targeted lesion, and the thermal diffusivity (κ) for the target vessel and the surrounding tissue. For cylindrical blood vessels the thermal relaxation time (t_r) time is a function of the vessel diameter (d) squared, $tr \cong d^2/16\kappa$, where κ is 1.3×10^{-3} cm^2/s.[8,10] Studies have shown that a selective mode of action with minimal thermal damage to the surrounding tissues can be achieved by selecting the laser pulse durations to be roughly equal to or less than the thermal relaxation time of the target vessels.[11,12]

Using the above formula the thermal relaxation time of various sized vessels can be calculated (Table 9.1). Port-wine stains have an average blood vessel size of 100 µm with a thermal relaxation time of < 5ms. The average vessel size in facial telangiectases is > 100 µm (150–300 µm), with an estimated thermal relaxation time of up to 50ms.[13]

Another important laser parameter is the fluence, or the amount of energy delivered per unit area, which is measured in J/cm^2. The fluence delivered by a laser, along with the pulse duration, should produce damage to the target while sparing the surrounding tissue. Various factors such as skin temperature and color affect the amount of energy delivered to the tissue. In darker skinned individuals epidermal melanin acts as a barrier which necessitates the use of higher energies in order to obtain clinical effect.[14,15]

In addition to wavelength, fluence and pulse duration, the different lasers used for the treatment of cutaneous lesions have various spot sizes. Studies have shown that the spot size greatly influences the amount of scattering of the laser beam. The use of larger spot sizes decreases the amount of peripheral scattering and allows for deeper penetration of the specific wavelength into the tissue.[12] Larger spot sizes also enable fewer pulses to be used, thereby decreasing the time needed to treat a given area. Understanding of the concept of selective photothermolysis and the relations between basic laser parameters enables a clinician to assess the multitude of different lasers that are available. The lasers that have historically been used in the treatment of facial vascular lesions differ based on the wavelength of action, pulse duration, power, and spot size. These variations result in wide range of clinical benefits and side-effects.

Table 9.1 Thermal relaxation times ($t_r \cong d2/16\kappa$)

Vessel diameter (µm)	Thermal relaxation time (ms)
30	0.43
50	1.2
70	2.35
100	4.8
150	10.8
200	19.2
250	30.0
300	43.3
350	58.9
400	76.9

ARGON LASER

The argon laser was one of the first lasers to be used in medical practice. The lasing medium is the argon-ion gas that emits a continuous wave of light at wavelengths of 488–514 nm. Approximately 80% of the light emitted is at 488 and 514 nm (blue-green), and 6% is at 476.5 or 496.5 nm. The remaining wavelength output is at 454.5 and 528.7 nm.[16] Based on the wavelengths produced by this laser, the target chromophores are oxyhemoglobin in the blood vessels and, therefore, melanin in the epidermis. The beam produced by the argon laser can be used in a continuous mode or it can be mechanically shuttered to produce different tissue exposure times. Parameters used with this laser include powers ranging from 0.8 to 2.9 W, spot sizes of 0.1, 1.0, and 2.0 mm in diameter, and pulse durations of 50 ms to 1.0 s.[17–19] The use of hexagonal robotized handpieces with spot beams of 3–13 mm in diameter have been used to treat facial telangiectasia with the argon laser.[20] Test-spot application with the argon laser is an important step in order to avoid scarring or considerable pigmentary changes. The test spot also allows the clinician to accurately assess the methods and laser parameters that are needed to obtain the best cosmetic response.[21] The site chosen for the test spot must be representative of the primary lesion being treated. For port-wine stains, a 1–2 cm area is treated using a 1.0 mm spot size at a low power. The handpiece is held perpendicular to the skin surface and moved slowly to produce minimal blanching of the treated area. Postoperatively, the treated area has a dusky-grayish discoloration with edema. The edema decreases over 1–2 days. Mild scabbing and crust formation is seen over the treated skin. Progressive lightening of the lesion is seen over the next several months.[22]

Treatment with the argon laser is associated with varying levels of discomfort, depending on the size of the lesion being treated. In the treatment of telangiectasia, the heat and burning sensation produced by the laser is usually tolerable without the need for anesthetics. Administration of local anesthetic can cause obliteration of the targeted vessels due to pressure induced by infiltration of the anesthetic material into the skin.[23] However, due to the level of pain associated with treatment of large lesions, administration of local anesthetic is often required.

Prior to the advent of newer lasers, such as the pulsed dye and the KTP lasers, the argon laser's absorption by oxyhemoglobin had made this laser the treatment of choice for vascular lesions such as port-wine stains and telangiectasia.[24] Many studies have demonstrated the clinical significance of the argon laser in the improvement of cutaneous vascular lesions; however, significant scarring and pigmentary changes have also been reported, with the incidence of scarring ranging from 5 to 40%.[12] One study cited a 38% incidence of scarring in children under 12-years old and a 22% incidence of scarring in adults

3–6 weeks after treatment for port-wine stains.[25] Permanent pigmentary changes, including hyper- and hypopigmentation, have also been reported in a high percentage of vascular lesions treated with this laser.[26] Sites such as the upper lip, nasolabial folds and the neck are at an increased risk of scarring.[25,27]

Histological study of sites treated with the argon laser demonstrate thermal damage to a depth of 1 mm in the dermis.[28] The epidermis shows coagulative necrosis extending down to the level of the papillary dermis. Electron microscopy shows vacuolization and denaturation of endothelial cells, keratinocytes, and fibroblasts. This nonspecific thermal damage, along with absorption by the melanin in the epidermis, results in the significant adverse effects seen with the argon laser.[29,30]

CARBON DIOXIDE LASER (CO_2)

The carbon dioxide (CO_2) laser operates in the infrared region of the spectrum at a wavelength of 10,600 nm. The targeting chromophore of this laser is the water molecule. Based on the intracellular and extracellular distribution of the target chromophore, the damage produced by CO_2 lasers is highly nonselective. The use of the CO_2 laser for the treatment of vascular lesions, specifically for facial port-wine stains, has been reported.[31] Many of these cases involve patients who had failed to show adequate improvement with the argon or the 577 nm pulse dye laser. In a study by Lanigan and Cotterill,[32] 40 patients (23 adults who had previously failed argon or continuous-wave dye laser therapy, and 17 children with pink port-wine stains) were treated with the CO_2 laser and followed for 12 months. Seventy-four per cent of adults and 53% of children responded positively, with no evidence of scarring or pigmentary changes; however, two of the children showed hypertrophic scarring and hyperpigmentation. Significant adverse effects seen with the use of the CO_2 laser include dyspigmentation, textural changes, and hypertrophic scar formation.[33] Histology of port wine stains treated with CO_2 lasers has shown vessel necrosis with significant damage to the surrounding dermis.[34] With the availability of other lasers, the CO_2 laser is no longer used for the treatment of facial vascular lesions.

COPPER VAPOR AND COPPER BROMIDE LASER

The copper vapor laser uses copper as the heavy metal vapor to emit light at 578 (yellow) and 510 nm (green) wavelengths; a filter is used to change between the two wavelengths. The power produced is dependent on the wavelength used, with the green wavelength adjustable to 3.0 W and the yellow beam to 1.3 W maximum. At 578 nm, the target chromophore for this laser is oxyhemoglobin within the blood vessels. This laser is a pulsed laser with a pulse duration of 20 ns. It is capable of emitting 10,000–15,000 pulses/s, which is seen as a continuous beam. As indicated earlier, facial telangiectasia have a diameter of 100–400 μm and a corresponding thermal relaxation times of 5–100 ms. A single pulse with a 20 ns pulse duration is unable to generate enough energy to produce clinical effect; however, the cumulative effect of multiple pulses can be useful in the treatment of facial vascular lesions. The spot size for the copper vapor laser varies from 100 to 800 μm, with 150 μm the most commonly used spot size for the treatment of telangiectasia.[35] Individual blood vessels are traced with the laser beam and the end-point of treatment is marked with blanching of the vessel.

Twenty patients with facial telangiectasia were treated with the copper vapor laser at a wavelength of 578 nm, a pulse duration of 20 ns, a pulse repetition rate of 15 KHz, and a shutter speed of 200 ms. Eighteen patients had a satisfactory clearance, three patients had postinflammatory hyperpigmentation that had resolved within 6–8 weeks after treatment, and one case showed depressed scarring.[35] In a similar study, 33 patients with facial telangiectasia were treated with the copper vapor laser. Laser parameters included a shuttered mode with pulse durations of 50–200 ms, and energy densities of 8–32 J/cm². Vessel-selective damage was seen with energy densities of 12 J/cm². Most of the patients, 69%, showed an excellent to good response, 12% with a fair, and 19% with a poor response in the improvement of the telangiectasia.[36] Side-effects with the copper vapor laser include scarring, and pigmentary and textural changes.[37] The incidence of adverse effects is higher in individuals with increased skin pigmentation, as well as in cases where greater energy intensities are produced by the laser.[38]

Histological studies of sites treated with the copper vapor laser show a subepidermal blister formation with degeneration of segments of the capillary and reticular dermis. The ectatic vessel walls appear 'shattered' and are replaced with fibrous connective tissue cords over 3–6 months.[39] It is this nonselective damage to the surrounding dermis that can lead to scarring.

Studies comparing the efficacy of the copper vapor laser and the 585 nm flashlamp pulsed dye laser in treating facial telangiectasia have shown similar improvements in lightening these cutaneous vascular lesions. Greater clearance was seen in the treatment of larger vessels with the copper vapor laser, while the pulsed dye laser was more effective in treating finer telangiectatic vessels. The pain associated with both lasers was comparable, without the need for local anesthetic. Postoperatively, minimal scabbing of the treated vessels and edema is seen with the copper vapor laser, while the 585 nm pulsed dye laser produces significant purpura and swelling.[40]

The copper bromide laser is a variant of the copper laser that also emits light in 578 (yellow) and 511 nm (green) wavelengths. Similar to the copper vapor laser, this laser produces a quasi-continuous wave system of a 30 ns pulse duration at 16 KHz that appears as a continuous beam. Mechanical shutters are used to provide pulse durations that range from 7 ms to 6 s. In treating facial vascular lesions, the 578 nm wavelength is used, which correlates best with the absorption peak of oxyhemoglobin. Two main advantages of this laser system include the ability to generate high output powers, and the production of variable exposure times to treat microvessels based on their thermal relaxation times. The average power output of the laser in the 578 nm wave spectrum is 2 W. The method of treatment is identical to the copper vapor lasers. The handpiece of the laser is used to trace individual blood vessels with the treatment end-point marked by disappearance of the vessels. It is important to avoid whitening of the skin during the treatment since whitening represents collateral damage to the surrounding tissues.[41]

In one study, 17 patients with facial telangiectasia were treated with the copper bromide laser. The pulse duration used in the study was 10–60 ms, with a spot size of 0.7 mm diameter. Large and medium sized vessels were treated with, on average, 19.8 and

17.8 J/cm² respectively. After an average of two treatments, one patient had excellent results showing 90–100% improvement, nine patients had 75–90% clearing and five patients 50–75% clearing. One patient had 25–50% clearance, and one patient < 25% clearance after only one treatment.[41] A larger study with 570 patients with facial telangiectasia were treated with the copper bromide laser and followed for a period of five years. Seventy per cent of patients had > 75% clearance, 17.4% of patients had 50–75% clearance, and 12.6% of patients showed < 50% clearance of facial telangiectases. Vessel size correlated with the level of response to treatment, with the copper bromide laser producing the best response for vessels 100–300 μm in diameter vessels.[42]

The pain associated with treatment with the copper laser has been minimal without any need for anesthetics. The postoperative response of treated vessels includes minimal erythema, and swelling with occasional scab and crust formation of the treated vessels. In the studies discussed above there was one report of scarring and atrophy when high intensity energy was used.[41,42]

KRYPTON LASER

The krypton laser is a gas medium, continuous-wave laser that emits light in the yellow (568 nm) and green (521 and 530 nm) region of the spectrum. The continuous wave produced by the laser can be shuttered to produce pulse durations as brief as 50 ms. The wavelengths of 530 and 568 nm emitted by the krypton laser correspond better with the 542 and 577 nm peak absorption bands of the target chromophore, oxyhemoglobin. The longer wavelength of 568 nm, compared to the 514 nm produced by the argon laser, allows for deeper penetration in to the dermis and less absorption by melanin in the epidermis. The krypton laser can be used in the 'yellow' spectrum, with the green light filtered out, or in the 'green' spectrum where all three wavelengths are combined. Two spot sizes used for the treatment of telangectasia are the 0.1 and the 1 mm:[43] the handpiece is used to trace individual telangiectases with the disappearance of the vessels being the treatment end-point. The power chosen is dependent on the wavelength used in order to avoid significant thermal damage to the surrounding tissue. Prominent blanching at the site treated with the laser is an indication of extensive dermal damage. Power settings of 0.7–0.8 W have been used with pulse durations of 50 ms (pulsed mode). The krypton laser in also used in the green spectrum with a 1 mm spot size, a pulse duration of 50 ms, and an energy fluence of 16 J/cm².[43] In a study by Thibault,[44] 64% of patients had significant clearance of facial telangiectasia with 84% reporting a good to excellent response. Thirty-eight per cent reported textural changes and 11% had atrophic scarring. Treatment with the krypton laser is associated with minimal pain; in fact the level of discomfort is less than that using the copper vapor laser. There is immediate post-therapy erythema that resolves within 48 hours. There have been reports of periorbital edema with extensive treatment of vascular lesions on the cheek. Adverse effects include scarring, textural changes, and hypo- and hyperpigmentation. In comparing the krypton laser with copper vapor laser, the incidence of scarring and hypopigmentation was lower for the krypton laser but the incidence of hyperpigmentation was the same for both lasers.[43,44]

ARGON-PUMPED TUNABLE DYE LASER (ATDL)

The argon-pumped tunable dye laser (ATDL) is a continuous-wave laser that can be mechanically shuttered to produce shorter pulse durations. The power source is an argon laser that utilizes dyes as the lasing medium to produce different wavelengths. Use of the rhodamine 6 G dye produces a wavelength of 577 nm that can be tuned to 590 nm with the use of a computer-controlled prism; these wavelengths are optimal to target the oxyhemoglobin chromophore in the blood vessels. Spot sizes used with this system vary from 0.1 to 6 mm. Individual blood vessels are traced, with the treatment end-point marked by vessel disappearance without whitening of the skin. The 0.1 mm spot size has been used for the treatment of facial telangiectasias with minimal risk of adverse effects.[45] In a study comparing the flashlamp-pumped pulsed dye laser (FPDL) with the ATDL for the treatment of facial telangiectasia, 17 patients with bilaterally symmetrical facial telangiectasia were treated with both lasers. Treatment parameters for the ATDL wavelength were 585 nm of a 13 mm hexagonal spot size, an energy fluence of 20–27 J/cm^2, and a pulse duration of 0.1 s, compared to a wavelength of 585 nm, of a 5 mm spot size, an energy fluence of 6.0–6.75 J/cm^2, and a pulse duration of 450 μs for the FPDL. The FPDL-treated telangiectasia demonstrated a 100% excellent response while 47% of the ATDL-treated telangiectasia side showed an excellent response and 53% had fair results. Although the FPDL was more effective in the clearance of the telangiectasia, the absence of bruising and decreased incidence of hyperpigmentation with the ATDL made this laser more acceptable to nearly 50% of the patients.[46]

FLASHLAMP-PUMPED PULSED DYE LASER (FPDL)

The flashlamp-pumped pulsed dye laser (FPDL), also referred to as the pulsed dye laser (PDL), has successfully treated many types of vascular lesions. The most extensive research in the use of this laser has been in the treatment of port-wine stains.[47,48] The mechanism of action of the FPDL is based on the concept of selective photothermolysis. The use of different dyes within the pulse dye chamber allows for emission of different wavelengths by the laser. Rhodamine dye produces a wavelength of 577 nm;[49] this coincides with the 577 nm absorption peak of oxyhemoglobin and allows for selective heat production in the blood vessels. The depth of penetration of the 577 nm wavelength is 0.5 mm in the dermis;[50] use of the 585nm wavelength increases the depth of dermal penetration to 1.5 mm.[51] Histologic study of skin biopsies from six patients with port-wine stains treated with both the 577 and 585 nm pulsed dye lasers reported the depth of vascular injury to be, on average 0.72 and 1.16 mm, respectively. This 50% increase in the depth of penetration allows for absorption by vessels present in the deeper dermis with improved clinical outcome.[52] A newer version of this laser operates at wavelengths up to 600 nm, giving even deeper penetration into the dermis. These new systems use a coolant spray and are able to generate very high energy fluences.

The appropriate pulse duration for the treatment of different vessels such as facial telangiectasia and port-wine stains have been studied extensively. As mentioned previously, the ideal pulse duration for the treatment of vascular lesions is determined by the thermal relaxation time and the diameter of the targeted vessels; for port-wine stains this has been calculated as 1–10 ms.[53,54] For the treatment of larger vessels, as seen in facial telangiectasia, the ideal pulse durations are ≥ 20–100 ms (Table 9.1). The 585 nm FPDL operates at either 450 μs or 1.5 ms pulse durations. The newer 595 and 600 nm lasers have adjustable pulse durations ranging from 1.5 to 40 ms, allowing deeper penetration in to the skin at the longer wavelengths, and are also able to operate at pulse durations that more closely coincide with the thermal relaxation time of larger sized vessels.[55]

The FPDL spot sizes include 2, 3, 5, 7, 10 and 2 × 7 mm handpieces. The combination of the spot size and the energy fluence determine the amount of energy that penetrates into the dermis; the energies produced by this system range from 3 to 25 J/cm^2. Purpura generally occurs with therapy but is minimized or eliminated at the longer pulse durations without causing damage to the epidermis. Histological studies of skin after treatment with the FPDL show formation of an intravascular coagulum with agglutination of erythrocytes, fibrin, and platelet thrombi extending to the mid-dermis. Electron microscopy reveals focal epidermal edema, destruction of the endothelium, periocytes, and perivascular collagen with marked inflammatory reaction with perivascular polymorphonuclear leukocytes. One month after the treatment procedure the abnormal vessels are replaced by normal caliber vessels with slightly thickened vessel walls.[56]

In treating facial telangiectasia, the individual vessels are traced with pulses overlapping by up to 13% to cover the desired area.[57] The energy fluence used ranges from 3 to 8 J/cm^2 depending on the skin type, the site of treatment, the spot size, and the tissue response. Post-laser therapy lightening is often seen after 6–10 weeks. Subsequent treatments are performed at 2–3 month intervals in order to allow maximum lightening to occur (Figure 9.1a, and 9.1b).[49] Most patients experience a transient burning or stinging sensation with each pulse, which has been described as being like the snap of a rubber band or

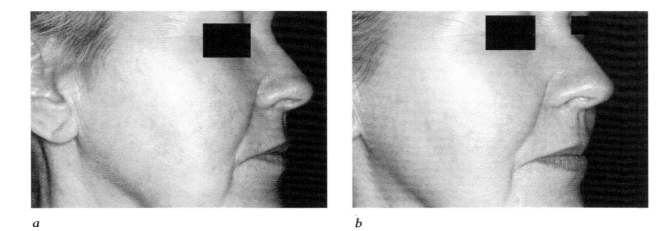

a   b

Figure 9.1 (A) Facial telangiestasia in a 55-year-old woman with multiple blood vessels on bilateral cheeks; (B) after two treatments with the pulsed dye laser at an energy fluence of 4 J/cm² with a 10 mm diameter spot size.

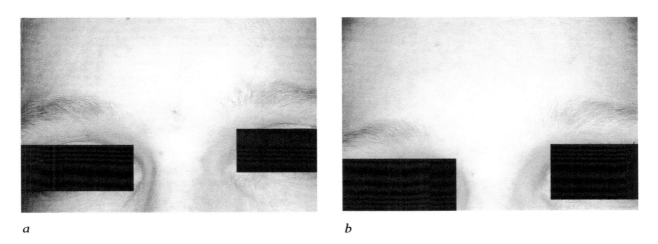

a   b

Figure 9.2 (A) Papular angioma in the glabella of a 31-year-old woman; (B) after one treatment with the pulsed dye laser at 6 J/cm² with a 5 mm spot size.

a pinprick. When treating adults for facial telangiectasia the discomfort is generally well tolerated without the need for anesthetics. In patients with increased sensitivity, use of topical anesthetics, cool compresses, cryogen spray to the skin surface, nitrous oxide, or local anesthesia may be beneficial.[58,59]

Multiple studies demonstrate the efficacy of the FPDL in treating facial vascular lesions. Ninety-two patients with facial telangiectases were treated with the 577 nm pulsed dye laser with a 5 mm spot size, a 300 μs pulse duration and an energy fluence of 6–8 J/cm². Ninety-one per cent of the patients

showed 76–100% clearing after one treatment; 9% showed 50–75% clearing after one treatment, and 94% clearing after two or three treatments. Spider and matted telangiectasias demonstrated 92–93% clearing compared to the linear telangiectasias with 77% clearing (Figure 9.2a and 9.2b).[60] In a similar retrospective study, 182 patients were treated for facial telangiectases at a wavelength of 585 nm with a 450 μs pulsed dye laser with a 5 mm spot size at energy fluences of 6–7.75 J/cm². Eighty-four per cent of the patients treated had a 76–100% response while 14% had 51–75% response rate. The clearance

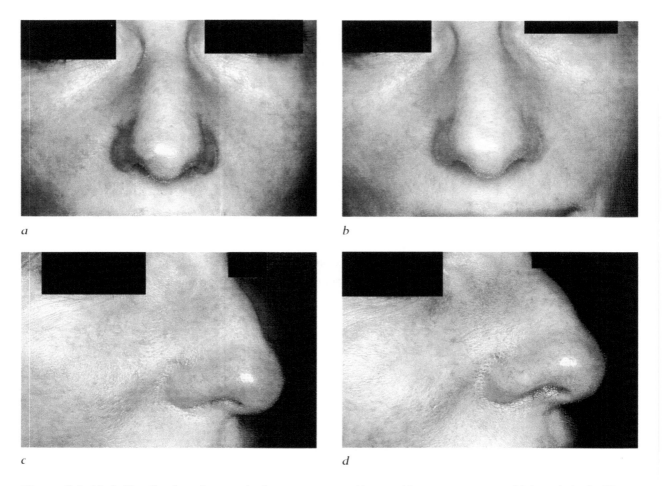

a   *b*   *c*   *d*

Figure 9.3 *(A) Diffuse facial erythema and telangiectasia in a 41-year-old woman on nose and bilateral cheeks (C); (B) after treatment with the pulsed dye laser (PDL) at an energy fluence of 6.5 J/cm² with a 5 mm spot size for the nasal tip; (D) after treatment with the PDL at an energy fluence of 9 J/cm² with a 2×7 mm spot size on bilateral cheeks.*

was greater with the use of higher fluences and increased number of treatments. The level of pain was described as moderate by 72% of the patients.[61] Use of the 2 mm spot size has been shown to be more effective for the treatment of superficial telangiectasia, with improved vessel clearance, decreased purpura and pain. This smaller spot size allows for use of higher energy fluences, with decreased incidence of adverse effects.[62] The use of the 595 nm, 1.5 ms pulsed dye laser has shown significant improvement in the treatment of vessels that have been less responsive to the traditional shorter pulsed dye lasers. Vessels in the nasolabial folds and cheeks measuring 1mm in diameter have been treated with the longer pulsed dye laser.[63]

Rosacea with diffuse erythema, facial telangiectases and erythematous papules is another condition that has shown improvement after treatment with the FPDL (Figure 9.3a–d, and 9.4a and b). In one study, use of energy fluences of between 6.0–7.5 J/cm² resulted in a decrease in the papular component of rosacea without any adverse effects in 59% of the patients.[64] There are many reports of treatment of poikiloderma of Civatte with the pulsed dye laser.[65–67] This term is used to describe a clinical picture comprised by atrophy, telangiectasia, and pigmentary changes.[68] One case report demonstrated an 80% improvement after four treatments, each one 8 weeks apart, with the use of the FPDL at a wavelength of 585 nm, a pulse duration of 450 µs and an energy

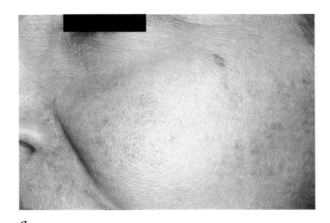 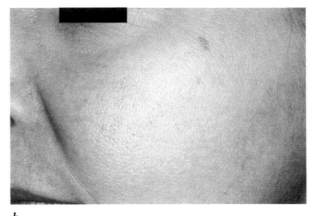

a   *b*

Figure 9.4 (A) *Facial telangiectasia and diffuse erythema on bilateral cheeks;* (B) *after treatment with a pulsed dye laser at an energy fluence of 3 J/cm² with a 10 mm spot size.*

fluence of 6.5 J/cm².[69] Other conditions with superficial small vascular lesions, such as telangiectasias in scleroderma,[70] Rothmund-Thomson syndrome,[71] focal dermal hypoplasia,[72] cutaneous lupus erythematosus,[73] and telangiectasia macularis eruptiva perstans,[74] have been treated using the pulsed dye laser. Caution must be adopted in the use of laser therapy for treatment of the photosensitive conditions mentioned above.

Adverse effects with the pulsed dye laser include hypo- and hyperpigmentation, and scarring.[75] In a study of 500 patients treated with the pulsed dye for port-wine stains, telangiectasias, and hemangiomas scarring was seen in < 0.1%, 1% with hyperpigmentation, and 2.6% with transient hypopigmentation.[76] In a retrospective study looking at 701 patients treated for port-wine stains the most common adverse effect was hyperpigmentation, occurring in 9.1% of patients, with gradual clearing over 6–12 months. Hypopigmentation was seen in 1.4% of patients. Other adverse effects included atrophic scarring (4.3%), and hypertrophic scarring (0.7%).[77] Epidermal damage is evident by blistering, crusting and scab formation. Thermal transfer from underlying vessels, as well as absorption by the pigment in the basal layer of the epidermis, are responsible for the thermal damage seen post-treatment.[78] Avoidance of sun is very important during the treatment course in order to minimize the adverse effects from increased absorption of energy by the epidermal melanin.[79] Keloid formation has also been noted with the use of the pulsed dye laser in patients on isotretinoin therapy.[80] In order to prevent unexpected clinical outcomes it is important to be aware that FPDL built by different manufacturers differ in the actual delivered spot size diameter and the beam profile, even though their emission wavelengths and spot size are thought to be identical.[81] The pulsed dye laser has greatly advanced the treatment of cutaneous vascular lesions by decreasing the adverse effects associated with treatments.[78]

POTASSIUM TITANYL PHOSPHATE LASER (KTPL)

The potassium titanyl phosphate laser (KTPL) is a solid-state frequency-doubled neodynymium-doped crystal of a yttrium–aluminum–garnet laser (Nd:YAG). In this laser the Nd:YAG crystal emits light at a wavelength of 1064 nm that is passed through a KTP crystal emitting a 532 nm (green) wavelength that is frequency doubled. The Nd:YAG laser functions in a continuous or pulsed mode; it may also produce a very rapid pulse in a Q-switch mode.[82] The target chromophore for the KTP is the oxyhemoglobin molecule, the 532 nm emission wave corresponding most closely with the oxyhemoglobin

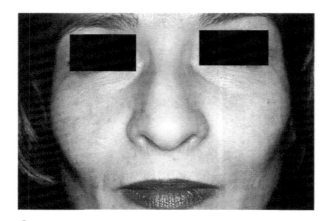
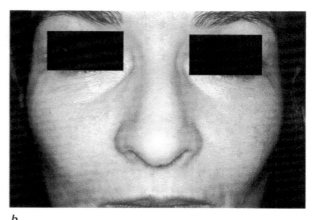

a   *b*

Figure 9.5 *(A) Facial telangiectasia in a 40-year-old woman; (B) after one treatment with the potassium titanyl phosphate laser at an energy fluence of 22 J/cm², a 1 mm spot size and a pulse duration of 20 ms.*

absorption peak of 542 nm. The depth of penetration at this wavelength is < 1 mm into the tissue, compared to the 1064 nm beam that penetrates up to 5–7 mm into the tissue. One of the main advantages of KTPL systems is the ease of use for the operator. Patients are usually placed in the supine position. In order to better visualize the vessels, magnifying optics may be used. The laser handpiece is traced along the course of the blood vessel, with the disappearance of the vessel as the end-point of treatment. Treatment is well tolerated without the need for anesthetics. Pain associated with the procedure is described as a stinging sensation. Treatment over sites such as the inferior nares and the columella are often associated with increased discomfort and pain (Figure 9.5a and b).

Multiple different pulsed KTPL with a 532 nm emission wavelength and variable pulse durations and spot sizes are marketed today. Some systems have a variable pulse duration of 2–10 ms, spot sizes ranging from 2 to 10 mm and frequencies of 1–6 Hz. This system utilizes a sapphire cooled 'chill tip' that is attached to the handpiece in order to cool the epidermis during treatment. The handpiece is placed in direct contact with the skin and the vessels are traced from the periphery to the center of the face. Others have an even more expanded pulse duration, ranging from 1 to 50 ms, pulse rates of up to 20 KHz, and a power output of 1–160 W. The spot sizes used in the

treatment of cutaneous vascular lesions include 0.25, 1, 2, and 4 mm handpieces.

Another frequency-doubled Q-switched Nd:YAG laser used in the treatment of facial vascular lesions is a diode-pumped system which uses a KTP crystal to produce a 532 nm wavelength beam similar to the KTPL already discussed. Finally, those that are Q-switched produce pulse durations from 10 to 50 ns, with pulse rate of 5–10 Hz, and spot sizes 2–6 mm in diameter (Figure 9.6a and b).[83]

The KTPL offers many advantages over previously used lasers. The variable pulse durations allow adjustments to be made depending on the size of the vessel being treated, and the machine is easy to use. When the pulse duration is comparable to the thermal relaxation time of the vessel then there is no postoperative purpura (unlike that seen with the pulsed dye laser). Post-operatively, patients present with minimal erythema that resolves within hours to a few days after treatment. Comparison of four KTPL showed similar clinical responses without evidence of scarring or pigmentary changes.[84]

In a study comparing a long-pulsed dye laser (590–595 nm wavelength and a 1.5 ms pulse duration) with the KTPL for the treatment of facial telangiectasias, all patients showed improvement regardless of the laser used. Twelve weeks after an equal number of treatments with either laser, the improvement with the long-pulsed dye system was

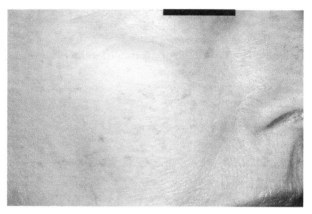
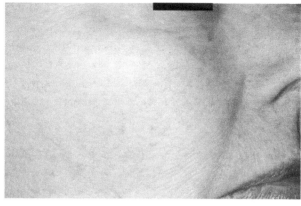

a   *b*

Figure 9.6 *(A) Multiple telangiectatic vessels on the outer bilateral cheeks in a 56-year-old woman; (B) after treatment with the diode laser at a wavelength of 532 nm, an energy fluence of 18 J/cm², a pulse duration of 47 msec, and a 1 mm spot size.*

better than that seen with the KTP laser. The superiority of the pulsed dye was seen in both facial and lower extremity telangiectasia. However, despite the level of clearance, the decreased pain associated with the treatment and the minimum postoperative findings with the KTPL, made this laser more desirable for the treatment of facial vascular lesions.[63] Another study of 40 patients using the KTPL for the treatment of facial telangiectasia, using energy fluences of 9.5–12.0 J/cm², spot sizes of either 3 or 4 mm, and a pulse duration of 10 ms showed 75% clearance of blood vessels measuring ≤ 1.5 mm in diameter after one treatment. A second treatment demonstrated a 90–100% clearance of blood vessels. Histologically, there was evidence of vessel wall damage and thrombosis but no epidermal damage.[85] Adverse effects associated with the KTPL include rare cases of mild linear crusting, hyper- and hypopigmentations and scarring.[85,86]

INTENSE PULSE LIGHT SYSTEMS (IPL)

Intense pulse light (IPL) systems produce a non-coherent light source with a broad spectrum that ranges from 500 to 1200 nm. Cut-off filters (515, 550, 570 and 590 nm) are designed such that each filter is capable of absorbing, and thus filtering out, all the wavelengths that are less than the wavelength designated to that filter; e.g. a 570 nm filter absorbs all wavelengths < 570 nm. Similar to previously discussed lasers, the IPL system functions based on the concept of selective photothermolysis. Dependent on the target chromophore and the depth at which this chromophore is present, different filters can be used to emit a wavelength that corresponds to the absorption peak of the specific target, and at the same time penetrate deep into the tissue to the level where the target chromophore is most abundant. Application of this light source also allows for specific adjustments based on the patient's skin type. For example, the shorter wavelengths can be filtered out in order to prevent absorption by the melanin chromophore that is present in a greater amount in the epidermis of darker skinned individuals. The pulse duration of the IPL system ranges from 2 to 25 ms. Another unique feature of this intense light source is the ability to produce trains of two or three pulses 10–500 ms apart. Fairly large spot sizes can be used with the intense light source that are generally rectangular in shape. The large spot size results in deeper penetration, decreased scattering of the light beam, and a decrease in the time needed for treatment of a given area. Energy fluences produced by these IPL systems can range from 3 to 90 J/cm². The cooling system of these units utilize a cooling gel that is applied directly to the skin surface being treated, both decreasing the burning sensation from the heat produced, and simultaneously removing excessive heat that may cause thermal damage to the epidermis and surrounding structures. The pain and discomfort associated with the use of IPL systems has been described as being like the snap of a rubber band or stinging. Treatment parameters are entered into the system and are adjusted based on the skin type, size, and depth of the vessel. The great versatility inherent to this light source enables its use in the treatment of various cutaneous lesions; conversely, this versatility produces difficulty in establishing the best parameter combinations in the treatment of cutaneous lesions.

The efficacy of IPL systems was studied in the treatment of 120 patients with different vascular lesions ranging from facial and leg telangiectasia to spider and cherry angiomas. Blue and red facial telangiectasia were treated with the 590 and 550 nm cut off filters, respectively. The blue telangiectasia showed a 90% clearance with treatment parameters set at 38–50 J/cm^2 energy fluences, and triple pulse times of 3.8, 3.1, and 2.6 ms. The red telangiectasia were treated with energy fluences of 30–34 J/cm^2 and pulse durations of either 10 or 20 ms, giving a 95% clearance. Minimal to no side-effects were seen, except pigmentary changes and blistering in the treatment of leg telangiectasia.[87] In a similar study, 200 patients with facial telangiectasia, hemangiomas, rosacea, and port-wine stains were treated with an IPL system. Of the 188 patients seen during follow-up period, 174 demonstrated 75–100% clearance. In the majority of the cases (128 of the 174) only one treatment was needed to obtain > 75% clearance. Fifty-one of the patients showed 50–75% clearance, while nine patients showed < 50% improvement after one treatment. There were no reports of scarring or permanent pigmentary changes in the patients treated.[88] The use of the IPL system has also been shown in the treatment of poikiloderma of Civatte. In a retrospective study, 82% of the patients demonstrated a 75–100% improvement after an average of three treatments. The incidence of adverse effects in this study was 5%, consisting of pigmentary changes.[89] Many studies have demonstrated the efficacy of the IPL system in the treatment of leg telangiectasia.[90]

However, a cautionary note must be sounded with the IPL system since the use of high energies can lead to surrounding thermal damage and blister formation that can readily produce scarring and pigmentary changes.[91] The IPL system may have some advantages over other laser systems in the treatment of vascular lesions but adjustment of all its different parameters are difficult, and require experience.

CONCLUSIONS

There has always been great interest in the treatment of cutaneous vascular lesions. With the development of new technologies the approach to treatment of patients with facial telangiectases has changed considerably. Even though each treatment plan must be tailored to the patient's skin type, and the size and location of the vascular lesion being treated, there are some general basic principles that can be followed. Appropriate laser systems for the treatment of minor facial telangiectasia include the KTPL, krypton, copper bromide, FPDL, and very careful application of the IPL systems, all used in a nonpostoperative purpura mode. In the treatment of diffuse facial redness and port-wine stains, the long-pulsed dye laser has demonstrated the highest efficacy, and especially safety. Facial telangiectases that have been resistant to therapy with the KTPL have also been successfully treated with the pulsed dye laser. The IPL system has also been effective in the treatment of diffuse background redness in addition to individual vessels. These recent advances have been beneficial for patients and the present authors anticipate that, with further modifications and developments in the laser field there will be even more advantageous therapeutic choices in the future.

References

1   Goldman MP, Bennett RG. Treatment of telangiectasia: a review. J Am Acad Dermatol 1987;17:167–82.

2   Goldman MP, Weiss RA, Brody HJ, et al. Treatment of facial telangiectasia with sclerotherapy, laser surgery, and/or electrodesiccation: a review. J Dermatol Surg Oncol 1993;19:899–906.

3   Redisch W, Pelzer RH. Localized vascular dilatations of the human skin: capillary

microscopy and related studies. Am Heart J 1949;37:106–14.

4 Kobayashi T. Electrosurgery using insulated needles: treatment of telangiectasias. J Dermatol Surg Oncol 1986;12:936–42.

5 Johannesson A. Razor blade surgery of large vessels on the nose. J Dermatol Surg Oncol 1988;14:617–18.

6 Lapins AN. Dermabrasion for telangiectasia. J Dermatol Surg Oncol 1983; 9:470–2.

7 Bodian EL. Techniques of sclerotherapy for sunburst venous blemishes. J Dermatol Surg Oncol 1985;11:696–704.

8 Anderson RR, Parrish JA. Selective photothermolysis: precise microsurgery by selective absorption of pulsed radiation. Science 1983;220;524–7.

9 Parrish JA, Anderson RR. Consideration of selectivity in laser therapy. In: Arndt KA, Noe JM, Rosen S, editors Cutaneous laser therapy: principles and methods. John Wiley & Sons, 1983: 41–52.

10 Anderson RR, Parish JA. Optical properties of human skin. In: Regan JD, Parrish JA, editors. The Science of Photomedicine. New York: Plenum; 1982:147–94.

11 Smithies DJ, Butler PH, Day WT, Walker EP. The effect of the illumination time when treating port-wine stains. Lasers Med Sci 1995;10:93–104.

12 Grossman DJ, Kauvar ANB. Selected clinical applications of lasers. Adv Dermatol 1999;14:141–65.

13 Anderson RR, Parish JA. Microvasculature can be selectively damaged using dye lasers: a basic theory and experimental evidence in human skin. Lasers Surg Med 1981;1:263–76.

14 Paul BS, Anderson RR, Jarva J, Parrish JA. The effect of temperature and other factors on selective microvascular damage caused by pulsed dye laser. J Invest Dermatol 1983;81:333–5.

15 Ashinoff R, Geronemus RG. Treatment of a portwine stain in a black patient with the pulsed dye laser. J Dermatol Surg Oncol 1992;18:147–8.

16 Levine VJ, Lee MS, Geronemus RG, Arndt KA. Continuous-wave and quasi-continuous wave lasers. In: Arndt KA, Dover JS, Olbricht SM, editors. Lasers in cutaneous and aesthetic surgery. New York: Lippincott-Raven, 1997:67–107.

17 Apfelberg DB, Maser MR, Lash H. Argon laser treatment of cutaneous vascular abnormalities: progress report. Ann Plast Surg 1978;1:14–18.

18 Arndt KA. Treatment techniques in argon laser therapy: comparison of pulsed and continuous exposures. J Am Acad Dermatol 1984;11:90–7.

19 Apfelberg DB, Maser MR, Lash H, Rivers JL. Progress report on extended clinical use of the argon laser for cutaneous lesions. Lasers Surg Med 1980;1:71–83.

20 McDaniel OH, Mordon SR. Hexascan: a new robotized scanning laser handpiece. Cutis 1990;15:300–5.

21 Cosman B. Experience in the argon laser therapy of port wine stains. Plast Reconstr Surg 1980;65(2):119–29.

22 Dover JS, Arndt KA, et al. Argon lasers. In: Dover JS, Arndt KA, et al., editors. Illustrated cutaneous laser surgery. A practitioner's guide. Connenticut: Appleton & Lange, 1990:73–106.

23 Arndt KA. Argon laser therapy of small cutaneous vascular lesions. Arch Dermatol 1982;118:220–4.

24 Noe JM, Barsky SH, Greer DE, Rosen S. Port wine stains and the response to argon laser therapy: successful treatment and the predictive role of color, age, and biopsy. Plast Reconstr Surg 1980;65:130–6.

25 Dixon JA, Huether S, Rotering R. Hypertrophic scarring in argon laser treatment of port-wine stains. Plast Reconstr Surg 1984;73(5):771–7.

26 Nanni CA, Alster TS. Complications of laser surgery. Dermatol Surg 1998;24:209–19.

27 Ratz JL. Posttreatment complications of the argon laser. Arch Dermatol 1985;121:714.

28 McBurney E. Clinical usefulness of the argon laser for the 1990s. J Dermatol Surg Oncol 1993;19:358–62.

29 Apfelberg DB, Kosek J, Maser MR, Lash H. Histology of port wine stains following argon laser treatment. Br J Plast Surg 1979;32:232–7.

30 Tan OT, Carney JM, Margolis R, et al. Histologic responses of port-wine stains treated by argon, carbon dioxide, and tunable dye laser. Arch Dermatol 1986;122:1016–22.

31 Ratz J, Bailin P. The case for the use of carbon dioxide laser in the treatment of port-wine stains. Arch Dermatol 1987;123:74–75

32 Lanigan SW, Cotterill JA. The treatment of port wine stains with the carbon dioxide laser. Br J Dermatol 1990;123: 229–235.

33 Garden JM, Geronemus RG. Dermatologic laser surgery. J Dermatol Surg Oncol 1990; 16; 156–168.

34 Buecker JW, Ratz JL, Richfield DF. Histology of port wine stains treated with carbon dioxide laser. J Am Acad Dermatol 1984;10:1014–19.

35 Key JM, Waner M. Selective destruction of facial telangiectasia using a copper vapor laser. Arch Otolaryngol Head Neck Surg 1992;118:509–13.

36 Neumann RA, Leonhartsberger H, Bohler-Sommeregger K, et al. Results and tissue healing after copper-vapour laser (at 578nm) treatment of port wine stains and facial telangiectaias. Br J Dermatol 1993;128:306–12.

37 Pickering JW, Walker EP, Butler PH, Halewyn CN. Copper vapor laser treatment of port-wine stains and other vascular malformations. Br J Plast Surg 1990;43:273–82.

38 Haedersdal M, Wulf HC. Risk assessment of side effects from copper vapor and argon laser treatment: the importance of skin pigmentation. Lasers Surg Med 1997;20:84–9.

39 Tan OT, Stafford TJ, Murray S, Kurban AK. Histologic comparison of the pulsed dye laser and copper vapor laser effects on pig skin. Lasers Surg Med 1990;10:551–8.

40 Waner M, Dinehart SM, Wilson MB, Flock ST. A comparison of copper vapor and flashlamp pumped dye lasers in the treatment of facial telangiectasia. J Dermatol Surg Oncol 1993;19:992–8.

41 McCoy S, Hanna M, Anderson P, et al. An evaluation of the copper-bromide laser for treating telangiectasia. Dermatol Surg 1996;22:551–7.

42 McCoy SE. Copper bromide laser treatment of facial telangiectasia: results of patients treated over five years. Lasers Surg Med 1997;21:329–40.

43 Patel BCK. The krypton yellow-green laser for the treatment of facial vascular and pigmented lesios. Sem Ophthalmol 1998;13(3):158–70.

44 Thibault PK. A patient's questionnaire. Evaluation of krypton laser treatment of facial telangiectases. Dermatol Surg 1997;23:37–41.

45 Orenstein A, Nelson JS. Treatment of facial vascular lesions with a 100–micron spot 577–nm pulsed continuous wave dye laser. Ann Plast Surg 1989;23:310–16.

46 Ross M, Watcher MA, Goodman MM. Comparison of the flashlamp pulsed dye laser with the argon tunable dye laser with robotized handpiece for facial telangiectasia. Lasers Surg Med 1993;13:374–8.

47 Polla LL, Tan OT, Garden JM, Parrish JA. Tunable pulsed dye laser for the treatment of benign cutaneous vascular ectasia. Dermatologica 1987;174:11–17.

48 Garden JM, Polla LL, Tan OT. The treatment of port-wine stains by the pulsed dye laser. Arch Dermatol 1988;124:889–96.

49 Garden JM, Tan OT, Parrish JA. The pulsed dye laser: its use at 577nm wavelength. J Dermatol Surg Oncol 1987;13:134–8.

50 Nagawaka H, Tan OT, Parrish JA. Ultrastructural changes in human skin after exposure to a pulsed laser. J Invest Dermatol 1985;84:396–400.

51 Tan OT, Murray S, Kurban AK. Action spectrum of vascular specific injury using pulse radiation. J Invest Dermatol 1982;92:868–71.

52 Tan OT, Morrison P, Kurban AK. 585nm for the treatment of port-wine stains. Plast Reconstr Surg 1990;86(6):1112–17.

53 Dierickx CC, Casparian M, Venugopalan V, et al. Thermal relaxation of port-wine stain vessels probed in vivo: the need for 1–10msec laser pulse treatment. J Invest Dermatol 1995;105:709–14.

54 Van Gemert JMC, Welch AJ, Amin AP. Is there an optimal laser treatment for port wine stains? Lasers Surg Med 1986;6:76–83.

55 Kauvar AWB. Long-pulse high energy pulsed dye laser treatment of port wine stains and hemangiomas. Lasers Surg Med 1997;9(Suppl):36–40.

56 Morelli JG, Tan OT, Garden J, et al. Tunable dye laser (577nm) treatment of port wine stains. Lasers Surg Med 1986;6:94–9.

57 Dinehart SM, Flock S, Waner M. Beam profile of the flashlamp pumped pulsed dye laser: support for overlap of exposure spots. Lasers Surg Med 1994;15:277–80.

58 Tan OT, Stafford TJ. EMLA for treatment of portwine stains in children. Lasers Surg Med 1992;12:543–8.

59 Arendt-Neilsen L, Bjerring P. Laser induced pain for evaluation of local analgesia: a comparison of topical application (EMLA) and local injection (lidocaine). Anesth Analg 1988;67:115–23.

60 Gonzalez E, Gange RW, Momtaz K. Treatment of telangiectases and other benign vascular lesions with the 577nm pulsed dye laser. J Am Acad Dermatol 1992;27:220–6.

61 Ruiz-Esparza J, Goldman MP, Fitzpatrick R, et al. Flash lamp-pumped dye laser treatment of telangiectasia. J Dermatol Surg Oncol 1993;19:1000–3.

62 Grekin RC, Flynn TC, Cooper D, Geisse J. Efficacy of a 2mm spot size lens for the treatment of superficial vascular lesions with a flashlamp-pumped dye laser. Int J Dermatol 1997;36:865–9.

63 West TB, Alster TS. Comparison of the long-pulse dye (590–595nm) and KTP (532 nm)lasers in the treatment of facial and leg telangiectasias. Dermatol Surg 1998;24:221–6.

64 Lowe NJ, Behr KL, Fitzpatrick R, et al. Flash lamp pumped dye laser for rosacea associated telangiectasia and erythema. J Dermatol Surg Oncol 1991;17:522–5.

65 Goldman L, Bauman WE. Laser test treatments for postsolar poikiloderma. Arch Dermatol 1984;120:578–9.

66 Geronemus R. Poikiloderma of Civatte. Arch Dermatol 1990;126:547–8.

67 Wheeland RG, Applebaum J. Flashlamp-pumped pulsed dye laser therapy for poikiloderma of Civatte. J Dermatol Surg Oncol 1990;16:12–16.

68 Fitzpatrick TB, Bernhard JD, Cropley TG. The structure of the skin lesions and fundamentals of diagnosis. In: Freedberg IM, Eisen AZ, Wolff K, et al., editors. Dermatology in general medicine. New York: McGraw-Hill, 1999:13–41.

69 Clark RE, Jimenez-Acosta F. Poikiloderma of Civatte. Resolution after treatment with the pulsed dye laser. North Carolina Med J 1994;55(6):234–5.

70 Ciatti SC, Varga J, Greenbaum SS. The 585nm flashlamp-pumped pulsed dye laser for the treatment of telangiectases in patients with scleroderma. J Am Acad Dermatol 1996;35(3):487–8.

71 Potozkin JR, Geronemus RG. Treatment of the poikilodermatous component of Rothmund-Thomson syndrome with the flashlamp-pumped pulsed dye laser: a case report. Pediatr Dermatol 1991;8:162–5.

72 Alster TS, Wilson F. Focal dermal hypoplasia (Goltz's syndrome): treatment of cutaneous lesions with 585nm flashlamp-pumped pulsed dye laser. Arch Dermatol 1995;131:143–4.

73 Nunez M, Boixeda P, Miralles ES, et al. Pulsed dye laser treatment of telangiectatic chronic erythema of cutaneous lupus erythematosus. Arch Dermatol 1996;132:354–5.

74 Ellis DL. Treatment of telangiectasia macularis eruptiva perstans with the 585nm flashlamp-pumped dye laser. Dermatol Surg 1996;22:33–7.

75 Swinehart JM. Textural change following treatment of facial telangiectasias with the tunable pulsed-dye laser. Arch Dermatol 1999;135(4):472–3.

76 Levine VJ, Geronemus RG. Adverse effects associated with the 577- and 585-nanometer pulsed dye laser in the treatment of cutaneous vascular lesions: a study of 500 patients. J Am Acad Dermatol 1995;32:613–17.

77 Seukeran DC, Collins P, Sheehan-Dare RA. Adverse reactions following pulsed tunable dye laser treatment of port wine stains in 701patients. Br J Dermatol 1997;136:725–9.

78 Garden JM. Bakus AD. Clinical efficacy of the pulsed dye laser in the treatment of vascular lesions. J Dermatol Surg Oncol 1993;19:321–6.

79 Hohenleutner U, Hilbert M, Wlotzke U, Landthaler M. Epidermal damage and limited coagulation depth with the flashlamp-pumped pulsed dye laser: a histochemical study. J Invest Dermatol 1995;104:798–802.

80 Bernstein LJ, Geronemus RG. Keloid formation with the 585nm pulsed dye laser during isotretinoin treatment. Arch Dermatol 1997;133:111–12.

81 Jackson BA, Arndt KA, Dover JS. Are all 585nm pulsed dye lasers equivalent? A prospective, comparative, photometric, and histologic study. J Am Acad Dermatol 1996;34:1000–4.

82 Fuller TA, Intintoli A. Laser instrumentation. In: Arndt KA, Dover JS, Olbricht SM, editors. Lasers in cutaneous and asthetic surgery. Philadelphia: Lippincott-Raven; 1997:52–64.

83 Goldberg DJ, Meine JG. Treatment of facial telangiectases with the diode-pumped frequency-doubled q-switched Nd:YAG laser. Dermatol Surg 1998;24:828–32.

84 Goldberg DJ, Meine JG. A comparison of four frequency-doubled Nd:YAG (532nm) laser systems for treatment of facial telangiectases. Dermatol Surg 1999;25:463–7.

85 Adrain RM, Tanghetti EA. Long pulse 532–nm laser treatment of facial telangiectasia. Dermatol Surg 1998;24:71–4.

86 Apfelberg DB, Bailin P, Rosenberg H. Preliminary investigation of KTP/532 laser light in the treatment of hemangiomas and tattoos. Lasers Surg Med 1986;6:38–42.

87 Schroeter CA, Neumann HAM. An intense light source. The photoderm VL-flashlamp as a new treatment possibility for vascular skin lesions. Dermatol Surg 1998;24:743–8.

88 Angermeier MC. Treatment of facial vascular lesions with intense pulse light. J Cutan Laser Ther 1999;1:95–100.

89 Weiss RA, Goldman MP, Weiss MA. Treatment of poikiloderma of Civatte with an intense pulsed light source. Dermatol Surg 2000;26:823–8.

90 Goldman MP, Eckhouse S. Photothermal sclerosis of leg veins. Dermatol Surg 1996;22:323–30.

91 Dover JS, Arndt KA. New approaches to the treatment of vascular lesions. Lasers Surg Med 2000;26:158–63.

COMBINATION TREATMENT (Nicholas J Lowe)

Indications	Potential combination treatments	Chapter reference
Telangiectasia	Topical photoprotection	1
Red face	Topical vitamin C agents	3
	Glycolic acid peels	6
Rosacea	Treatment for rosacea	
Poikiloderma (necks)		

10. Erbium:YAG laser rejuvenation

Roland Kaufmann and Daniel Fleming

INTRODUCTION

As an early alternative to dermabrasion, continuous-wave CO_2 laser technology had been used for rapidly vaporizing larger skin surface areas. However, despite the practical gain of a non-bleeding wound surface, the coagulation necrosis turned out to be a major drawback with regard to healing time and risks of unwarranted complications, thus making these systems of limited value for cosmetic skin surgery.[1] The subsequent development of short-pulsed, high-energy and scanned CO_2 laser systems contributed to a much better control of thermal side-effects and to a safer approach. As a consequence, skin vaporization using such devices became very popular among dermatologists and plastic surgeons, especially for rejuvenation purposes in cosmetic indications, such as photodamaged skin, wrinkles and acne scars.[2–5]

Nevertheless, even with pulsed CO_2 lasers, a significant amount of thermal injury within adjacent tissue structures, along with an immediate dermal shrinkage and consecutive fibrosis after wound healing, is observed. Moreover, repetitive pulsing tends to further enhance the cumulative depth of tissue necrosis after each pass without adding much to deeper skin vaporization, thus increasing the risk of unjustifiable side-effects. Several long-term complications have also been observed, including keloid formation after deeper vaporization. In addition to early pigmentary changes, fibrosis and scarring, prolonged erythema and late occurrence of depigmentation may also be common, especially with more aggressive therapy.[6–9]

Therefore, attempts have been initiated to search for alternatives avoiding uncontrolled heat damage in resurfacing procedures and to allow for a better depth control in sites critical for mechanical dermabrasion. In fact, 'cold' ablation by other pulsed mid-infrared lasers was originally developed with the intention of replacing dermabrasion by a technique offering maximal control over depth whilst enabling highly precise and circumscribed work in skin areas at risk; it was also hoped to avoid the disadvantages of hazardous heat production seen with predominantly thermal CO_2 laser vaporization.

After initial attempts using diverse ultraviolet and infrared systems,[10,11] this aim has been reached by the results obtained at wavelengths emitted by pulsed erbium:yttrium–aluminium–garnet (Er:YAG) or YSSG lasers, absorbed many folds stronger by tissue water as compared to the emission line of CO_2 lasers.[12–14] The Er:YAG laser was introduced in 1987 for medical use, initially in experimental ophthalmology for corneal surgery.[15,16] Thereafter, it was used for performing skin ablation and skin incisions with minimal heat injury and excellent healing, firstly in in vivo experiments.[10,13,14] However, technical difficulties with limited fluences and low repetition rates turned out to be unfavorable for most dermatological applications.[11,12] Within the last several years, major advances in Er:YAG laser technology have made this instrument a highly effective tool for skin resurfacing purposes, since it is able to ablate very narrow layers of tissue with only minimal residual thermal damage, thus ensuring an extremely precise control of tissue ablation.

FUNDAMENTALS OF ER:YAG LASER–TISSUE INTERACTIONS

Er:YAG laser characteristics

The Er:YAG laser is a pulsed flashlamp-excited mid-infrared system with a crystal of yttrium–aluminium–garnet (YAG) dotated with erbium (Er) gas as an active laser medium that is cooled by a closed-circuit water system with forced air. The 2.94 μm beam is usually delivered through articulated mirror arms with a coaxial red aiming beam. The temporal profile of the pulses in the free-running mode shows the typical spike formation of flashlamp-pumped solid-state lasers.[17] Within each single laser pulse of c. 250–300 μs bandwidth, a number of very short spikes of 1 μs in duration follow on from each other, the number and height of which depend on the energy of the flashlamp pumping laser. Recently, many companies have introduced their own pulsed Er:YAG systems, offering a wide range of high powered machines (up to 20 W) with spot sizes of 1–10 mm and repetition rates of mostly up to 10–15 Hz and also modifications in pulse width (see below).

Ablation characteristics

Owing to an extremely high absorption of its invisible 2.94 μm wavelength in organic materials, the Er:YAG laser has become an ideal tool to ablate both soft (e.g. skin) and hard (e.g. bone, cartilage, teeth) tissues.[17,18] Efficient ablation of soft tissues largely depends on the ability of a given laser to deliver sufficient energy at a wavelength appropriate to vaporize intracellular water. As with the 10.6 μm CO_2 laser, the major tissue chromophore that absorbs the 2.94 μm wavelength of the Er:YAG laser is tissue water. However, when compared to other mid-infrared lasers, the wavelength of the Er:YAG laser is absorbed best – 15 times more efficiently than the wavelength of the 10.6 μm CO_2 laser – which is due to the fact that the 2940 nm Er:YAG laser corresponds almost exactly to the 3000 nm water absorption peak (Figure 10.1). The more than 10-fold higher absorption has dramatic effects on the tissue ablation threshold, the residual thermal damage and the ablation efficacy, as compared to CO_2 laser resurfacing.[10,19] Moreover, the wavelength of the Er:YAG

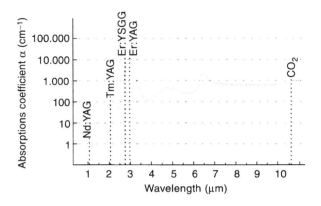

Figure 10.1 *Absorption coefficient of water in the infrared spectral range (modified from Kaufmann et al).*[14] *Note absorption peak c. 3 μm matching the emission lines of Er:YAG and Er:YSSG lasers, whereas CO_2 laser light is at least 10–fold less absorbed.*

laser is close to an absorption band for collagen, thus providing a further target within the connective tissue supporting the deeper dermal ablation process.

To limit the amount of adjacent heat damage to the surrounding tissue, laser energy should be delivered in a time shorter than the thermal relaxation time of skin, which is c. 1 ms. For laser resurfacing, the conventional CO_2 laser was modified so that ultrashort pulses (< 1 ms) are used together with high energy fluences. When fluences typically applied are used, the initial pass of such a laser ablates c. 20–50 μm of tissue and creates an additional 20–30 μm zone of thermally damaged tissue; further passes increase the thermal injury up to 150 μm.[2,20]

Pulsed Er:YAG lasers typically have pulse durations of 250–350 μs, which is much shorter than the 1 ms thermal relaxation time of skin. The extinction length of this laser is c. 3 μm much shorter than that with pulsed CO_2 lasers. This shallower extinction length along with the shorter pulse duration of the Er:YAG laser limits the amount of non-specific thermal damage to the surrounding tissue. For Er:YAG laser skin ablation, the threshold energy per tissue volume to cause ablation was calculated to be below the energy necessary to evaporate the same volume of pure water (2.7 J/cm³). Thus, it is assumed that the tissue is not vaporized completely but is ejected in the form of small particles by mechanical forces, which in clinical use can be seen as whitish grey tissue debris covering the freshly ablated surface. The ablation

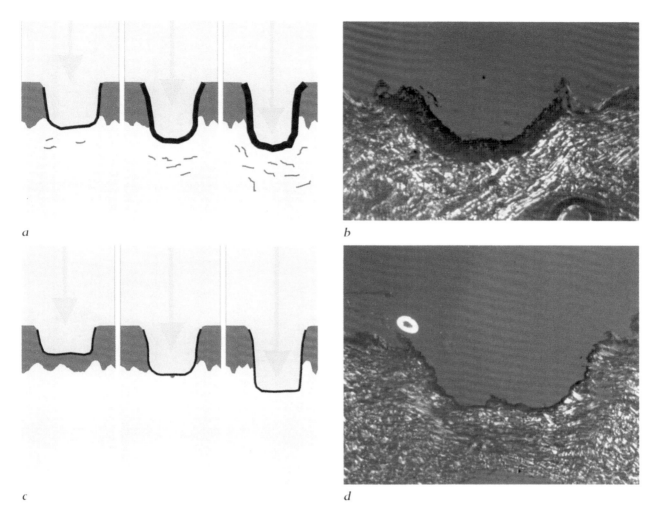

Figure 10.2 *Typical ablation craters after pulsed CO_2 (A and B) and Er:YAG laser (C and D) skin ablation. Schematic display in (A) exhibits cumulative thermal necrosis with repetitive pulsing in CO_2 vaporization, whereas in Er:YAG laser craters (C) the coagulation zone at the crater depth remains of constant width.*

threshold of c. 1.5 J/cm² is much lower than for CO_2 laser vaporization (c. 5 J/cm²). Once this threshold is exceeded, ablation crater depth per pulse increases linearly with the radiant exposure (energy fluence). Several investigators have confirmed this linear relationship of ablation depth to energy fluence in Er:YAG laser surgery, so that c. 4–5 μm of tissue is ablated per 1 J/cm² of energy delivered per pulse.[10,17,18,21,22]

In in vivo test cuts, in ablation craters as well as in resurfaced areas, damage zones are found at the lesional bottom that are largely unaffected by the laser parameters used and the healing process is comparable to that of cold-knife surgery (i.e. punch holes versus laser craters, scalpel cuts versus laser cuts, dermabrasion versus resurfaced areas).[14] In

particular, the overall heat damage zone at the bottom of the ablated area does not increase with further pulses, even in deeper crater holes such as in recipient sites of hair grafting or when ablating deeper lesions, e.g. syringomas. In contrast, the CO_2 laser beam produces increasing amounts of thermal injury, adding up to c. 150 μm with additional laser passes, and the desiccated carbonized surface interferes with further etching of the surface (Figure 10.2). For practical purposes, a single pulse of the Er:YAG laser at an energy fluence of 5 J/cm² will ablate c. 20–25 μm of tissue with an additional 5–10 μm zone of thermal necrosis; an energy fluence of 10 J/cm² will remove 40–50 μm of tissue, down into mid-epidermis, leaving the same amount of thermal

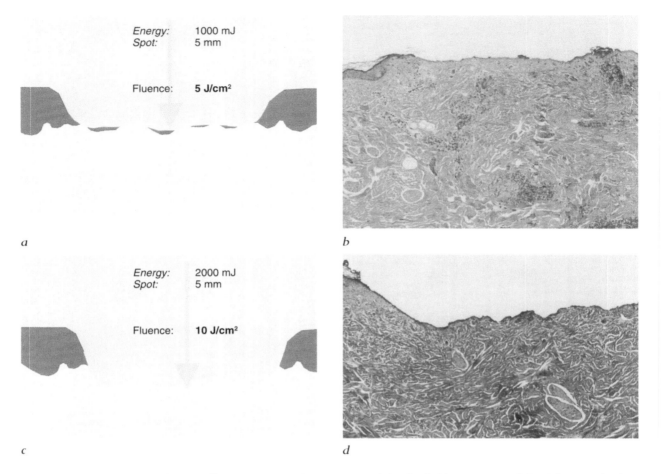

Figure 10.3 *Correlation of energy fluence, pulse number (passes) and depth of ablation: (A) and (B) Schematic display and histology, respectively, after four pulses at 5 J/cm² with removal of the entire epidermis; (C) and (D) doubling the pulse number and the energy fluence ablates the papillary dermis.*

damage at the bottom. To ablate a thin epidermial layer of c. 125 μm thickness, complete de-epithelialization would be expected after delivering an energy fluence of c. 25 J/cm² (Figure 10.3). Even in facial areas, where the average thickness at the cheek or in the forehead region can reach up to 150–200 μm but the minimal thickness between the rete ridges can be much lower, occasional pinpoint bleeding will occur after exposing the capillary loops within the upper papillary dermis in such spots (Figure 10.4).

Variations in pulse application mode

In its original version, the Er:YAG laser provided pulse lengths of typically c. 250–300 μs producing clean and precisely controlled ablation craters. However, in order to achieve haemostasis, even with pulses emitted at

2.94 μm wavelengths, several modifications have been introduced, e.g. prolonging the pulse lengths and addition of serial subablative low-fluence pulses following each ablative pulse.[23–27] Both types of modification lead to an increase in the amount of adjacent heat damage with subsequent tissue coagulation that allows capillary haemostasis or immediate tissue shrinkage. This results in an even more versatile use of such systems, providing either a purely ablative mode or a coagulative one (Figure 10.5).

An alternative approach to achieve both goals was to combine an ablative Er:YAG laser with a vaporizing pulsed CO_2 laser. Some surgeons have preferentially chosen this approach in order to facilitate a clean surface etching by Er:YAG laser ablation on the one hand and to permit additional coagulation by CO_2 pulses when required. Conversely, also Er:YAG laser

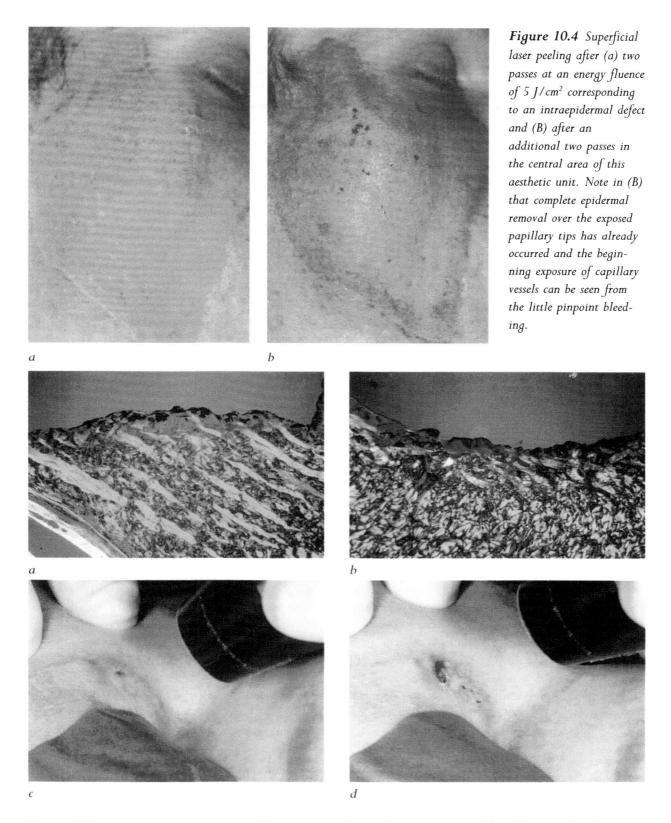

Figure 10.4 *Superficial laser peeling after (a) two passes at an energy fluence of 5 J/cm² corresponding to an intraepidermal defect and (B) after an additional two passes in the central area of this aesthetic unit. Note in (B) that complete epidermal removal over the exposed papillary tips has already occurred and the beginning exposure of capillary vessels can be seen from the little pinpoint bleeding.*

a

b

a

b

c

d

Figure 10.5 *Laser–tissue interaction in dual mode Er:YAG laser work. (A) Histology of the ablative mode with minimal necrosis; (B) coagulative mode with an additional subablative pulse series following the ablative pulse, showing significant amount of underlying necrosis; (C) ablative mode in clinical application (Xanthelasma); (D) coagulative mode showing dark coloured thermal carbonization.*

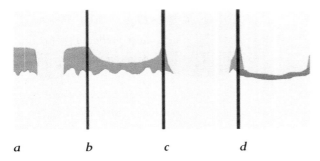

Figure 10.6 *Schematic display of Er:YAG laser skin removal. (A) Deep ablation crater; (B) superficial laser peel; (C) deeper laser resurfacing; (D) combined ablation plus coagulation.*

pulses were added after CO_2 resurfacing in order to remove excessive surface necrosis.[28-33]

Hence, today apart from purely ablative Er:YAG lasers, several dual mode Er machines (Superb laser, Fidelis CO_3 laser, Sciton Contour™ laser) and also a combined Er–CO_2 laser (Derma™ K laser, Lumenis) are available, so that a choice among different options can be made depending on individual demands and the spectrum of indications treated. Therefore, modern Er:YAG laser systems, equipped with high pulse energies, high pulse repetition rates and the option of additional thermal application modes, offer high flexibility for laser surgeons (Figure 10.6), enabling the performance of pure ablation craters (e.g. in hair transplants or punctual lesions), rapid superficial laser abrasion of larger surfaces (laser peeling, laser resurfacing) or the addition of controlled coagulation when desired (e.g. removal of rhinophyma, warts or blepharoplasty). However, in the present authors' view, for the vast majority of cosmetic indications, where a maximum of tissue sparing is essential in order to avoid the risk of unpleasant early or late adverse effects, any additional thermal damage is best be avoided. Therefore, a purely ablative mode of laser action is preferred in order to provide the highest safety along with the most satisfying results.

GENERAL RECOMMENDATIONS AND TECHNICAL ASPECTS

Preoperative aspects

Basically, the preoperative considerations are more or less identical to those in patients undergoing

dermabrasion. As in dermabrasion, the overall depth of skin removal and the type and location of treated skin are of the utmost importance for the final outcome, and in the risk of scar formation and other complications.[1,34] Re-epithelialization of an Er:YAG laser ablated skin surface largely depends on intact adnexal structures. Therefore, areas with thin or atrophic skin, as the dorsum of the hands in elderly persons or in those with atrophic disorders, should be treated with caution.[35] In such cases, the possibility of a highly controlled and very superficial laser ablation ('laser peeling') by using only limited pulse series leading merely to de-epithelialization (or even partial de-epithelialization) without further dermal damage is a great advantage of the controlled etching provided by Er:YAG laser pulses. Nevertheless, in critical areas, test treatments should be performed.

Since capillary bleeding may be disadvantageous in the purely ablative mode of resurfacing, especially when treating atrophic sundamaged skin of aged people or when resurfacing larger areas and certain indications, such as multiple actinic keratoses, patients should be advised to avoid aspirin and non-steroidal anti-inflammatory drugs for at least 10 days preoperatively. As with dermabrasion, patients who have been treated with isotretinoin may show atypical scarring following deeper laser treatment It is therefore recommended to wait for 1 year after discontinuing this type of medication prior to the resurfacing of acne patients. However, preoperative treatments with topical tretinoin and with vitamin C for a 2 week period have been used to improve the postoperative re-epithelialization rate. Based on the present authors' recent experience preoperative application of retinaldehyde instead of retinoic acid is preferred. Retinaldehyde is much less irritating and can also be applied postoperatively immediately after re-epithelialization has occurred (8–10 days after surgery) without prolonging the erythema.[36]

Topical pretreatment with hydroquinone or azelaic acid does not seem to have a significant enough influence on postoperative hyperpigmentation to generally justify its use, especially in less aggressive treatments.[35,37] However, postoperative use can shorten postinflammatory hyperpigmentation and a pretreatment in patients with Fitzpatrick skin types III and higher should be considered, especially in superficial ablations, since deeper adnexal melanocytes remaining after more aggressive ablation would not be suppressed by pretreating the skin surface.

Use of anaesthetics

The perception of pain is again largely dependent on the depth, the pulse frequency and the extent of the procedure. Circumscribed small lesions, such as solitary senile lentigines (flat seborrhoic keratosis) can be removed without any anaesthesia. Also, very superficial procedures that will remove only parts of the epithelium (laser peeling) can be performed using a eutectic mixture of lidocaine and prilocaine (EMLA). It has to be ascertained that this cream is applied under occlusive dressings for at least 1 hour prior to the procedure; injuries to the cornea of the eye have been reported in periocular applications of this cream.[38] Also, the topical combination of tetra-caine and lidocaine (LaserCaine®) may be used for superficial resurfacing procedures; anaesthesia occurs more rapidly and no occlusion is required.

However, in all deeper or more extended proce-dures, Er:YAG laser ablation will become a painful procedure. Therefore, local anaesthetics are used for infiltration anaesthesia, the concentration and type being dependent on the depth and site of lesion. When resurfacing circumscribed aesthetic units, regional nerve blocks of the respective areas (supra- or infraorbital, mental) can be used in conjunction with infiltration anaesthesia of the treatment field in order to provide adequate anaesthesia. In full-face procedures, many surgeons prefer to work with an anaesthesiologist providing appropriate intravenous sedation or general anaesthesia as necessary.

Treatment techniques

The aesthetic areas to be ablated are marked out with a skin pencil, including special targets such as wrinkles or scars. Prior to the resurfacing process, the skin surface is treated with an antiseptic and gently cleansed using normal saline. Surrounding tissue and hairs are protected with wet gauze. Flammable materials, including oxygen, should be excluded from the treatment field. In all treatments the eyes should be protected by appropriate safety glasses and if the eyelid area is to be rejuvenated,

appropriate intraocular stainless-steel eyeshields are recommended.

The laser impact produces a loud cracking noise due to explosive tissue removal and photoacustic effects, and with higher repetition rates and energy fluences this can be quite distressing. The noise from these explosions has been measured at the ear of the operator as 122 dB using a 5 mm spot, 5 J/cm² at 8 Hz. This is equivalent to a pneumatic drill and, with repeated exposure, can cause permanent loss of hearing. Noise-reducing earplugs should be worn by staff in the operating area. As with vaporizing techniques, the plume of generated laser smoke has to be carefully removed by appropriate suction devices.

Due to the high absorption of the Er:YAG laser light in water, the targeted surfaces should be kept more or less dry, since any superfluous water could interfere with the tissue ablative process. The thin zone of thermal necrosis in wound surfaces created by Er:YAG laser ablation, while advantageous for wound healing, may be problematic for achieving haemostasis, since the narrow rim of necrosis is not sufficient to coagulate the superficial dermal capillaries. Pinpoint bleeding is therefore observed clinically after several passes, indicating penetration into the papillary dermis (Figure 10.4b). Since residual blood on the skin will absorb irradiated laser energy, care must be taken to maintain the surface free of fresh blood. This is not a problem in rapidly creating deep ablation crater lesions with high pulse repetition rates penetrating faster into the tissue than the ensuing bleeding, as in hair grafting procedures.[39] Also, in larger areas, the problem of intermittent capillary bleeding can usually been overcome by covering the surface with normal solution saline-soaked gauzes in between the pulse series. Wiping away the white-coloured proteinaceus tissue debris from the wound surface is usually not necessary and rather will induce fresh bleeding.

Depending on the manufacturer, most available Er:YAG lasers can be used with beam diameters of 1–10 mm. Laser treatment takes place by the delivery of slightly overlapping patterns over the targeted area. Each pulse series is a 'pass' of the laser over the affected skin. To minimize a visible border between resurfaced and untreated skin feathering or blending can blur the boundaries. For resurfacing crucial sites (e.g. lower eyelid) the authors prefer the freehand or single-spot technique, in which the treated area is ablated with a 20–30% overlap of spots (Figure 10.9b). Treating a given aesthetic unit, or the whole face, evenly with several pulse series is usually the appropriate and safest approach and can be followed by fine sculpting of areas particularly more pronounced and inhomogenous acne scars. In deeper procedures, residual blood is gently removed from the tissue before the next pass using saline-soaked gauze. Goldman described the dermabrasion technique, in which sections of the face are resurfaced first in a vertical pattern, followed by a horizontal pattern and finally by oblique patterns, thus minimizing extra overlapping. In the infraorbital area and the upper eyelid, curvilinear passes alternating with vertical passes are used from the eyelid crease to the lash line.[40]

Scanning devices may facilitate and accelerate the treatment procedure but, in contrast to CO_2 laser vaporization, they are not essential for safe resurfacing over larger areas. Whereas in CO_2 laser resurfacing an uncontrolled overlap of pulses should be strictly avoided in order to prevent cumulative heat damage and unacceptable cosmetic results, this is not the case with Er:YAG lasers. With Er-YAG lasers, even after accidental overlapping exposure, no additional necrosis will occur at the wound bottom. Also with lower energy fluences (c. 5 J/cm^2), as preferred by the present authors, each impact will ablate c. 25 μm so the consequence of an impact overlap would be only this additional ablation depth; with larger areas and more passes, at the end of treatment there will be some averaging of uneven overlaps, ultimately resulting in a sufficiently even injury so as never to cause visible stripiness or relevant chequerboarding.[41] Nevertheless, scanning systems with variable overlap patterns ranging from −30 to +30%, similar to the computer pattern generators used in CO_2 lasers, have been developed, allowing a rapid and more uniform ablation of the skin, especially when treating larger areas.[42] However, this again carries a special risk of over treatment in areas of interscan overlap due to high fluences associated with small spot sizes. Therefore, even with scanners, lower fluences and multiple passes are still advised.

With CO_2 vaporization, the end-point can be defined by the number of passes and the typical type of tissue discoloration, the procedure will also be more or less limited after a certain amount of dermal necrosis and desiccation has occurred; however, the situation is entirely different in Er:YAG laser skin ablation. In Er:YAG ablation, the depth of penetration is closely related to the number of pulses and the energy fluence used and deep ablation holes can be created by continuous pulsing. However, the total depth of injury can be calculated by understanding the tissue interactions, by knowing the exact parameters used and the ablation rates for each pulse, e.g. 20–25 μm with a 5 J/cm^2 pulse. At this energy fluence, in most areas of facial skin, after c. 100 μm (about four pulse series or 'passes') complete de-epithelialization will be reached, corresponding to a superficial 'laser peel'. In some areas, early pinpoint bleeding will indicate spots where penetration of the papillary dermis and exposure of the capillary vessels has occurred, whereas more profuse bleeding is possible after penetrating into deeper levels of the papillary dermis.

INDICATIONS FOR ER:YAG LASER SKIN ABLATION

Overview

The Er:YAG laser has rapidly become an extremely versatile instrument for skin ablation and has been used in the last decade for a growing number of indications in dermatological surgery. Regardless of the indication, Er:YAG laser ablation is of special value in all critical anatomical sites and, in addition, enables highly controlled laser peeling of the skin surface. Above all, the skin around the eyelids, on the neck, the chest and at the dorsa of the hands, where deeper damage should be avoided, is better suited for a gentle ablation in all types of resurfacing procedures. In these areas, the skin in elderly patients is not only atrophic and thin but in contrast to the facial areas, contains less abundant adnexal structures, that can serve as islands for re-epithelialization after deeper damage.

Basically, all indications formerly treated by dermabrasion can now be removed by laser resurfacing.[43] They comprise such diverse procedures as the removal of osteoma cutis[44,45] or see urchin spikes (unpublished data), the ablation of psoriatic plaques or aquired lymphangioma, and resurfacing in Darier's disease.[46–48] Table 10.1 summarizes most of the indications in which Er:YAG laser skin ablation can be considered as a useful treatment option.[49–53]

In all superficial skin disorders spreading over large areas or composed of papules aggregated in

Table 10.1 *Preferential indications for Er:YAG laser ablation*

Pigmented lesions	
Epidermal nevi	+++
Congenital nevomelanocytic nevi	++
*Scars**	
Keloids	+
Hypertrophic scarring	+
Acne scars	++
Rejuvenation of photoaged skin	
Superficial rhytides	+++
Senile lentigines	+++
(including superficial seborrhoic keratosis)	
Favre-Racouchot	+++
Actinic keratosis	++
Actinic cheilitis	+**
Miscellaneous	
Superficial multicoloured tattoos	+
Darier disease	++
Hailey-Hailey disease	+++
Syringoma	++
Xanthelasma	++
Viral warts	+
Adenoma sebaceum	++
Epithelioma adenoides	++
Osteoma cutis	++
Rhinophyma	++**

+, Can be considered; ++, well suited; +++, very well suited; *
in combination with other techniques; ** in combination with
thermal mode or CO_2 lasers.

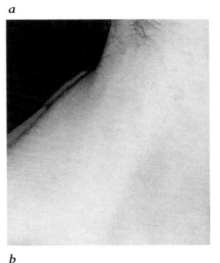

a

b

Figure 10.7
Er:YAG laser
ablation of
an epidermal
nevus at the
neck: (A)
preoperative
view; (B)
after complete
removal.

larger plaques, as in epidermal nevi, rapid and stepwise laser ablation is an excellent treatment modality (Figure 10.7). Moreover, in punctual lesions, which might even be situated in the dermis, such as in syringomas of the eyelids, use of a focused beam to produce tiny ablation craters is well suited for the removal of such disorders and to confine the damage strictly to the lesional sites (Figure 10.8).

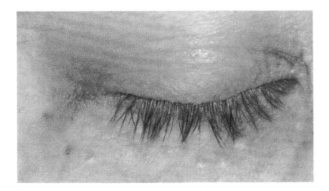

a

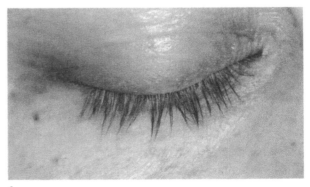

b

Figure 10.8 *Er:YAG laser ablation of syringoma at the lower lid area: (A) preoperative view; (B) after removal.*

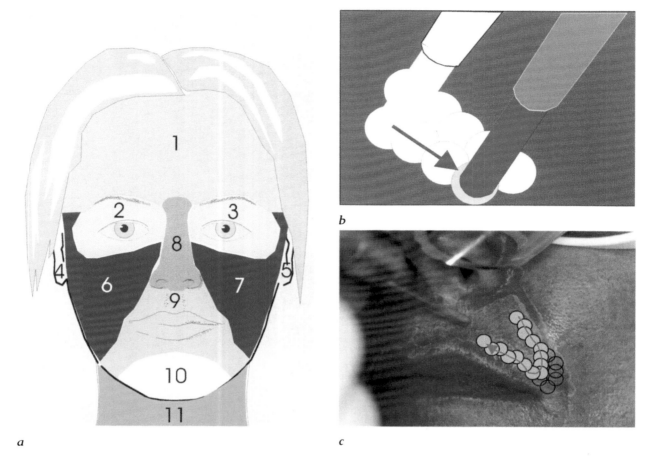

Figure 10.9 Resurfacing in the face and neck area: application mode of pulses. (A) Aesthetic units of the face and neck according to Gonzales-Ulloa et al.;[77] (B) freehand mode with 30% overlapping of pulses; (C) blending of the bounderies and stepwise increase of pulse numbers from the out most border inwards and towards the shoulder of wrinkles.

The role of the Er:YAG laser in resurfacing acne scars

For the present authors, for many years the Er:YAG laser has replaced dermabrasion in treating various types of pitted scars of the face such as acne or chickenpox scars; others have also reported beneficial effects in using this laser for treatment of acne and other types of depressed scars.[37,54,55] In particular, in critical perioral areas and along the mandibula much more controlled and homogeneous removal of the skin is possible with this laser, and a stepwise decrease in the pulse number at the overlapping edges adjacent to the non-ablated skin surface around a demarcation line. Also, the precision in sculpturing the scars, due to excellent visual control and minimal heat damage,

can make this approach for superior to CO_2 laser treatment.[56] Moreover, thermal damage to follicles and sebaceous glands can be avoided, so that acne flare ups, as reported after CO_2 laser vaporization are not a problem.

Clinical outcome is not usually significant after only one treatment session (Figure 10.10), so a deeper and more aggressive treatment or additional thermal modes of action (dual mode Er:YAG lasers, combinations with CO_2 lasers) are used. However, as with dermabrasion, patient satisfaction is usually much higher than expected from the clinical outcome assessment. Nevertheless, by performing repetitive treatment sessions and combining the procedure with other techniques, such as punch elevations or fine excisions and subcisions, a stepwise improvement can

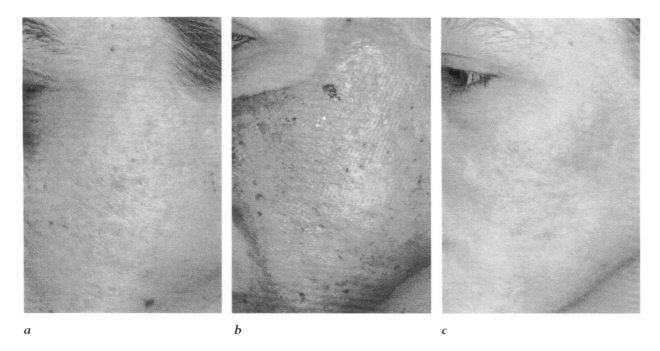

a   *b*   *c*

Figure 10.10 *Superficial Er:YAG laser peel in acne scars (four passes at an energy fluence of 5 J/cm², ablating c. 100 µm of the surface. (A) Preoperative view; (B) aspect 1 day after surgery; (C) result 3 months postoperatively with minimal smoothing effect.*

be achieved and unwarranted side-effects are avoided. As with rejuvenation procedures in other cosmetic indications, it is always much easier to retreat a patient whose result has been suboptimal rather than to later have to deal with severe or long-lasting complications. In younger patients in particular, it is best to remain on the side of caution with regard to long-term or irreversible side-effects such as additional scarring or persistent depigmentations.

Kye resurfaced 21 acne patients with pitted scars using up to six passes at 500 mJ with a 2 mm spot size and found an average improvement of 40% after 3 months of treatment.[37] Weinstein reported on the treatment of 63 patients with mild to moderate scarring and those with darker skin type V.[42] In 15 pronounced cases a combined Er and CO_2 modality was used (Derma K laser) in order to achieve a dry surface, based on the assumption that it was felt difficult to perform deeper ablation into the reticular dermis with the Er:YAG laser alone in such cases, since the visual 'end-points' might be obscured and the ablation efficiency might decrease due to ensuing exsudation and bleeding. All patients experienced fair

(50–70%) or good (70–90%) corrections. The mean time to re-epithelialization was 7.3 days with Er alone and 9.6 days in the dual mode; also, erythema lasted longer with the combined approach (mean 7.3 weeks versus 5.8 weeks). All patients were satisfied with their results and, in most cases, as with the present authors' patients, the outcome exceeded their expectations.

The role of the Er:YAG laser in resurfacing photoaged skin

Basically, Er:YAG laser resurfacing can be indicated in all manifestations of photoaged skin. The present authors have successfully used this technique to improve cutaneous elastosis in the condition of Morbus Favre-Racouchot (Figure 10.11), evening out superficial and even less moderate wrinkles (Figures 10.12 and 10.13) or to remove solar lentigines and solar keratoses.

With the introduction of CO_2 laser resurfacing dermabrasion had already fallen out of favour in these indications for practical reasons (e.g. ease of handling) and due to the more predictable damage caused by

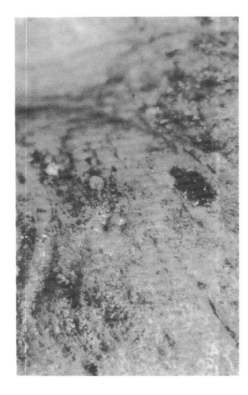

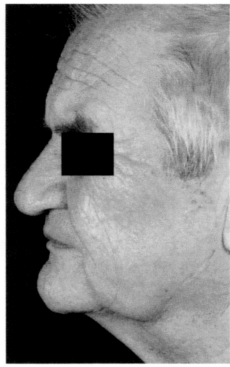

Figure 10.11 Deeper resurfacing of severe facial elastosis in Morbus Favre-Racouchot. (A) Exposure of cysts and comedones after ablating down into the papillary dermis; (B) aspect 3 weeks following surgery with mild residual erythema due to deeper ablation.

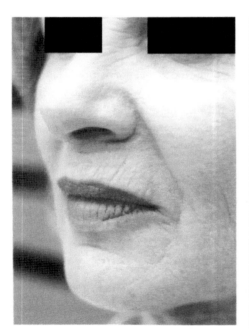

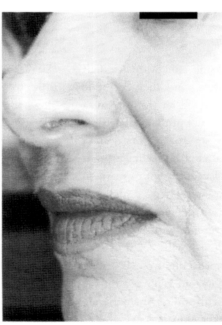

Figure 10.12 Er:YAG laser resurfacing of upper lip wrinkles preoperative view; (A) and (B) 6 weeks after the procedure.

lasers as compared to the major disadvantages of dermabrasion, e.g. technical difficulties, risk of mechanical injury, little control in critical areas and potential exposure to aerosoled blood-borne pathogens. Moreover, immediate 'shrinkage' and flattening of the skin, as a result of heat injury to collagen, was more obvious immediately after CO_2 laser treatment, and both prolonged oedema and later formation of dermal fibrosis contributed to the convincing aspect of a tightened skin surface. With

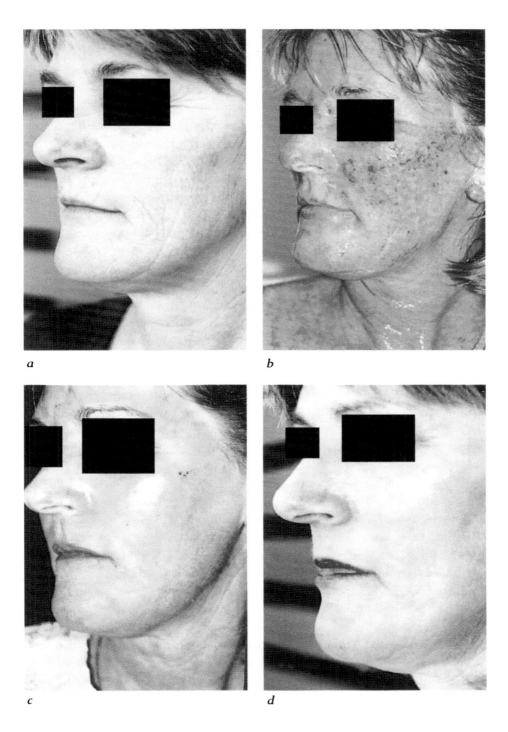

a

b

c

d

Figure 10.13 Full-face and neck resurfacing in photodamaged skin with fine wrinkles: (A) preoperative views; (B)–(D) 24 hours, 7 days and 3 months after the procedure, respectively.

more aggressive treatments even long-lasting improvements can be achieved in many cases, but the risk of side-effects is also increased. Therefore, in using laser rejuvenation treatment, a more conservative approach has been advised by limiting the number of passes and avoiding any unnecessary injury to the wound surface.[57] Interestingly, by comparing the cosmetic outcome and adverse effects of mechanical dermabrasion and superpulsed CO_2 laser treatment of perioral rhytides, of 15 volunteers treated in a half-and-half fashion it was shown that both dermabrasion and CO_2 laser resurfacing were equally effective in the majority of cases.[58] Though there was a trend towards greater improvement in rhytide scores with the CO_2 laser treatment, in 50% of the cases no difference was discernible between the two sides. Dermabrasion resulted in cleaner wounds that re-epithelialized more quickly than the CO_2 laser ones. However, it was not determined whether or not the two sides were treated with a comparable overall depth of injury. As with CO_2 laser resurfacing, a thickened zone of horizontally arranged new collagen can be detected many years after dermabrasion,[59] and dermal procollagen was found to be strikingly increased 12 weeks after dermabrasion.[60]

Also, with Er:YAG laser ablation, which produces wound surfaces that are in many aspects comparable to those produced by dermabrasion, some degree of tissue tightening can be observed. Hughes[61] examined skin contraction following Er:YAG laser resurfacing using solar lentigines as markers. He demonstrated an immediate 4% linear tightening after two to three laser passes that subsequently increased to 14% contraction after 4 months. In a recent comparitive study of patients treated for actinic skin damage it was found that resurfacing using the CO_2 laser produced the greatest thickness of neocollagen, the highest neocollagen density and the greatest decrease in elastosis, but took the longest time for healing and resolution of erythma and inflammation (up to 6 months).[62] The Er:YAG laser used alone produced the least collagenesis but the most rapid resolution of erythema (within 10 days). The CO_2 laser followed by the Er:YAG produced effects that were intermediate and it was concluded that blended CO_2–Er:YAG regimens provide an optimal combination. This result is not unexpected, due to the different depths of total injury produced, leading to more or less dramatic initial and late effects; however, it remains unclear what the difference would be if the skin could be ablated by the Er:YAG laser alone to the same total depth as that produced by the combined approach. Comparative half-and-half results so for available (albeit assessed at the same depth by the operator) at least indicate that they are not that different at all, given that an appropriate depth has been reached also by Er:YAG ablation.

In contrast to CO_2 resurfacing, the narrower zone of thermal necrosis created by the Er:YAG laser allows the skin to re-epithelialize more quickly with a shorter period of postoperative erythema. Re-epithelialization will usually occur within an average range of only 5–8 days, and postoperative erythema can last up to six weeks but will resolve mostly within 1–3 weeks (or less) depending on the location and the depth of injury produced.[14,35,41,62] Above all, when comparing dermabrasion or Er:YAG laser skin removal with CO_2 resurfacing at the same total depth of injury, it becomes clear that outcomes are more or less comparable. Therefore, it might be concluded that it is generally the amount of injury to the skin and not the modality per se that determines the efficacy and the risk of complicatons of the treatment.[41] However, the question remains as to whether the additional heat injury of pulsed CO_2 lasers, together with its lack of control and the impact on immediate wound care, pain and oedema, as well as prolonged duration of erythema and increase in hypopigmentation is really required and justifiable.

The results obtained with six different Er:YAG laser treatments were compared in a prospective, randomized trial.[63] Each half of the face was treated with one of six Er:YAG lasers at energy fluencies of 5 J/cm^2 and using three passes, corresponding to a shallow injury of c. 60 μm per ablation. With each of the lasers a similar 50% clinical improvement was achieved, despite this being a superficial intraepidermally treatment.[63] To achieve a visual lessening of wrinkles Teikemeier and Goldberg[64] found a clinical improvement in 20 patients resurfaced with only one to three passes with a maximum spot size of 5 mm and an energy fluence of 600–800 mJ (3–4 J/cm^2). Perez et al[65] also treated his patients with a 5 mm spot size at energy fluences of 800–1000 mJ (4–5 J/cm^2) with the number of passes ranging from two to three (periorbital) up to five to seven (chin, forehead, cheeks). Erythema resolved within 3–6 weeks and improvement was seen in all patients. Also, Weiss et al[66] reported on moderate to good results in 50 patients treated with only three Er:YAG laser passes for wrinkles.

In a further half-and-half study comparison was made of treatment with the CO_2 laser on one half of the face and the Er:YAG laser on the other half in six patients.[35] The number of passes using each laser varied in order to treat both sides of the face to a similar depth of vaporization (determined clinically by the investigator). Re-epithelialization of the Er:YAG-treated side occurred within 5–7 days, whereas re-epithelialization of the CO_2–treated side occurred after 7 to 14 days. Erythema was largely resolved on the Er:YAG-treated side within 7–21 days, whereas erythema routinely lasted 1–3 months on the CO_2–treated side. With respect to clinical improvement of the rhytides, both the Er:YAG laser and the CO_2 laser were effective, although a greater number of passes was required with the Er:YAG laser to achieve a similar clinical outcome as the CO_2 laser. Kathri et al.[67] compared the side-by-side effects of an UltraPulse® CO_2 Laser (Coherent; 3 mm spot size, energy fluences of 3.5–6.5 J/cm², and two to three passes), with an Er:YAG laser (5 mm spot size), 300 µs pulse width, energy fluences of 5–8 Jcm², and more then three passes until bleeding occured). In subjects receiving more than five pulse series of the Er:YAG laser, improvement scores did not significantly differ from what achievable using CO_2 rejuvenation, however, erythema and hypopigmentation was less on the Er:YAG side. Similar results have been reported by other workers for cases where the total depth of injury was comparable.[41] Another study compared the Er:YAG laser (5 mm spot size, at an energy fluence of 1 J/cm², 12–15 passes for the upper lip and, 5–7 passes for the periocular area) producing deeper ablation wounds (140–300 µm) with the wounds created by CO_2 resurfacing of the periocular and perioral skin leading to less dramatic differences in postoperative side-effects.[24] Whereas the CO_2 effect was superior in patients with moderate to deep wrinkles the difference was not distinguishable in those with more superficially located damage.

Nevertheless, several investigators believe in the benefits of thermal interactions for rejuvenational procedures, leading to an improved tightening of the skin by inducing collagen shrinkage and consecutive dermal fibrosis. On the other hand, others recommend the combined use of both CO_2 and Er:YAG (Derma K) lasers, or dual-mode Er lasers (Sciton, CO_3, Superb), to minimize thermal damage by removing the zones of necrosis following CO_2 or by adding thermal injury to lesions, aiming at improved results. Studies have been made both in patients with photodamaged skin and acne scars, where prolonged erythema and delayed wound healing are common adverse sequelae following pulsed CO_2 laser treatment alone.[31,32,62,68–70] Goldman et al[32] investigated whether removal of residual thermal necrosis from the wound bottom with an Er laser could decrease these adverse effects. For this purpose, patients were treated in a half-and-half comparison study, with the CO_2 laser alone on one half of the face and with both the CO_2 and Er:YAG lasers on the other half. In fact, it was shown that combining Er:YAG laser resurfacing decreased the incidence of side-effects. Although the degree of wrinkle improvement was identical on both sides of the face, erythema following combined laser treatment resolved much more quickly than CO_2 laser treatment alone (2–3 weeks versus 8 weeks postoperatively, respectively).[32] A reduction in the duration of postoperative crusting, swelling and ichting by the addition of Er:YAG laser pulses following CO_2 laser resurfacing was also found by McDaniel et al.[68] It has also been shown that a variable pulse Er:YAG laser combining an ablative and coagulative mode when compared to CO_2 laser resurfacing of upper lip wrinkles produced fewer side-effects but did not equal the benefit seen with CO_2 treatment.[71] It has also been demonstrated that a long-pulsed Er:YAG laser produces a thicker zone of thermal damage, giving similar effects to CO_2 lasers in moderate to deeper facial rhytids.[72] It was concluded, that a greater degree of heat injury in the dermis may underlie the benefit in the treatment of ageing skin. However, the discrepancy between the conclusions drawn from different investigators, i.e. the fact that some investigators can achieve improvements equal to CO_2, and others cannot, suggests that Er:YAG resurfacing of deep rhytids is more technique-dependant than CO_2 and disproves the notion that Er:YAG cannot achieve the same degree of improvement in such patients.

Apart from the controversial discussion about the role of each of such resurfacing procedures, and the need for themal collagen damage in photoaged skin, there is no doubt that the Er:YAG laser has significant advantages in the treatment of perioral and periorbital skin, and in resurfacing critical anatomic areas other than the face, such as the neck, the chest or the dorsa of the hands.[73,74] These particular regions have always been difficult to improve surgically, regardless whether using dermabrasion or CO_2laser vaporization. The high precision and control provided by the Er:YAG laser, which ablates only 20–25 µm of skin surface per pass (or even less depending on the energy fluence), is definitely unique and can neither been accomplished by dermabrasion nor by CO_2 vaporization. Since even a single pass of a pulsed-CO_2 laser of these areas is associated with a significant risk of scarring or textural changes, the Er:YAG laser has been recommended as a superior choice in treating photodamaged skin of these particularly challenging anatomical sites.[30,35] In general, fewer passes are used in these areas, where the skin is usually thinner than on the remaining aesthetic units of the face (Figures 10.9 and 10.12). Laser resurfacing of the neck attempts to blend the colour and the texture of the skin of the neck with that of the face and chest by entirely removing the epidermal layer within the upper one-third of the neck and an even more gentle intraepidermal ablation of the lower neck. Goldberg and Meine[75] resurfaced 10 patients with neck wrinkles, using a 5 mm spot size with energy fluences of 600–800 mJ and a total of four passes, with only minimal overlap of 10%. Without wiping of debris, further passes were added over the involved wrinkle areas until initial bleeding started. No adverse effects were seen after 6 months but the wrinkles were at least 25% improved in all patients.

In theory, deeper rhytides can also be ablated, as with dermabrasion, despite the onset of bleeding that might interfere with the procedure, especially after attempting to vigorously wipe away the debris in between each new laser pass; however, they are not considered a good indication and the risk of side-effects will increase in such patients, regardless of what procedure has been chosen. Instead, superficial to moderate wrinkles are treated more effectively by this method as in sundamaged skin of younger individuals (Figure 10.13).

As with dermabrasion, Fitzpatrick skin types I–III are the best candidates for treatment with the Er:YAG laser. Though, patients with skin types IV and V have also been treated with a lower incidence of postinflammatory hyperpigmentation because of the minimal thermal damage compared to that of pulsed-CO_2 laser resurfacing, where patients with pigmented skin are prone to long-lasting hyperpigmentations.[76,77] Twenty-one patients with wrinkles and 10 patients with acne scars of Asian skin types underwent resurfacing (5 mm spot size, 1000 mJ per pulse, energy fluences of 20–30% overlap, and four to 12 passes).[78] An 80% improvement in wrinkles was reported and post-treatment erythrema lasted only

up to a maximum of 8 weeks. Postinflammatory hyperpigmentation started in the second week and resolved at 4–8 weeks. Though a lower incidence of postinflammatory hyperpigmentation after Er:YAG resurfacing in patients with darker skin types, or with oriental skin types, has been reported, results are conflicting. This makes sense when the problems with dermabrasion are recalled, i.e. the risk in such patients is related to the depth of abrasion. Also, in Er:YAG resurfacing a higher likelihood of pigmentary changes has to be expected in deeper and more aggressive procedures. However, especially in skin types prone to hyperpigmentation one can at least aim at very superficial and careful ablations, thus minimizing such side-effects.

In summary, the advantages of pulsed Er:YAG lasers for facial and non-facial skin rejuvenation in acne scars or manifestations related to an actinic damage are mainly related to:

- the precision and control of the ablation process;
- the possibility of a very superficial tissue removal;
- the absence of unnecessary heat injury to adjacent tissue structures

These unique features help to:

- facilitate resurfacing in areas prone to side-effects;
- enable rejuvenation in skin types at higher risks of postinflammatory pigmentary changes;
- shorten wound healing in many superficial cosmetic procedures.

POSTOPERATIVE TREATMENT GUIDELINES

Smaller and more superficial wounds created by Er:YAG laser ablation can be treated by an antiseptic ointment until re-epithelialization has occurred. After superficial rejuvenation procedures (Er:YAG 'laser peel') with only partial or complete removal of the epidermal layer, healing will be usually much faster than that observed with the necrotic wound areas created by CO_2 laser resurfacing procedures. In such cases, expected oedema, exsudation and erythema are usually short-lived and are not severe. In deeper and larger wound surfaces, as after more aggressive full-face procedures, postoperative care can be managed following the procedures described for CO_2 resurfacing. In the acute exsudative phase, wounds are either managed by an open or closed technique, the latter being mostly preferred in outpatient settings and by the present authors. The open method (e.g. fat–moist combination dressings) involves the application of ointments every couple of hours. The excess exsudate build-up is bathed with saline and weak vinegar solutions or cool tap water until reepithelialization has occurred. The closed technique involves the use of an occlusive sterile dressing (hydrogel, polymer film or composite foam) applied in the operating theatre and left for 24–48 hours, depending on the exsudation. Initially, for both methods, the patients should sleep with the head elevated and ice packs should be applied to reduce oedema and discomfort. After re-epithelialization has occurred (3–8 days postoperatively, depending on the extent and depth of the procedure) a regular emollient should be applied over itchy areas – this can contain 1% hydrocortisone for short-term use and later on retinaldehyde and hydrochinone can be used, depending on the skin type. Make-up can help to minimize erythema. Sun exposure has to be strictly avoided for at least as long as the erythema lasts and during that period a high-factor broad spectrum sunscreen must be applied daily.

SIDE-EFFECTS

Though in recent CO_2 laser dominated years many of the risks in laser resurfacing have been attributed to the amount of thermal damage, the type and severity of complications seems to be related to the overall deepness of tissue damage (i.e. to the total amount of vaporization depth and underlying thermal damage zone). That is why, with few exceptions (e.g. bullous reactions, linear streaks, vascular proliferations), all of the complications known from CO_2 resurfacing have more or less already been observed following aggressive and deeper dermabrasion, without necessarily being thermally mediated.[1] Therefore, for Er:YAG skin ablation, similar early and late occurring side-effects as with dermabrasion or thermal laser damage of the same total depth of injury have to be considered;[53,79] they are listed in Table 10.2. Apart from early symptoms associated with skin wounding

Table 10.2 Potential side-effects of Er:YAG skin rejuvenation

	Superficial	Deep
Early:		
Oedema	+	++
Burning/pain	+	++
Superinfections	+++	
Acne flare-up	–	+
Postoperative erythema	+	++
Temporary hyperpigmentations*	+	+
Pruritus	+	+
Hyperreagibility/fragility	+	+
Intermediate:		
Persistent erythema	+	+
Hyperpigmentations	+	++
Milia	+	+
Late:		
Persistent hypo-/depigmentation	+	++
Atrophies	+	+
Keloids	–	+

* depending on skin type; – not observed; + little risk; ++ high risk.

(exsudation, oedema or erythema) and irritation, major early complications are related to secondary infections (viral, bacterial, fungal), intermediate adverse effects are related to the risk of scar formation and postinflammatory hyperpigmentation, and late complications are related to depigmentation.

The risk of infection is comparable to dermabrasion of equal depth and extent; however, since less thermal necrosis occurs than in CO_2 laser burned wound surface and the critical period until reepithelialization has occurred is shorter, this risk should be decreased. None the less, it is still advisable to protect patients from bacterial and, especially, viral infections, particularly in larger or deeper procedures such as full-face resurfacing in acne patients or extended rejuvenation procedures in those with sundamaged skin. We combine oral antibiotics (covering Pseudomonas aeruginosa species) together with oral anti-herpetic drugs is generally recommended for up to 10 days postoperatively, starting one day prior to the procedure. However, these recommendations are more critical with closed techniques of

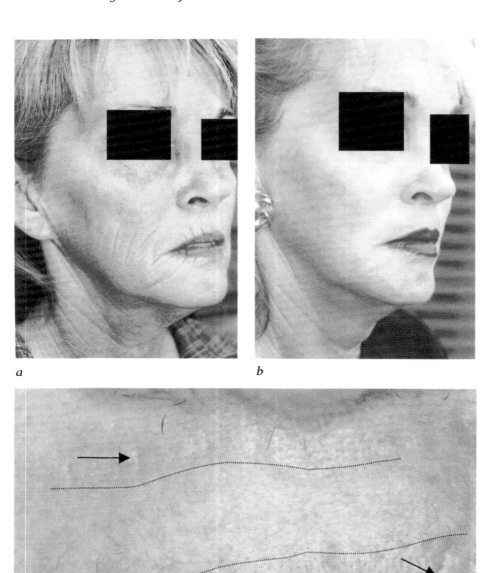

a   b

c

Figure 10.14 *Risk of late depigmentation after deeper ablation. Full-face rejuvenation: (A) of photoaged skin pretreatment; (B) perioral depigmentation due to deeper Er:YAG laser resurfacing in this area. (C) Identical side-effect seen in a different patient treated by deep mechanical dermabrasion of the upper lip, in between the dotted lines, where the wrinkles have disappeared; however, in the more superficially treated outer borders normal pigmentation is still present but the wrinkles (arrows) have completely reappeared.*

wound care, and when using open methods we have not yet observed any pseudomonas infection, even when using cephalosporins not covering this bacterium.

Though the Er laser avoids unnecessary thermal damage to the wound surface, the risk of postinflammatory hyperpigmentation cannot be completely avoided, even after pretreatment with topical bleaching agents. As with dermabrasion, it is highest in patients with Fitzpatrick skin types III–IV and

increases with deeper procedures, such as in acne patients. Though none of the laser-ablated patients were pretreated with hydroquinone, mild postinflammatory hyperpigmentation at 3 months postoperatively was observed in only two out of 30 patients with Fitzpatrick skin types III and IV treated for facial scars.[37] In contrast, late onset hypo- or depigmentation is usually a persistent problem and is now more frequently reported as a late complication after CO_2 laser rejuvenation;[7] however, it has also been seen after deep dermabrasion and has likewise to be considered after more aggressive Er:YAG rejuvenation procedures (Figure 10.14).

Finally, when comparing side-effects between CO_2 resurfacing, Er:YAG resurfacing and dermabrasion, the major difference is that Er:YAG technology is able to aid the avoidance of such side-effects in the first place by: choosing a more superficial approach; having a better control in critical anatomical sites; and in protecting the wound bottom from additional thermal injury.

References

1 Kaufmann R, Landes E. Dermatologische Operationen. 2nd edition. Stuttgart: Thieme; 1992.

2 Fitzpatrick RE, Goldman MP, Satur NM, Tope W. Pulsed carbon dioxide laser resurfacing of photoaged facial skin. Arch Dermatol 1996;132:395–402.

3 Jordan R, Cummins C, Burls A. Laser resurfacing of the skin for the improvement of facial acne scarring: a systematic review of the evidence. Br J Dermatol 2000;142:413–23.

4 Shim E, Tse Y, Velaquez E, et al. Short-pulse carbon dioxide laser resurfacing in the treatment of rhytides and scars. Dermatol Surg 1998;24:113–17.

5 Sawcer D, Lee HR, Lowe NJ. Lasers and adjunctive treatments for facial scars: a review. J Cutan Laser Ther 1999;1:77–85.

6 Fulton JE. Complications of laser resurfacing: methods of prevention and management. Dermatol Surg 1998;24:91–9.

7 Laws RA, Finley EM, McCollough ML, Grabski WJ. Alabaster skin after carbon dioxide laser resurfacing with histologic correlation. Dermatol Surg 1998;24:633–6.

8 Nanni CA, Alster T. Complications of carbon dioxide laser resurfacing. An evaluation of 500 patients. Dermatol Surg 1998;24:315–20.

9 Ragland HP, McBurney E. Complications of resurfacing. Sem Cutaneous Med Surg 1996;15:200–7.

10. Kaufmann R, Hibst R. Pulsed erbium:YAG and 308 nm UV-Excimer laser: an in vitro and vivo study of skin-ablative effects. Lasers Surg Med 1989;9:132–40.

11. Hibst R, Kaufmann R. Treatment of superficial skin lesions with the Er:YAG laser. In: Kao MC, editors. Proceedings of the 8th Congress of the International Society for Laser Surgery and Medicine, Volume II. Taiwan: Taiwan University Press; 1990:1322–8.

12 Kaufmann R, Hibst R. Pulsed 2.94 µm erbium–YAG laser skin ablation: experimental results and first clinical application. Clin Exp Dermatol 1990;15:389–93.

13 Kaufmann R, Hibst R. Pulsed UV- and mid-infrared laser skin ablation: experimental and first clinical results. In: Steiner, R Kaufmann R, Landthaler M, Braun-Falco O, editors. Lasers in Dermatology. Berlin: Springer; 1991:130–46.

14 Kaufmann R, Hartmann A, Hibst R. Cutting and skin-ablative properties of pulsed mid-infrared laser surgery. J Dermtol Surg Oncol 1994;20:112–18.

15 Peyman GA, Katoh N. Effects of an erbium:YAG laser on ocular structures. Int J Ophthalmol 1987;10:245–53.

16 Peyman GA, Badaro RM, Khoobehi B. Corneal ablation in rabbits using an infrared (2.9 microns) erbium:YAG laser. Ophthalmology 1989;96:1160–70.

17 Hibst R, Kaufmann R. Fundamentals of pulsed UV and mid-infrared laser skin ablation. In: Steiner R, Kaufmann R, Landthaler M, Braun-Falco O, editors, Lasers in Dermatology, Berlin: Springer; 1991:102–15.

18 Hibst R, Kaufmann R. Effects of laser parameters on pulsed erbium:YAG laser skin ablation. Lasers Med Sci 1991;6:391–7.

19 Walsh JT, Flotte TJ, Deutsch TF. Er:YAG laser ablation of tissue: effect of pulse duration and tissue type on thermal damage. Lasers Surg Med 1989;9:314.

20 Ross EV, Naseef GS, McKinlay JR, et al. Comparison of carbon dioxide laser, erbium:YAG laser, dermabrasion, and dermatome: a study of thermal damage, wound contraction, and wound healing in a live pig model: implications for skin resurfacing. J Am Acad Dermatol 2000;42:92–105.

21 Hohenleutner U, Hohenleutner S, Baumler W, Landthaler M. Fast and effective skin ablation with Er:YAG laser: determination of ablation rates and thermal damage zones. Lasers Surg Med 1997;20:242–7.

22 Walsh JT, Deutsch TF. Er:YAG laser ablation of tissue: measurement of ablation rates. Lasers Surg Med 1989;9:327–37.

23 Hibst R, Stock K, Kaufmann R. Ablation and controlled heating of skin with the Er:YAG Laser. Lasers Surg Med 1997;9:40(abstract).

24 Adrian RM. Pulsed carbon dioxide and erbium-YAG laser resurfacing: a comparitive clinical study. J Cutan Laser Ther 1999;1:29–35.

25 Majaron B, Srinivas SM, Huang He, Nelson JS. Deep coagulation of dermal collagen with repetitive Er:YAG laser irradiation. Lasers Surg Med 2000;26:215–22.

26 Pozzner JM, Goldberg DJ. Histologic effect of a variable pulsed Er:YAG laser. Dermatol Surg 2000;26:733–6.

27 Zachary CB. Modulating the Er:YAG laser. Lasers Surg Med 2000;26:223–6.

28 Weinstein C. Modulated dual mode erbium/CO_2 lasers for the treatment of acne scars. J Cutan Laser Therapy 1999;1:203–8.

29 Millman AL, Mannor GE. Combined erbium:YAG and carbon dioxide laser skin resurfacing. Arch Facial Plast Surg 1999;1:112–16.

30 Goldman MP. Laser resurfacing of the neck with the erbium:YAG laser. Dermatol Surg 1999;25:164–8.

31 Goldman MP, Marchell N, Fitzpatrick RE. Laser skin resurfacing of the face with a combined CO_2/Er:YAG laser. Dermatol Surg 2000;26:102–4.

32 Goldman MP, Manuskiatti W, Fitzpatrick RE. Combined laser resurfacing with the UltraPulse carbon dioxide and Er:YAG lasers. In: Fitzpatrick RE, Goldman MP, editors. Cosmetic laser surgery, St. Louis: Mosby; 2000:88–103.

33 Weinstein C. Simultaneously combined Er:YAG and carbon dioxide laser (derma K) for skin resurfacing. Clin Plast Surg 2000;27:273–85.

34 Fulton JE. Dermabrasion, chemabrasion, and laserabrasion. Historical perspectives, modern dermabrasion techniques, and future trends. Dermatol Surg 1996;22:619–28.

35 Tse Y. Use of the erbium :YAG laser in skin resurfacing. In: Fitzpatrick RE, Goldman MP, editors. Cosmetic laser surgery. St. Louis: Mosby, 2000:71–87.

36 Sachsenberg-Studer EM, Ochsendorf FR, Mengeaud V, et al. Laser skin resurfacing and retinaldehyde: a double blind study. JEADV 2000:14(Suppl 1):85–6.

37 Kye YC. Resurfacing of pitted facial scars with the Er:YAG laser. Dermatol Surg 1997;23:880–3.

38 Eaglstein F. Chemical injury to the eye from EMLA cream during erbium laser resurfacing. Dermatol Surg 1999;25:590–1.

39 Podda M, Spieth K, Kaufmann R. Er:YAG laser-assisted hair transplantation in cicatricial alopecia. Dermatol Surg 2000;26:1010–14.

40 Goldman MP. Techniques for erbium:YAG skin resurfacing: initial pearls from the first 100 patients. Dermatol Surg 1997;23:1219–21.

41 Fleming D. Controversies in skin resurfacing: the role of the erbium. J Cutan Laser Ther 1999;1:15–21.

42 Weinstein C. Computerised scanning with erbium:YAG laser for skin resurfacing. Dermatol Surg 1998;24:83–9.

43 Kaufmann R. Klassische Dermabrasion versus Laserverfahren. In: Plettenberg A, Meigel WN, Moll I. editors. Dermatologie an der Schwelle zum neuen Jahrtausend. Aktueller Stand von Klinik und Forschung. Berlin: Spinger; 2000:669–72.

44 Ochsendorf FR, Kaufmann R. Erbium:YAG laser assisted treatment of miliary osteoma cutis. Br J Dermatol 1998;138:371–2.

45 Hughes PSH. Multiple miliary osteoma cutis of the face ablated with the erbium:YAG laser. Arch Dermatol 1999;135:378–80.

46 Boehncke WH, Ochsendorf F, Wolter M, Kaufmann R. Ablative techniques in psoriasis vulgaris resistant to conventional therapies. Dermatol Surg 1999;25:618–21.

47 Beier Ch, Kaufmann R. Erbium:YAG laser ablation of Darier's and Hailey-Hailey's disease. Arch Dermatol 1999;135:423–7.

48 Ochsendorf FR, Kaufmann R, Runne. Erbium:YAG laser ablation of acquired vulval lymphangioma. Br J Dermatol 2001;144:in press.

49 Kaufmann R, Hibst R. Clinical evaluation of Er:YAG Lasers in cutaneous surgery. Lasers Surg Med 1996;19:324–30.

50 Kaufmann R. Stellenwert der Lasertherapie bei Pigmentläsionen. In: Landthaler M, Hohenleutner U, editors. Operative Dermatologie im Kindes- und Jugendalter. Berlin: Blackwell; 1997:23–8.

51 Kaufmann R. Comparison of different procedures for the treatment of benign and malign skin tumors. Min Invas Ther Allied Technol 1998;7:511–17.

52 Kaufmann R. The role of lasers in the treatment of nevocellular nevi. Lasermedizin 2000;15:168–73.

53 Lanigan SW. Lasers in Dermatology. London: Springer; 2000.

54 Kaufmann R, Beier C. Narben-Korrekturmöglichkeiten mit dem Laser. In: Mang WL, Kokoschka EM, editors. Ästhetische Chirurgie, Volume II, Reinbek: Einhorn Presse Verlag; 1998;20–5.

55 Kwon SD, Kye YC. Treatment of scars with a pulsed Er:YAG laser. J Cutan Laser Ther 2000;2:27–31.

56 Dover JS. Roundtable discussion on laser skin resurfacing. Dermatol Surg 1999;25:639–53.

57 Lent WM, David LM. Laser resurfacing: a safe and predictable method of skin resurfacing. J Cutan Las Ther 1999;1:87–94.

58 Holmkvist KA, Rogers GS. Treatment of perioral rhytides: a comparison of dermabrasion and superpulsed carbon dioxide laser. Arch Dermatol 2000;136:725–31.

59 Benedetto AV, Griffin TD, Benedetto EA, Humeniuk HM. Dermabrasion: therapy and prophylaxis of the photodamaged face. J Am Acad Dermatol 1992;27:439–47.

60 Nelson BR, Majmudar G, Griffith CE, et al. Clinical improvement following dermabrasion of photoaged skin correlates with synthesis of collagen I. Arch Dermatol 1994;130:1136–42.

61 Hughes PS. Skin contraction following erbium:YAG laser resurfacing. Dermatol Surg 1998;24:109–11.

62 Greene D, Egbert BM, Utley DS, Koch RJ. In vivo model of histologic changes after treatment with the superpulsed CO_2 laser, erbium:YAG laser, and blended lasers: a 4- to 6-month prospective histologic and clinical study. Lasers Surg Med 2000;27:362–72.

63 Alster TS. Clinical and histological evaluation of six erbium:YAG lasers for cutaneous resurfacing. Lasers Surg Med 1999;24:87–92.

64 Teikemeier G, Goldberg DJ. Skin resurfacing with the erbium:YAG laser. Dermatol Surg 1997;23:685–7.

65 Perez MI, Bank DE, Silvers D. Skin resurfacing of the face with the erbium:YAG laser. Dermatol Surg 1998;24:653–9.

66 Weiss RA, Harrington AC, Pfau RC, et al. Periorbital skin resurfacing using high energy erbium:YAG laser: results in 50 patients. Laser Surg Med 1999;24:81–6.

67 Kathri K, Ross V, Grevelink J, et al. Comparison of erbium:YAG and carbon dioxide lasers in resurfacing of facial rhytides. Arch Dermatol 1999;135:392–7.

68 McDaniel DH, Lord J, Ash K, Newman J. Combined CO_2/erbium:YAG laser resurfacing of peri-oral rhytides and side-by-side comparison with carbon dioxide laser alone. Dermatol Surg 1999;25:285–93.

69 Goldman MP, Manuskiatti W. Combined laser resurfacing with the 950–microsecond pulsed CO_2 + Erbium:YAG lasers. Dermatol Surg 1999;25:160–163.

70 Utley DS, Koch RJ, Egbert BM. Histologic analysis of the thermal effect on epidermal and dermal structures following treatment with the superpulsed CO_2 laser and the erbium:YAG laser: an in vivo study. Lasers Surg Med 1999;24:93–102.

71 Adrian RM. Pulsed carbon dioxide and long pulse 10-ms erbium:YAG laser resurfacing: a comparative clinical and histologic study. J Cutan Laser Ther 1999;1:197–202.

72 Newman JB, Lord SL, Ash K, McDaniel DH. Variable pulse erbium:YAG laser resurfacing of perioral rhytides and side-by-side comparison with carbon dioxide laser. Laser Surg Med 2000:26:208–14.

73 Jimenez G, Spencer JM. Erbium:YAG laser resurfacing of the hands, arms, and neck. Dermatol Surg 1999;25:831–4.

74 McDaniel DH, Ash K, Lord J, et al. The erbium:YAG laser: a review and preliminary report on resurfacing of the face, neck and hands. Aesth Surg 1997;17:157–63.

75 Goldberg DJ, Meine JG. Treatment of photoaged neck skin with the pulsed erbium:YAG laser. Dermatol Surg 1998;24:619–21.

76 Ho C, Nguyen Q, Lowe NJ. Laser resurfacing in pigmented skin. Dermatol Surg 1995;21:1035–7.

77 Kim JW, Lee JO. Skin resurfacing with laser in Asians. Aesth Plast Surg 1997;21:115–17.

78 Polnikorn N, Goldberg DJ, Suwanchinda A, Ng SW. Erbium:YAG laser resurfacing in Asians. Dermatol Surg 1998;24:1303–7.

79 Kaufmann R, Beier C. Fehler und Risiken der Hautablation. In: Bull HG, Mang WL, editors. Ästhetische Chirurgie, Volume III. Reinbek: Einhorn Presse Verlag, 2001; in press.

COMBINATION TREATMENT (Nicholas J Lowe)

Indications	Potential combination treatments	Chapter reference
Facial aging	Photoprotection	1
Periorbital	Topical therapy	2,3
Perioral lines	Glycolic peels	6
Neck (caution)	Combination chemical peels	7
	Facial pigment treatment	8
	Vascular laser treatment	9
	Botulinum toxin A	13–15
	Fillers	16,17
	Implants	18,19
	Endoscopic surgery	20
		13
	Non-ablative lasers	12

11. Laser skin resurfacing

Nicholas J Lowe, Philippa Lowe, Paul Yamauchi and Gary P Lask

CARBON DIOXIDE (CO_2) LASER RESURFACING

The initial observations on the potential use of CO_2 lasers for skin rejuvenation were reported in 1989.[1]

The critical goal of laser resurfacing depends on targeted laser delivery for tissue vaporization. Excessive laser effect is associated with a risk of unwanted thermal injury to the surrounding dermis and adnexal structures. Advances in rapidly pulsed lasers and flashscan techniques allow more precise control of tissue ablation, reducing the risk of scarring.[2-7]

Laser skin resurfacing removes layers of damaged skin and replaces them with more youthful skin. It also offers a clinical advanatage in the treatment of superficial skin lesions for which surgery may leave scars. It has also been claimed that pulsed CO_2 lasers offer advantages over cold-steel surgery for incisional procedures such as blepharoplasty these techniques discussed in Chapter 24.

Types of CO_2 lasers

Several CO_2 lasers are available. These can be divided into two groups: pulsed laser systems and continuous-wave scanned systems. Table 11.1 shows features of some different CO_2 laser systems.

The UltraPulse® 5000C CO_2 laser (Coherent, Palo Alto, CA) produces high-energy pulses of very short duration, which allows controlled tissue ablation with a thermal injury depth of c. 70 µm, depending on the laser settings. It has a pulse width of < 1ms and a pulse energy of up to 500 mJ. The energy is delivered through an articulated handle connected to a computer-controlled scanner. This scanner allows the user to select different shapes, densities and sizes of laser skin treatment target.[3-6]

The Sharplan Surgilase was another type of pulsed laser. It produced a double pulse in 1.8 ms but each pulse is within the limit of the thermal relaxation time. The first pulse partially ablates the tissue and, during the resting period that follows, steam, debris

Table 11.1 *Some CO_2 laser systems used for skin resurfacing*

Laser	Pulse width	Pulse energy (mJ)	Collimation	Type of laser delivery system
Clearpulse	6 ms	500	Yes	Pulsed
FeatherTouch	300 ps	500	No	Scanned
NovaPulse	800 ps	500	No	Pulsed
SilkTouch	600 ps	500	No	Scanned
Surgilase	1.8 ms	400	Yes	Pulsed
Tru-Pulse	65 ps	500	No	Pulsed
UltraPulse	1 ms	500	Yes	Pulsed

and thermal build-up from the first pulse are dispersed. Subsequently, the second pulse is fired, completely vaporizing the tissue.[2] This laser is currently not often used.

Luxar Corporation introduced the NovaPulse® CO_2 laser (Lumenis Ltd., Yokneam, Israel), which allowed the delivery of a laser beam through a lightweight, flexible, hollow fibre arm. The NovaPulse superpulsed laser delivers laser energy to tissue in high-amplitude, short-duration pulses of 800 ps. Each pulse is followed by a laser period of off-time, which allows the tissue to cool down. This minimizes unwanted charring and thermal necrosis. In addition, the NovaPulse features a 'top hat' beam geometry, providing even distribution of laser energy up to 500 mJ, unlike the Gaussian beam distribution of other pulsed laser systems.

The Clearpulse laser produced by LaserSonics delivers single pulses of 500 mJ. Unlike other pulsed laser systems, the Clearpulse laser has a pulse duration of 6 ms, which is six times that of the thermal relaxation time. However, the manufacturer states that the 'histological testing has shown that the Clearpulse laser effectively ablates the epidermis to a level of 100 j~tm, with collateral damage limited to only 25~tm.'

One addition to the pulsed system is the Tru-Pulse™ CO_2 laser by Tissue Medical Lasers, Inc., (Albuquerque, NM, USA). The Tru-Pulse laser was specifically designed to reduce postoperative erythema and expedite healing time after laser resurfacing. Erythema due to thermal damage is minimized through use of a pulse width of only 65 ps. The ability to deliver high energies, up to 500 mJ, rapidly may account for the shorter healing time and less erythema. However, the amount of tissue removed per pass may also be less, so more passes are required for areas of deep rhytides.

The Sharplan SilkTouch laser, unlike the pulsed laser system, is an optomechanical device, is microprocessor controlled and consists of mirrors rotating at rapid speeds, resulting in a spiral scan beam.[2] The resulting dwell time of the laser beam at any particular point is less than the thermal relaxation time. The time for one cycle of beam rotation ranges from 0.2 to 0.45 s, and the spot sizes vary from 2 to 16 mm. The SilkTouch device can be adapted to a conventional continuous-wave CO_2 laser. Later,

Sharplan added the FeatherTouch to its flashscanner devices. The FeatherTouch laser has a shorter dwell time than the SilkTouch, which allows more superficial ablation of the epidermis and reduces postoperative erythema. By switching between the SilkTouch and FeatherTouch modes, the user can select the depth of skin resurfacing in accordance with the depth of the rhytid or scar.[7]

Laser–skin interactions with CO_2 lasers

The CO_2 laser emits a beam of infrared light with a wavelength of 10,600 nm. This light is absorbed by all biological tissues containing water, its target chromophore. Approximately 90% of the laser energy is absorbed by 30 ~tm of tissue, resulting in intracellular boiling to 100°C and therefore vaporization. In earlier use of the CO_2 laser in the continuous mode, the tissue became progressively desiccated and heat accumulated to a temperature of 600°C. This heat would then conduct away from the treating site, leading to a surrounding zone of thermal necrosis 200 ~im to 1 mm thick. The non-selective thermal damage can leave scars and discoloration.[8,9]

Newer laser systems can reduce the collateral thermal injury by shortening the duration that the laser beam spends on the target site. According to Beer's law, laser energy heats a critical volume of tissue until the temperature exceeds the vaporization threshold. This threshold for human skin – the thermal relaxation time, defined as the time required for the heated tissue to lose 50% of its heat through surrounding diffusion – is c. 695–950 ~tsec. Thus, if the laser energy is delivered in less than the thermal relaxation time, heat dissipates rather than accumulates around the treatment area. The current type of CO_2 lasers (pulse or scanned) allow the tissue dwell time, or exposure time, to be less than the thermal relaxation time.[3–12]

General considerations

The energy density, or fluence needed to ablate tissue has been estimated to be 4.5–5.0 J/cm^2. By using a laser system with an energy fluence > 5 J/cm^2 and a pulse duration <1 ms, an effective depth of 30 μm of tissue can be vaporized, leaving a shallow residual zone of thermal damage of 40–100 ~tm. This zone of necrosis is responsible for the sealing of small

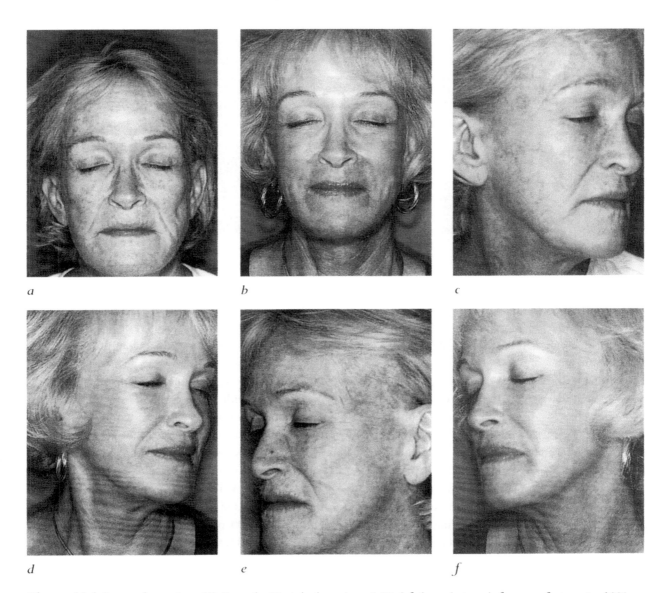

Figure 11.1 *Severe photoaging. (A) Frontal, (C) right lateral, and (E) left lateral views before resurfacing. An 80% improvement is noted on (B) frontal, (D) right lateral, and (F) left lateral views 6 months after resurfacing of the face and neck. Two passes were done on the face: for the first pass settings were 300 mJ with a density of 5 and for the second pass, 250 mJ with a density of 4. One pass was done on the neck; the settings were 250 mJ with a density of 3. Coherent UltraPulse CO_2 laser.*

blood vessels, resulting in hemostasis. It has been hypothesized that collagen shrinkage also takes place below this zone, which accounts for the skin tightening effect seen during laser surgery.[3–6]

Recent clinical and histologic comparisons among pulsed CO_2 lasers, medium-strength trichloroacetic acid (TCA) peels, and dermabrasion have shown comparable results, with the exception of Baker's phenol peel, which may give deeper dermal injury.[11] Healing from medium-strength TCA peels and dermabrasion was similar to that

after one to three passes of pulsed laser treatment. The phenol treatment caused a deeper wound and required a longer recovery time.[13]

Neck resurfacing

In the past, most studies were performed on facial skin Caucasian phototypes I and II. There have been few reports on the use of these lasers for the rejuvenation of photoaged neck skin. The neck is often

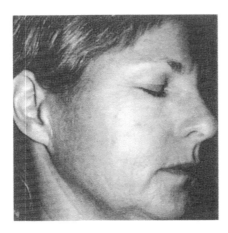 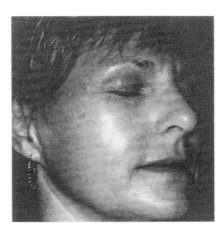

Figure 11.2 *Moderate photoaging. (A) Before resurfacing, (B) a 60% improvement noted 6 months after resurfacing. Two passes were done with settings at 300 mJ and 60 W with a density of 5. Coherent UltraPulse CO_2 laser.*

considered to be an area of potential complication with treatments such as dermabrasion and some chemical peels. In a recent study, 200 patients with facial photoaging and 40 patients with neck skin photoaging, skin types I–IV were treated. All patients were treated with an Ultrapulse CO_2 laser with a CPG handpiece. An energy setting of 225 or 250 W/cm^2 was used with a low-density CPG setting of 3, using a single pass, and no wiping technique.[4,14,15]

One of the present authors (NJL) routinely treats the upper part of the neck using these parameters to provide a graded 'feathering' of the neck skin, so avoiding a line of demarcation between treated and untreated skin.

Facial photoaging was improved by 50–75% with a single treatment; occasionally a second treatment was given. The result after a single treatment continues to improve for 6 months to 2 years.

Successful rejuvenation of the neck skin is very dependent on single passes of appropriate low-density settings, and the skill and caution of the laser surgeon. Figures 11.1 and 11.2 show examples of CO_2 laser neck resurfacing.

Preoperative preparation

For optimal results with laser skin resurfacing, carefully selected skin-care regimens are needed both before and after treatment, particularly in the treatment of patients with darker complexions.[12,13] One pretreatment regimen consists of the use of daily broad-spectrum sunscreens, application of bleaching agents such as hydroquinone or azelaic acid, and nightly application of tretinoin cream or glycolic acid cream. This regimen is usually started after the initial consultation, c. 2–4 weeks before the procedure is performed.[3,4,7,14]

The day before laser surgery, the patient is started on therapy with oral antibiotics and antiherpes medications. Use of these drugs is continued for 5–7 days postoperatively. One of the present authors (NJL) only now uses 'open' postoperative laser skin care. Wound care consists of solid vegetable shortening (Crisco, USA; Trex, UK) applied for 2 weeks (NJL reports no cases of skin irritation or contact dermatitis in over 5000 patients treated with this regime), iced water or diluted acetic acid soaks up to day 7 if pustulation occurs, and soap-free wash (e.g. Aquanil, Cetaphil) thereafter (Figure 11.3). A sunscreen, skin lightening and tretinoin cream regimen is started again 2–4 weeks after treatment, depending on rate of healing and other factors such as skin phototype.

Complications of CO_2 laser resurfacing

Complications of laser surgery include infection, contact dermatitis, swelling, prolonged erythema, depigmentation and scarring. Recurrence of herpes infections can be prevented with prophylactic medication. Topical antibiotic use is no longer recommended because of the common occurrence of contact dermatitis. Postoperative swelling, especially around periorbital areas, is managed with ice compresses or a short course of systemic corticosteroid. Prolonged erythema can last from several weeks to several months (Figure 11.4). Postinflammatory hyperpigmentation sometimes

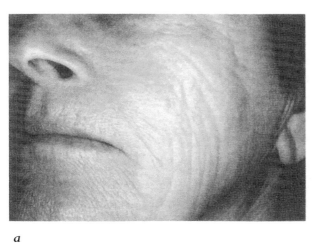
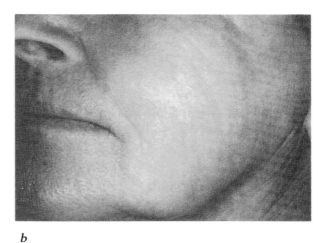

a   b

Figure 11.3 Severe photoaging. (A) Before resurfacing. (B) Twelve months after resurfacing. Two passes were made with settings of 300 mJ and 60 W with a density of 5. Density was set at 4 for a third pass on the cheeks. Coherent UltraPulse CO_2 laser.

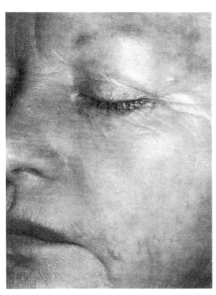
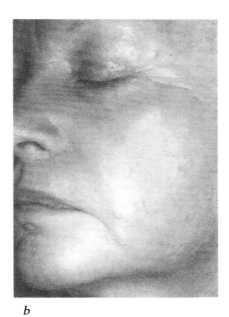

Figure 11.4 Moderate photoaging. (A) Before resurfacing, (B) twelve months after resurfacing. Two passes were done. Settings for the first pass were 300 mJ and 60 W with a density of 5; settings for the second pass were 250 mJ and 60 W with a density of 4. Coherent UltraPulse CO_2 laser.

a   b

follows the erythema, so all patients with prolonged erythema are treated with bleaching agent. Hyperpigmentation is most common in the infraorbital areas, where direct sunlight exposure can play a role. Hypopigmentation can also occur and tends to be delayed, occurring 6 months to 1 year after the procedure; it is possible that this is partially pigment loss and partially reduced dermal vascularity. Although laser skin resurfacing can be precise, thermal damage accumulates with multiple passes of the laser and hypertrophic scars

have been reported. Scarring is related to the depth of resurfacing as well as to the location of treatment. The perioral areas usually require more passes and a few incidences of scarring have been reported.[12]

Laser techniques

Anaesthesia
Anaesthesia for separate cosmetic units (e.g. perioral, periorbital or malar areas) can be achieved with topical

ELA-max® (Ferndale Laboratories, Ferndale, Michigan, USA) cream applied at least 1 hour because the nerve blocks (infraorbital or mental), using lidocaine 1% with 1:100,000 epinephrine. Additional ring blocks are usually necessary for the periorbital and lateral face areas, since these are innervated by more than one nerve branch. Topical anaesthesia can be sufficient for up to two laser passes for a full-face procedure.[14] Sedation with 5 mg of diazepam (Valium) or an intramuscular injection with 50 mg meperidine (Demerol) is necessary in some patients. For patients with a low pain threshold, sedational anaesthesia is required with appropriate monitoring by an anaesthetist (anaesthesiologist). Many laser surgeons prefer sedational over topical anaesthesia because of the pain patients experience during large area laser resurfacing.[5,10,14]

The technique for treating rhytides consists of laser ablation of a particular cosmetic unit. A series of multiple side-by-side laser impacts with minimal overlap is laid down. The areas are subsequently wiped off with saline-soaked gauzes. Repeated passes are made, emphasizing the shoulders of the deep rhytides. In general, it takes three or four passes to achieve significant improvement of the perioral rhytides. The periorbital areas, in contrast, require fewer laser passses because the dermis is thinner. Treatment of icepick scars sometimes necessitates punch excisions of these scars 1 month before laser resurfacing. Feathering of the margins of the treated areas can be performed by decreasing the power or decreasing the density of the scanner pattern to reduce the obvious change of skin texture and colour during the healing phase.[3–7,14]

It can be helpful to use the visual signs of laser depth penetration to decrease the chance of scarring. If used inappropriately, even char-free ablation lasers can cause scars, despite their minimal thermal injury. The signs of depth penetration of the skin are suggested as follows:

(1) pink, erythematous appearance – ablating of the epidermis with effacing of the papillary dermis;
(2) yellow chamois cloth appearance – deep papillary dermis.

However, this feature may be altered by the presence of solar elastosis. One of the present authors (NJL) does not wipe the final laser pass as he has found

removal to lead to more prolonged erythema. These are helpful guides but are not always consistent and should not be used as the sole end-point determination.

Summary of CO_2 laser resurfacing for the face and neck

Skin resurfacing with CO_2 lasers is an effective form of skin rejuvenation (Figures 11.5–11.10). One of the present authors (NJL) uses an Ultrapulse 5000C CO_2 laser with a CPG of either pattern 3 (for most areas of the face and neck) or pattern 5 (for the neck and perioral skin). For the central and main areas of the face, the maximum size setting was 9, with the density setting either 5 or 6, depending on the degree of photodamage. For the subsequent laser pulses on the face, the settings were 250 mJ and 60 W with patterns 3 or 5 determined as above. Laser settings for neck rejuvenation were as follows: a single pass of the laser; energy settings of 225 Mj and 100 W; a density setting of 3 (Table 11.2). For the face, the vaporized skin was wiped after each pass, except for the final pass that was left unwiped. For the neck treatment, no wiping of the vaporized skin was performed after the single low-density CPG laser ablation.

Table 11.2 Laser settings at different skin sites using Coherent UltraPulse 5000 CO_2 lasers

Treatment site	Laser nergy settings	CPG density
Cheeks	300 mJ	4–6
	60–100 W	
Perioral	300 mJ	5–6
	60–100 W	
Acne scars	300 mJ	5–6
Cheeks/forehead	60–100 W	4–6
Eyelids	250 mJ	3–5
	60–100 W	(two passes)
Neck	250 mJ	2–3
(no wiping)	60–100 W	(one pass)

In skin types III and IV, transient hyperpigmentation may last up to 7–9 months in some patients' rejuvenation on the neck, and it is advisable that the laser be tested in a small area before general treatment is undertaken.

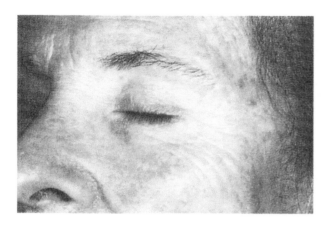
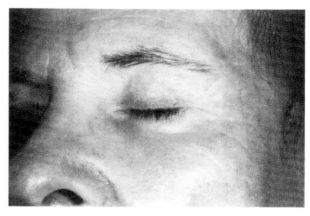

a   b

Figure 11.5 *Moderate photoaging. (A) Before resurfacing. (B) A 70% improvement is noted 6 months after resurfacing. Two passes were done. Settings for the first pass were 250 mJ and 60 W with a density of 5; settings for the second pass were 225 mJ and 60 W with a density of 4. Botox® injections to the "crows feet" before and three months after laser treatment.*

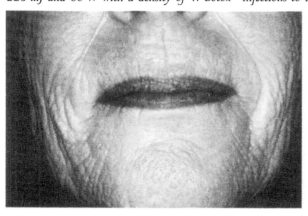
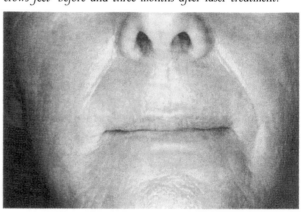

a   b

Figure 11.6 *Severe photoaging. (A) Before resurfacing. (B) The postreatment image was taken 18 months after the initial resurfacing and 6 months after a second treatment. Three passes were done for the first resurfacing; settings were 300 mJ and 60 W with a density of 5. Two passes were done for the second resurfacing; settings for the first pass were 300 mJ and 60 W with a density of 5 and settings for the second pass were 250 mJ and 60 W with a density of 4.*

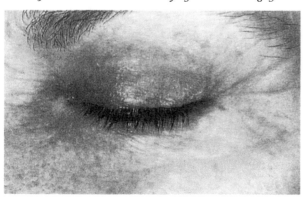
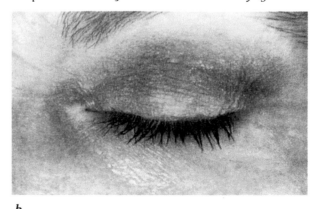

a   b

Figure 11.7 *Moderate aging in the periorbital region. (A) Before resurfacing. (B) Six months after resurfacing. Two passes were done. Settings for the first pass were 300 W and 60 W with a density of 4; settings for the second pass were 2350 mJ and 60 W with a density of 4.*
(All above using coherent UltraPulse 5000 CO₂ laser)

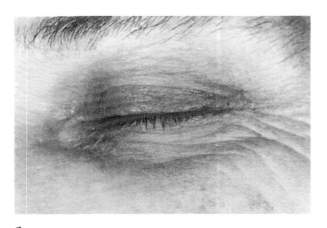
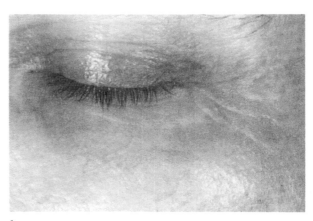

a   *b*

Figure 11.8 *Moderate aging in the periorbital region. (A) Before resurfacing. (B) Twelve months after resurfacing. Two passes were done. Settings for the first pass were 300 mJ and 60 W with a density of 5; settings for the second pass were 250 mJ and 60 W with a density of 4.*

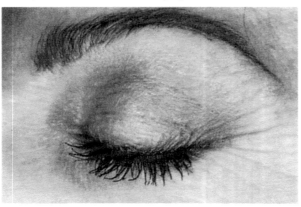
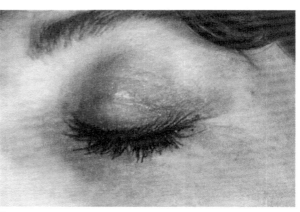

a   *b*

Figure 11.9 *Mild periorbital lines. (A) Before resurfacing. (B) Twelve months after resurfacing. Two passes were done. Settings for the first pass were 250 mJ and 60 W with a density of 5; settings for the second pass were 225 mJ and 60 W with a density of 4.*

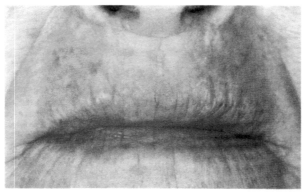
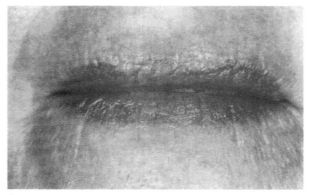

a   *b*

Figure 11.10 *Severe perioral lines. (A) Before resurfacing. (B) An 80% improvement is noted 12 months after resurfacing. Three passes were done. Settings for the first pass were 300 mJ and 60 W with a density of 5; settings for the second pass were 250 mJ and 60 W with a density of 5; settings for the third pass were 250 mJ and 60 W with a density of 5. The patient also had a SoftForm implant to the upper lip at the time of resurfacing.*
(All above using Coherent UltraPulse 5000 CO_2 laser)

For superficial facial resurfacing the following laser settings were used: a single superficial pass; energy setting of 250 mJ and 100 W; a density of 3 or 4; no wiping. This led to a rapid 5–8 days of initial healing.

In one of our studies, results of the treatment of facial photoaging was 50–75% improvement achieved 12–24 months after a single laser treatment. A number of patients were treated completely or partially with a second laser treatment and in these patients the final improvement was 25–50% improved over the first treatment. In general, the patients received fewer passes during their second treatment than during their first.[4]

The global responses after a single neck rejuvenation treatment varied between 40 and 75% improvement. The neck is at much greater risk for scarring than the face. The risk increases the more inferior one goes, in part because of the decreasing number of adnexal structures. The temporary side-effects were exudation, scaling, erythema, and discomfort. After days 7–10, complete re-epithelization was seen. A smaller percentage of patients had postoperative erythema that lasted up to 6 months. After the second month, however, this was generally of a relatively mild degree and was frequently more pronounced after exercise or exposure to hot weather.[15]

Improvement from laser skin rejuvenation was observed to last during the entire study period for these patients.[4] For patients who have severe photo-damage (e.g. perioral rhytides), it is perhaps best to treat a second time to avoid an overaggresive single treatment. The patients treated for a second time showed a significant improvement. Potential mechanisms of action include in vivo dermal collagen shrinkage and remodelling. In addition, it is likely that the epidermal proliferative regrowth seen after laser skin rejuvenation also releases a variety of growth factors that aid the formation of new dermal connective tissue.

Recent observations on the successful treatment of photodamaged neck skin are encouraging, but the advice given here about superficial use and low-density laser settings should be heeded. Further studies are needed before laser neck rejuvenation can be considered safe and effective.[16]

ERBIUM:YAG LASER

In the past few years, there has been significant development and use of the erbium:yttrium–aluminium–garnet (Er:YAG) laser for skin resurfacing.[17–19] The Er:YAG laser has created much interest because of its ability to deliver superficial skin resurfacing.

The Er:YAG laser has a high affinity for water absorption. The wavelength of 2940 nm is at the peak of water absorption and is 10 times greater than the CO_2 laser. The Er:YAG laser will ablate tissue at relatively low energy fluences of c. $0.5–1.5 \text{ J/sm}^2$. Because of this property, there is much less residual thermal damage to the skin than with the CO_2 laser. Approximately 2–4 µm of tissue are vaporized for each J/cm^2 delivered. Initial studies have shown than a single pass with some Er:YAG lasers ablates 20–25 µm of epidermis.[17,18]

The older generation Er:YAG lasers have a pulse duration of 250–350 µs. The minimal thermal damage of Er:YAG lasers has been claimed to allow quicker healing times and less erythema than CO_2 lasers. This is entirely dependent on the aggressiveness of laser resurfacing. However, with the superficial degree of ablation into the papillary dermis and the small amount of coagulation inherent at these short pulse durations, bleeding can pose a significant problem. Excessive bleeding will prevent further tissue vaporization because the laser beam will be absorbed by the wet field. More passes are required to attain adequate depth for clinical improvement and the excess blood must be wiped off between passes.

There has been much discussion and debate as to whether the Er:YAG laser is equal in efficacy to the CO_2 laser in the treatment of rhytides. Because of the ablative properties of the Er:YAG laser, there is associated lack of residual thermal damage. Many laser surgeons claim that this is associated with a lack of heat-induced collagen tightening that is inherent with the use of CO_2 laser. Consequently, immediate visible tissue contraction is absent with the Er:YAG laser.

Recent advances have led to the development of new generation Er:YAG lasers with longer pulse widths and a combination of both ablative and coagulative capabilities. This allows for much deeper vaporization while allowing for control of haemostasis. Three laser systems will be discussed below.

The Derma™ K (Lumenis) is a hybrid laser system that combines a conventional Er:YAG laser with the coagulating CO_2 laser at low power. The Derma K can be programmed to deliver a low energy fluence subablative CO_2 pulse immediately following the ablative Er:YAG pulse. The CO_2 pulse may fill part or all of the time between Er:YAG laser pulses. For example, a 50% CO_2 cycle pulse would fill half of the time between Er:YAG pulses and a 100% CO_2 pulse would fill the whole time. The energy fluence of the CO_2 laser can also be changed. In most situations, many laser surgeons tend to use at least a 50%, and often a 100%, CO_2 pulse between Er:YAG pulses. This allows for some control of haemostasis and contactility of tissue.

The CO_3 system (Cynosure Inc, Chelmsford, MA) is a variable pulse Er:YAG laser that delivers single pulses of variable lengths from 500 μs to 10 ms. Short pulses will produce more ablation and longer pulses will be more coagulative. It should be noted that this laser does not employ any features of a CO_2 laser. There is evidence that a reduction in photodamaged skin can be achieved with this laser.

The Contour™ (Sciton, Palo Alto, CA) system is a dual-mode laser that comprises two Er:YAG laser heads, providing both short-pulse ablative and long-pulse coagulative properties. The Contour employs a technology termed optical multiplexing in which stacks of individual Er:YAG pulses are grouped to produce either short ablative pulses at high energy fluences or coagulative micropulses at low energy fluences. The optical multiplexing allows the laser to be used either in an ablative mode, a combined ablative and coagulative mode, or a purely coagulative mode. The ablative mode is comprised of a short 200 μs pulse; the ablative–coagulative mode is achieved by an ablative pulse followed immediately by a longer subablative pulse; and the coagulative mode consists of a series of subablative pulses.

There are advantages in using the dual-mode and longer-pulsed Er:YAG lasers over conventional lasers. The dual-mode systems allow for superficial and deep vaporization while simultaneously providing controlled coagulation. With the conventional Er:YAG laser, there is efficient superficial ablation but little coagulation. A recent study demonstrated that a dual-mode Er:YAG laser provides similar histologic findings over depth of ablation when compared with short-pulsed Er:YAG lasers.[6] In addition, the same histological thermal effect desired from CO_2 lasers could be observed when such a system is used with longer Er:YAG laser pulses.[19] Good correlation was seen between the chosen laser parameters and histological findings after a first pass of either a longer-pulsed thermal damaging Er:YAG laser alone or in combination with a shorter-pulsed ablative Er:YAG laser.

In another study, the variable pulse Er:YAG laser was compared with the CO_2 laser in the treatment of upper lip rhytides. There was an overall reduction in the duration of crusting from 7.7 days with the CO_2 laser to 3.4 days with the Er:YAG laser. Chromometer measurements demonstrated decreased postoperative erythema. There was a 63% improvement in upper lip rhytides for the CO_2 treatment site and 48% improvement in the variable pulse Er:YAG site. No cases of permanent hyperpigmentation, hypopigmentation, or scarring were reported in this study. Longer-term follow-up would be valuable.

The long-pulsed Er:YAG laser may be of some benefit in the treatment of acne scars in Asian skin. Patients with Fitzpatrick skin types III–V who had pitted facial acne scars were treated with a long-pulsed Er:YAG laser. A 5 mm handpiece at a setting of 7.0–7.5 J/cm^2 with a 10 ms pulse duration was used. The results of long-pulsed Er:YAG laser resurfacing for pitted facial acne scars were excellent in 36%, good in 57% and fair in 7% of patients. Erythema occurred in all patients after laser treatment and lasted > 3 months in 54% of the subjects. Postinflammatory hyperpigmentation occurred in 29% of the patients but disappeared within 3 months. The long-pulsed Er:YAG may be an effective tool in the treatment of acne scars in higher skin types provided that conservative settings are utilized to minimize postoperative complications.

The Er:YAG laser is potentially of benefit in areas of high risk for scarring such as the neck and dorsum of the hands. In dealing with deeper rhytides and extensively sun-damaged skin, investigators are evaluating variations in parameters, scanning patterns and repetition rates that will allow them to increase penetration and thermal damage when necessary.

Table 11.3 Typical laser settings and passes for Er:YAG lasers (250–350 ms) at different skin sites

	Each pass laser settings	Number of passes
Cheeks	700–900 mJ	5–10
Perioral	700–900 mJ	5–10
Periorbital	500–900 mJ	2–4
Acne scars (cheeks, forehead)	700–900 mJ	5–10
Eyelids	500 mJ	Usually 3
Neck	500 mJ	Usually 3

One study comparing the Er:YAG laser with the UPCO$_2$ laser found seven passes with the former and three passes with the latter produced tissue vaporization of 50–80 μm. Residual thermal damage was 0–20 μm with the Er:YAG laser and 80–150 μm with the CO$_2$ laser. Regardless of the number of passes, the Er:YAG laser resulted in more rapid re-epithelization and decreased erythema than the CO$_2$ laser. However, with an equal number of passes, the CO$_2$ laser resulted in greater wrinkle improvement.

In addition to the lasers used, the outcome of laser skin rejuvenation depends on many factors, including the laser settings and pre- and post-treatment skin care produced (Table 11.3).

The depth of skin injury with both ultrapulsed CO$_2$ laser or Er:YAG lasers is entirely dependent on the laser settings and operator technique. It is possible to produce superficial rapid healing resurfacing with both laser types. It is also possible with overly aggressive technique to produce short and late complications of scarring and pigment changes with both lasers.

SUMMARY

The rapidly advancing technological development in the area of laser resurfacing, makes this a constantly evolving area. Physicians require frequent updates to perform the most efficacious and safest procedures possible. The combination of laser resurfacing with reduction of dynamic rhytides using botulinum toxin is frequently being employed by the present authors.

However, the technique of laser skin resurfacing is not without side-effects and these are outlined in Table 11.4.

In addition to photoaged skin, numerous other skin lesions can be treated with resufacing lasers, including a variety of benign and malignant skin lesions that are often associated with ageing skin (Table 11.5). Their removal with lasers offers another aspect of rejuvenation of the ageing face.[20–22]

Table 11.4 Laser skin resurfacing side-effects

Early side-effects	Delayed side-effects
Pain	Persistent erythema
Crusting	Hyperpigmentation
Exudation	Hypopigmentation
Bacterial infection	Skin whitening (vascular)
Herpes simplex infection	Scars: atrophic
	keloid
	erythematous
	ectropion

Beware of treating patients who have had oral isotretinoin within a 1-year period prior to laser treatment.

Table 11.5 Skin lesions treatable with CO$_2$ or Er:YAG laser

Epidermal lesions	Actinic keratosis, seborrheic keratosis, verrucae, epidermal naevi
Skin tumours	Superficial basal cell carcinoma, Bowen's diseae, benign pigmented naevi
Dermal lesions	Syringomata, sebaceous hyperplasia, xanthelasma, neurofibroma, adenoma sebaceum, trichoepithelioma
Rhinophyma	

In some cases CO$_2$ lasers preferable, in others Er:YAG lasers are preferable.[16–21]

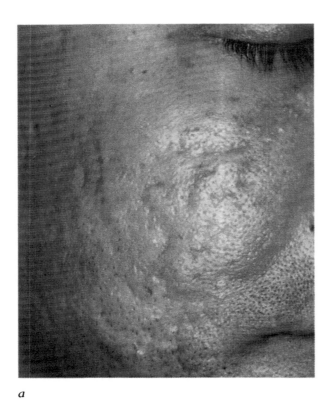

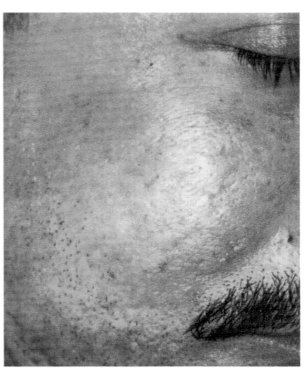

a

b

Figure 11.11 *(A) Severe acne scarring before treatment. (B) Following scar subcision, fat transfer and UltraPulse CO_2 laser resurfacing.*

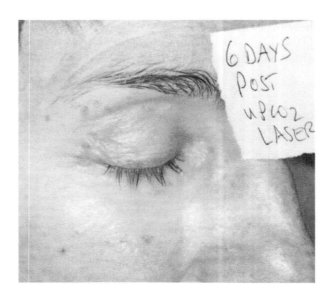

Figure 11.12 *Rapid healing 6 days after periorbital CO_2 laser resurfacing. A single pass setting, 225 mJ 100 W, CPG density 3, no wiping, 6x daily application of vegetable shortening cream (Trex UK).*

SOME COMPLICATIONS AND PROBLEMS

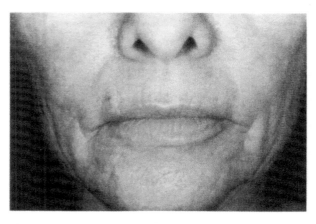

a

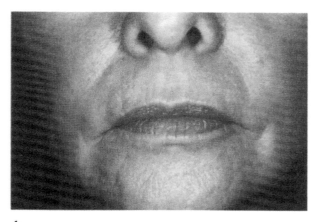

b

Figure 11.13 Moderate to severe photaging. (A) Before resurfacing. (B) Twelve months after resurfacing of the perioral region and lower face. Two passes were done. Settings for the first pass were 300 ml and 60 W with a density of 5; settings for the second pass were 250 mJ and 60 W with a density of 5. Note whitening of upper lip.

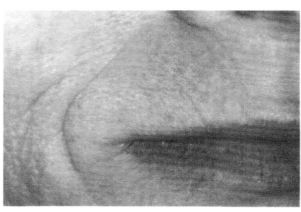

a

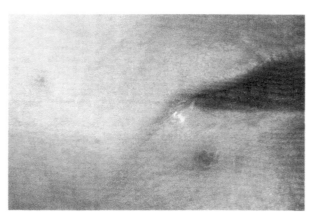

b

Figure 11.14 Severe photoaging. (A) Before resurfacing. (B) Acneiform lesions and scattered telangiectasia are seen 3 weeks after resurfacing.

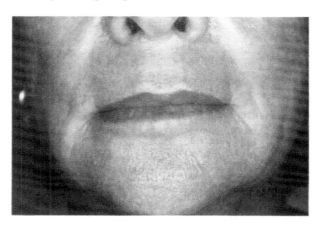

Figure 11.15 Erythema and mild skin whitening have developed 6 months later.

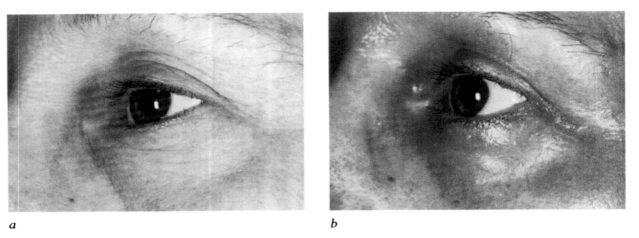

a *b*

Figure 11.16 *Moderate photoaging. (A) Before resurfacing. (B) Moderate erythema has developed 2 weeks after treatment. Settings for the two passes were 300 mJ with a density of 5 and 225 mJ with a density of 4, respectively.*

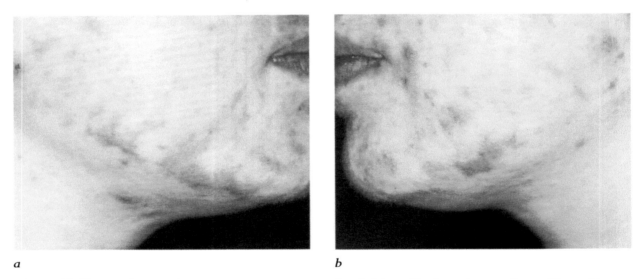

a *b*

Figure 11.17 *Severe hypertrophic scarring in a patient treated with Erbium-Yag laser skin resurfacing. This problem may occur with any resurfacing laser and is technique-dependent*

References

1. David LM, Lask GP, Glassberg E et al. CO_2 laser ablation for cosmetic and therapeutic treatment of facial actinic damage. Cutis 1989;43:583–7.

2. Fitzpatrick RE, Ruiz-Esparza J J, Goldman MP. The depth of thermal necrosis using the CO_2 laser: a comparison of the superpulsed mode and the conventional mode. J Dermatol Surg Oncol 1991;17:340–4.

3. Fitzpatrick RE, Goldman MP. Advances in carbon dioxide laser surgery. Clin Dermatol 1995;13:35–47.

4. Lowe NJ, Lask G, Griffin ME et al. Skin resurfacing with the ultrapulsed carbon dioxide laser: observation on 100 patients. Dermatol Surg 1995;21:1025–9.

5. Hruza G. Skin resurfacing with lasers. Clin Dermatol 1995;3:38–41.

6. Waldorf HA, Kauvar A, Geronemus RG. Skin resurfacing of fine to deep rhytides using a char-free carbon dioxide laser in 47 patients. Dermatol Surg 1995;21:940–6.

7. Lask G, Keller G, Lowe N et al. Laser skin resurfacing with the SilkTouch flashscanner for facial rhytides. Dermatol Surg 1995;21:102–4.

8. Trust D, Zacheri A, Smith M. Surgical laser properties and their tissue interaction. Chicago: Mosby Year Book;1992:131–62.

9. McKenzie AL. How far does thermal damage extend beneath the surface of CO_2 laser incisions? Phys Med Biol 1983;28:905–12.

10. Hobbs E, Bailin P, Wheeland R, Ratz J. Superpulsed lasers: minimizing thermal damage with short duration high irradiance pulses. J Dermatol Surg Oncol 1987;13:9.

11. Verschueren RCJ, Koudstaal I, Oldhoff I. CO_2 laser surgery. In: Hilleneamp F, Pratesi R, Sacni CA, eds. Lasers in biology and medicine. New York: Plenium;1980.

12. Von Gernen MJC, Welch AL. Time constants in thermal medicine. Lasers Surg Med 1989;9:405.

13. Fitzpatrick RE, Tope WD, Goldman MP et al. Pulsed carbon dioxide laser, trichloroacetic acid, Baker–Gordon phenol, and dermabrasion: a comparative clinical and histological study in a porcine model. Arch Dermatol 1996;132:469–71.

14. Lowe NJ, Lask O, Griffin ME. Laser skin resurfacing: pre and posttreatment guidelines. Dermatol Surg 1995;21:1017–19.

15. Ho C, Nguyen Q, Lowe NJ et al. Laser resurfacing in pigmented skin. Dermatol Surg 1995;21:1035–7.

16. Lowe NJ, Maxwell CA, Lowe P et al. Skin resurfacing. In *Lasers in Cutaneous and Cosmetic Surgery*. Ed. Lask GP, Lowe NJ. Churchill Livingstone, Philadelphia, 2000.

17. Kaufman R, Hirbot R. Pulsed erbium:YAG laser ablation in cutaneous surgery. Laser Surg Med 1996;19:324.

18. Hirst R, Stock K, Kaufman R. Ablation and controlled heating of skin with the Er:YAG laser. Laser Surg Med 1997;9(Suppl):40.

19. Khatri K, Russ V, Grevelink I et al. Comparison of erbium:YAG and CO_2 lasers in wrinkle removal. Laser Surg Med 1997;9(Suppl):37.

20. Apfelberg DB, Maser MR, Lash H et al. Superpulsed CO_2 laser treatment of facial syringomata. Laser Surg Med 1987;7:533.

21. Roenigk RK, Ratz IL. CO_2 laser treatment of cutaneous neurofibromas. J Dermatol Surg Oncol 1987;13:187.

22. Wheeland RG, Bailin PL, Kantor OR et al. Treatment of adenoma sebaceum with carbon dioxide laser vaporization. J Dermatol Surg Oncol 1985;13:149.

COMBINATION TREATMENT (Nicholas J Lowe)

Indications	Potential combination treatments	Chapter reference
Photodamage	Photoprotection	2
Solar elastosis	Topical therapy	3
Dyspigmentation	Depigmentary agents	8
Periorbital rhytides	Botox	13–15
Perioral rhytides	Botox fillers and fillers	13–19
Benign skin lesions	Topical therapy	3

12. Non-ablative lasers for skin rejuvenation

Teresa T Soriano, Paul S Yamauchi and Gary P Lask

INTRODUCTION

Various techniques have been used for the improvement of cutaneous changes seen with photoaging. These include dermabrasion, chemical peels, and lasers. They attain varying degrees of clinical improvement of rhytides, dyschromia, and textural irregularities. For optimal results, laser choices for attenuation of rhytides have been limited to the CO_2 and Er:YAG lasers. These systems ablate the epidermis leading to a protracted recovery period. Prior to re-epithelialization, the initial phase of postoperative healing can be associated with significant morbidity, including serous discharge, erythema, bleeding, pain, and infection. In addition, treatments can result in complications, including hypopigmentation, hyperpigmentation, persistent erythema, and scarring.[1–9] Non-ablative laser and light sources have recently been introduced as an alternative modality for skin rejuvenation.

BACKGROUND

The mechanisms underlying the clinical improvement seen with traditional treatments are not well understood. Photoaging from repeated sun exposure has been characterized by reduced amounts of type I collagen and decorin, and by increased amounts of elastin, fibrillin and versican.[10,11] Members of the matrix metalloproteinase family have been suggested to play a role in the degradation of dermal collagen seen in photoaged skin.[12] Topical applications of tretinoin and alpha-hydroxy acids lead to increased papillary dermal collagen and diminished rhytides.[13] Increased deposition of new collagen has been reported following CO_2 laser resurfacing, dermabrasion, and chemical peels.[14–17] It has been suggested that tissue ablation, leading to collagen shrinkage and new collagen deposition contributes to the clinical results after traditional laser resurfacing.[18–20] In addition, changes in long-term wound healing and associated dermal remodeling are likely to play a role in sustained improvement. Dermal wounding and new collagen deposition have been observed after use of non-ablative laser devices. Several non-ablative systems have become available and these will be discussed in this chapter.

THE 1064 NM Q-SWITCHED ND:YAG LASER

The 1064 nm Q-switched neodymium:yttrium–aluminum–garnet (QS Nd:YAG laser was used in one of the earliest clinical investigations in non-ablative rejuvenation. This laser has been widely used in cosmetic dermatology for several years for the removal of tattoos and other unwanted pigmented lesions. Using the 1064 nm wavelength, greater light penetration to the required depth for collagen remodeling is permitted. In addition, its short nanosecond pulse duration limits tissue destruction from heat diffusion.

Following initial reports of improvement of facial rhytides and acne scars using the QS Nd:YAG laser with ablative parameters,[21] Goldberg and Whitworth[22] investigated the use of a QS Nd:YAG laser in the ablative mode for improvement of perioral and periorbital class I and II rhytides. Eleven patients with skin types I or II received unilateral QS Nd:YAG treatments at 5 J/cm^2 and 3 mm spot size. The contralateral side was treated with char-free CO_2 resurfacing. Complete re-epithelialization occurred 6–9 days after CO_2 resurfacing, whereas QS Nd:YAG treatment required 3–5 days. Patients were evaluated 3 months after treatment. All CO_2-treated sites showed clinical improvement. Nine of the 11 QS Nd:YAG treated areas displayed some improvement: three of these nine areas showed improvements thought to be comparable with those seen after CO_2 resurfacing; the remaining six patients exhibited improvement but this was not to the degree as that seen with CO_2 resurfacing. Prolonged erythema was seen in all CO_2-treated areas; however, only three of the 11 QS Nd:YAG treated sites had erythema at 1 month after treatment. Of note, these same three patients experienced clinical improvement of their rhytides comparable to that seen in CO_2-treated areas. At 3 months after treatment, all erythema was resolved. Although the QS Nd:YAG laser did not uniformly attain the improvement seen with CO_2 resurfacing, this pilot study showed that the QS Nd:YAG laser may minimize facial rhytides with faster healing times and fewer adverse effects.

Goldberg and Metzler[23] followed with a larger study using a QS Nd:YAG laser in a non-ablative mode. They used a low energy fluence QS Nd:YAG laser potentiated by the use of a topical C-assisted solution. They treated 242 sites on 61 patients with the following parameters: energy fluence of 2.5 J/cm^2, pulse duration of 6–20 ns, and a spot size of 7 mm. These sites were evaluated at 32 weeks for skin texture, skin elasticity, and rhytid reduction. Unlike the previous study, epidermal ablation was not seen in any of the treated sites when low energy fluences were used. In addition, the main adverse effects were limited to mild and transient erythema. The authors reported improvement in all clinical parameters at 8 months after treatment. This early study suggests that the QS Nd:YAG laser may be a safe and effective system for non-ablative skin rejuvenation.

Another small study further investigated the efficacy and safety of multiple QS Nd:YAG laser treatments as a non-ablative modality in the treatment of facial rhytides.[24] The authors treated eight patients with Fitzpatrick skin types II–IV at 3-month intervals with a QS Nd:YAG laser. Parameters of the treatment included two passes with energy fluences of 7 J/cm^2 and a spot size of 3 mm. The investigators sought petechiae as the typical visible end-point. At 3 months after the last treatment, six of the eight patients were noted to show clinical improvement. The majority of patients reported no pain 1 day after the treatment. Erythema, purpura, and pigmentary alterations were not observed at 1 month after each treatment and 3 months after the last treatment. This study supports the potential of using the QS Nd:YAG laser for non-ablative rejuvenation. However, the post-treatment petechiae seen may be unacceptable in some patients; thus, further studies are needed to determine optimal treatment parameters to achieve cosmetic improvement with minimal adverse effects.

THE 1320 NM LONG-PULSED ND:YAG LASER

The 1320 nm long-pulsed Nd:YAG laser is a non-ablative laser that has been used for facial rejuvenation. It has a pulsed waveform composed of three 300 μs duration pulses delivered at a 100 Hz pulse repetition frequency; thus yielding a 20 ms duration macropulse containing three micropulses. It has energy fluences ranging from 25 to 35 J/cm^2. This laser allows penetration of 100–500 μm depth into dermal tissue. The current handpiece carries the laser beam of a 5 mm diameter spot size, a dynamic cooling system and a thermal-feedback sensor. In order to protect the epidermis, the dynamic cooling system releases a cryogen spray to the epidermis immediately prior to the pulsed laser exposure, i.e. by tens of milliseconds. Animal studies have shown that short cryogen bursts did not offer enough epidermal protection at higher energy fluences and longer spray times led to a cryogen burn on the skin.[25] Optional cryogen spray times have been determined to avoid epidermal disruption while allowing dermal heating with the production of procollagen I. The thermal sensor aids the use in adjusting the energy fluence to maintain ideal therapeutic temperatures for thermal injury to the dermis and

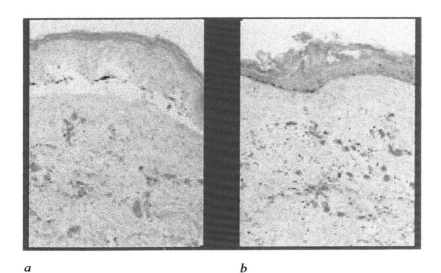

Figure 12.1 CoolTouch laser treatment: (A) without cryogen; (B) with cryogen.

a   b

protection of the epidermis. Ideal epidermal temperatures have been determined to be between 40 and 60°C, corresponding to dermal heating c. 25°C higher in the dermis.

Kelly et al.[26] investigated the use of the 1320 nm Nd:YAG laser for improvement of periorbital rhytides.

Thirty-five patients received three bilateral treatments at 2-week intervals. All patients received EMLA applied 1 hour prior to the procedure. Pre- and post-treatment photographs were evaluated. The authors reported the following results: no improvement in patients with mild rhytides, mild improvement in those

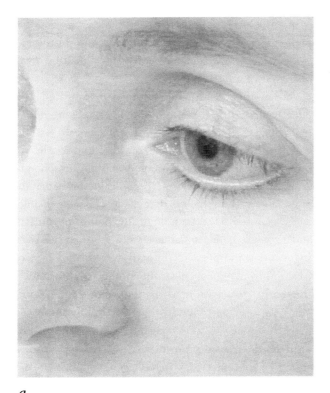

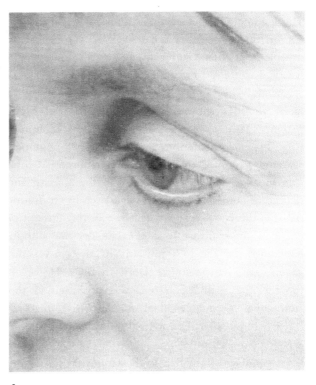

a   b

Figure 12.2 Periorbital area: (A) before treatment; (B) after three CoolTouch laser treatments. (Courtesy of Robert Weiss MD.)

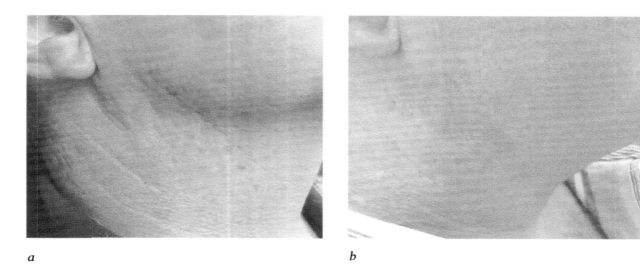

a   *b*

Figure 12.3 *Neck acne: (A) before treatment; (B) after CoolTouch laser treatment. (Courtesy of Robert Weiss MD.)*

with moderate rhytides, and significant improvement in those with severe rhytides. Patients developed transient post-treatment erythema. Four sites developed blisters, with two sites resulting in pinpoint scars. The etiology of blistering is unclear; however, the authors suggest that failure to release cryogen spray capable of providing sufficient epidermal cooling could have led to this adverse effect.

A study by Menaker et al.[27] on 10 patients with facial rhytides showed improvement in only four patients. Three patients experienced postinflammatory hyperpigmentation, and three had pinpoint scarring 3 months after treatment. In three patients, skin biopsies showed an increase in the amount and degree of homogenization of dermal collagen. In one patient, there was a slight decrease in the amount of collagen. In contrast to other studies, the authors concluded that the 1320 nm Nd:YAG system was not an effective treatment for facial rhytides. However, the thermal-feedback system was not used in this study, which could explain the adverse effects in some patients, and the minimal improvement seen in others.

A number of smaller studies followed, using the 1320 nm Nd:YAG laser for collagen remodeling. Goldberg[28] treated class I–II rhytides on 10 patients with sessions every 4 months using the 1320 nm Nd:YAG laser.[28] Laser pulsing was delivered 40 ms after a dynamic cryogen cooling was applied to the epidermis for 30 ms. Peak epidermal temperatures ranged from 40 to 48°C. Eight of the 10 patients showed improvement and there were no blisters. At 6 months after treatment no erythema, scarring or pigmentary alterations were noted, and histologic evidence of new dermal collagen formation was observed in all 10 subjects.

In another study, the authors investigated the effectiveness of the 1320 nm Nd:YAG laser in inducing collagen tightening and neocollagenesis.[29] They treated three to four areas on the inner arm or buttock of 10 subjects. No epidermal disruption was seen either clinically or microscopically. Immediately after laser treatment, no detectable collagen shrinkage was noted. Histopathologically, plump fibroblasts and a zone of collagen damage were seen. The authors suggest that the presence of activated fibroblasts may have led to neocollagenesis. In another study, Alster[30] treated patients with mild rhytides with the 1320 nm Nd:YAG laser and found progressive, slow improvement over a 26-week period. Side-effects were limited to transient erythema. Histologic studies showed slight increases in collagen contents at the end of the study. Other investigations have led to reports of some improvement of striae distensae[31] and acne scars[32] with the use of the 1320 nm Nd:YAG laser. These studies support the consistent safety and

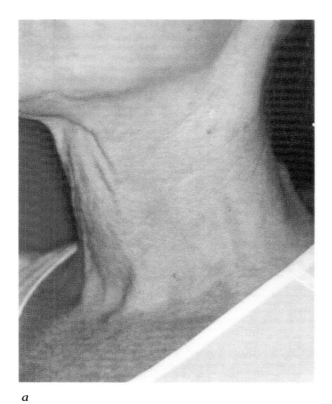
a

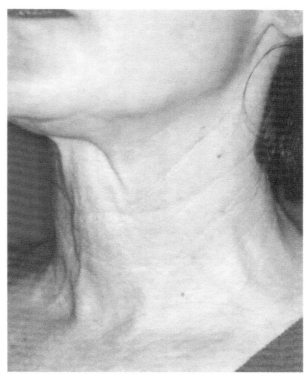
b

Figure 12.4 *Neck area: (A) before treatment; (B) after three CoolTouch laser treatments. (Courtesy of Robert Weiss MD.)*

some efficacy of this laser with dynamic cooling for dermal remodeling.

A recent study evaluated the 132Q nm Nd:YAG laser for full-face rejuvenation:[33] patients were treated using energy fluences below the threshold of pain. The patients received an average of 28 treatments, twice a week, for 3 months. The author reported modest improvements compared with traditional ablative resurfacing. Seventeen patients displayed increased skin turgor and 14 patients showed improvement of rhytides. Skin biopsies from five patients were taken before treatment and 6 months after the last treatment. Post-treatment biopsies showed more homogenous and eosinophilic collagen, and increased dermal thickness. This study demonstrated the use of the 1320 nm Nd:YAG laser for full-face rejuvenation without the need for anesthesia or convalescence. The number and frequency of treatments may be disadvantages of this protocol; however, this may be balanced by the absence of pain and morbidity experienced by the patients.

Table 12.1 *CoolTouch laser*

- Parameters
    25–32 J/cm^2
    Cooling: 20–30 and 30–40 ms
    Pattern-adjacent spots
    Passes
- Adjunctive treatment
    May be effective for longer
    Corrects more effectively

Table 12.2 *Dynamic cooling properties of the CoolTouch laser*

- Precisely pulsed cryogen spray (20–40 ms)
- Reduces surface temperature, protecting epidermis from damage
- Permits light to effectively target collagen
- Reduces patient discomfort
- Patented technique available only through Laser Aesthetics

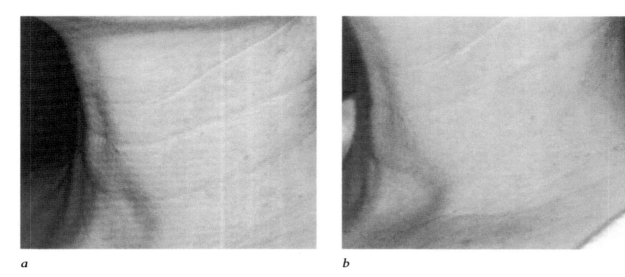

a　　　　　　　　　　　　　　　　　　　　　　*b*

Figure 12.5 *Neck area: (A) before treatment; (B) after three CoolTouch laser treatments. (Courtesy of Robert Weiss MD.)*

Table 12.3 *Newer non-ablative laser systems*

• Vascular chromophores	Sclerolaser
	N-lite
• Pigment chromophores	Ruby
	Alex
Others:	
• Epilight	Nd:YAG

PULSED DYE LASERS

Pulsed dye lasers (PDL) emit yellow light at wavelengths of 577–600 nm, i.e. well absorbed by hemoglobin. The systems having a pulse duration of 450 μs to 1.5 ms have been used for several years to treat vascular lesions by providing enough energy and short pulse durations to specifically target blood vessels with minimal damage to the epidermis and surrounding tissue. At 577 nm, light penetrates to a depth of 0.5 mm but increasing the wavelength to 585 or 595 nm allows a greater depth of penetration. POL have a low incidence of scarring; however, depending on the parameters used, this technique can produce cosmetically unacceptable purpura. Newer PDL systems have been developed with longer pulse durations that may possibly decrease the incidence of post-treatment purpura. Potential benefits of PDL for skin rejuvenation stemmed from reports of dermal collagen remodeling after treatment of striae, hypertrophic scars and keloids.[34–36]

Following reports of improvement of acne scars[37] and mild rhytides[38] with PDL, Zelickson et al.[39] treated facial rhytides on 20 patients using this method. Side-effects, including purpura and edema lasting 1–2 weeks, were universal; two patients had postinflammatory hyperpigmentation. Half of the patients – 90% of patients with mild to moderate wrinkling and 40% of patients with moderate to severe wrinkling – demonstrated clinical improvements 6 months after treatment. Histopathological examination of treated areas showed a band of well-organized elastin and collagen fibers in the superficial dermis, as well as increased cellularity and mucin deposition.

Zelickson and Kist[40] further investigated the concept of collagen remodeling after PDL treatment. Seven patients received one PDL treatment to an area of photodamage and biopsies were taken 6 weeks later. Increases in the following dermal proteins were observed: procollagen and collagen I in 71.4% of samples; collagen III, collagenase, and elastin in 85.7% of samples; and hyaluronate receptor in 57.1% of samples. These results suggest a process of dermal remodeling that translates into the clinical improvement of rhytides seen after PDL treatment.

Bjerring et al. studied the use of another pulsed dye laser (N-Lite™, SLS Ltd, Llanelli, Wales, UK) for non-ablative skin rejuvenation.[41] Thirty subjects with

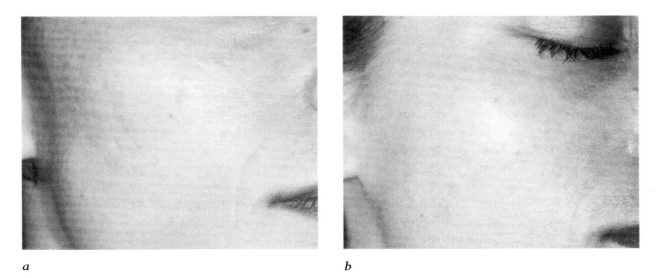

a   b

Figure 12.6 *An example of CoolTouch laser for mild facial scarring. (A) before and (B) after 4 treatment sessions, 6 weeks apart. Thermal probe reading 41 to 43° C each treatment.*

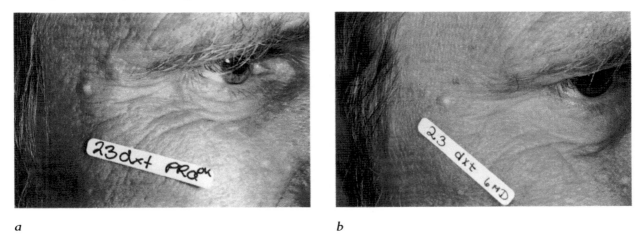

a   b

Figure 12.7 *Periorbital area of 58-year-old male: (A) before treatment; (B) 6 months after single laser treatment. (Courtesy of Bjerring et al.[41])*

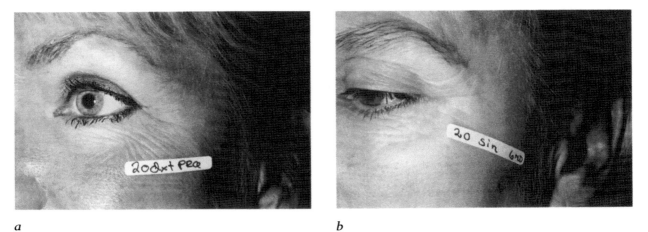

a   b

Figure 12.8 *Periorbital area of a 44-year-old female: (A) before treatment; (B) 6 months after single laser treatment. (Courtesy of Bjerring et al.[41])*

periorbital rhytides received one laser session with the following parameters: wavelength of 585 nm, pulse duration of 350 µs, energy fluence of 2.4 J/cm^2 and a spot size of 5 mm. Patients had minimal intraoperative discomfort; there was no post-operative pain, purpura or pigmentary change. The authors reported clinical improvement in all patients. In addition, in 10 other subjects, forearm areas were treated using the above parameters: one area received one pass, another received two passes, and a third served as the control. Suction blisters were raised 72 hours after laser treatment. The fluid was analyzed to determine the concentration of aminoterminal propeptide of type III procollagen (PIIINP). A significant increase in PIIINP at the sites receiving a single pass of treatment was seen; however, no significant difference was observed between the control and double-treated sites. The authors suggest that the lower increase in procollagen production at the double-treated sites may indicate that the additional energy dosage has a negative effect. They further postulate that this may be the reason why cosmetic improvement of rhytides has not been reported with PDL treatments of vascular lesions, as these lesions are usually treated at higher energy fluences compared with those used in their trial. In addition, the authors hypothesize that interaction with the vasculature, not just direct thermal injury to dermal collagen, may contribute to the mechanism of dermal remodeling. They suggest that PDL light is absorbed in the blood vessels at intensities too low to cause vessel rupture, but sufficient to induce the release of inflammatory mediators by endothelial cells. These mediators stimulate fibroblast activity to promote dermal remodeling. Further investigationis required to confirm this concept and to elucidate the underlying mechanism of dermal remodeling following PDL treatment.

INTENSE PULSED LIGHT SYSTEMS

Intense pulsed light (IPL) systems employ a non-laser light source that has reported uses in removing pigmented and vascular lesions, and unwanted hair.[42,43] It emits a non-collimated, non-coherent light at wavelengths of 550–1200 nm. The device has various filters that are chosen to selectively block shorter wavelengths. In addition, it can deliver various pulse durations over single, double or triple micropulses with variable delay times. IPL systems have been reported to improve diffuse facial erythema seen with rosacea and systemic lupus erythematosus, and pigment irregularities resulting from photodamage.[44,45] The shorter wavelengths from this device have been shown to improve vascular and epidermal pigmented lesions. The longer wavelengths are probably necessary for skin rejuvenation. IPL systems have been investigated for non-ablative treatment of isolated cosmetic units as well as full-face rejuvenation.

Bitter and Goldman[46] reported the use of an IPL system in improving the cutaneous changes associated with photoaging. In one study, 30 patients received five full-face IPL treatments at 3-week intervals. The investigators aimed to use subpurpuric parameters as follows: a 550 nm filter, energy fluences of 30–36 J.cm^2, and double 2.4–4.0 ms pulses. Transient erythema lasting for only a few hours was observed. Less than 2% of patients were reported to have purpura or swelling, requiring a 1–3 day recovery period; no scarring was reported. Clinical results from patient questionnaires revealed some subjective improvement: 49% of patients reported ≥ 75% overall improvement in the appearance of their skin; 73% reported ≥ 25% improvement of fine wrinkles; 36% reported ≥50% improvement of fine wrinkles. In addition, patients noted improvement of skin smoothness, pore size, and erythema. This early observation demonstrates the potential use of lPL systems for non-ablative rejuvenation with minimal to no patient downtime.

In another study, Goldberg and Cutler[47] reported mild to moderate improvement of some rhytides without epidermal ablation using an IPL system. The investigators treated 30 subjects with skin types I and II and class I–Il facial rhytides. One to four treatments were performed at 2-week intervals over a 10-week period. Parameters included a cut-off filter of 645 nm, and energy fluences of 40–50 J/cm^2 delivered over triple pulses of 7 ms with a 50 ms interpulse delay. At 6 months, nine of 25 patients showed substantial improvement of their rhytides. The authors reported that 25 subjects showed some improvement in skin quality and facial rhytides. All patients experienced transient post-treatment erythema; no erythema, pigmentary changes, or scarring was seen at 6 months after treatment.

Goldberg[48] followed this investigation with another study to evaluate the histological changes seen after multiple IPL treatments. Facial rhytides of four patients with skin types I and II were treated over a 10-week period using a filter of 645 nm and energy fluences of 40–50 J/cm² with triple 7 ms pulses and a 50 ms delay. Pretreatment skin biopsies showed solar elastosis. Skin biopsies taken 6 months after the last treatment demonstrated some degree of superficial papillary dermal fibrosis with an increased number of fibroblasts scattered in the dermis. The author concluded that the IPL system is the first non-laser light source to display clinical and histological evidence of new collagen formation.

Zelickson and Kist[40] examined the effects of PDL on dermal remodeling with the effects of IPL on various dermal proteins. Periorbital sun-damaged sites on two patients were treated with a single session of IPL. Skin biopsies at 6 weeks displayed increased amounts of collagen type I and III, elastin, procollagen, and hyaluronate receptor. One of the two specimens also showed an increase in collagenase. This study suggests a process of dermal repair and production of extracellular matrix proteins underlying the clinical reduction of rhytides seen after IPL treatments.

OTHER SYSTEMS

Muccini et al.[49] tested the effectiveness of a 980 nm diode laser in treating photoaging.[94] They noted epidermal preservation with tissue shrinkage equivalent to multiple passes of a CO_2 laser. A biopsy 3 weeks later revealed new collagen deposition and an abundance of young elastin fibers.

Ross et al.[50] investigated using an infrared laser coupled with a sapphire-surface cooling device as a non-ablative resurfacing system. The postauricular areas of nine patients were treated using various parameters. Histological examination showed epidermal preservation and zones of fibroplasia from 500 to 150 μm deep in the dermis. The authors concluded that this system is capable of selective dermal heating with new collagen deposition. However, suboptimal cosmetic benefit was seen at certain treatment parameters, possibly due to the depth of dermal damage. The authors suggested more superficial dermal zones (100–400 μm) of heating should be targeted to attain clinical improvement.

Finally, other systems have been shown to induce collagen remodeling in animal studies. Kelley et al.[51] demonstrated the use of the Er:YAG laser in non-ablative rejuvenation. They administered multiple laser pulses with subablative energy fluences and cryogen spray cooling to Sprague–Dawley rats, and evaluated histological sections of skin for epidermal injury and dermal remodeling. Examination performed 1 hour after treatment revealed minimal damage to the epidermis and dermal coagulation to a depth of > 100 μm. Biopsies at 4 and 8 weeks after treatment showed hypercellularity and compact collagen. Mordon et al.[52] evaluated a 1540 nm glass YAG laser with contact cooling on hairless rats using variable energy fluences and cooling temperatures. They found clinical improvements that were both energy fluence and temperature cooling dependent and also noted new collagen synthesis marked by fibroblastic proliferation.

CONCLUSIONS

Traditional ablative resurfacing has been shown to be effective in improving photoaged skin. These methods often require a protracted recovery period that can be accompanied by significant morbidity. In addition, they can lead to long-term adverse effects, including erythema, pigmentary changes, and scarring. Non-ablative dermal remodeling techniques have recently been developed to induce dermal damage without epidermal disruption. This can be achieved when the following requirements are met. First, the laser wavelength and radiant exposure must be sufficient to create selective dermal wounding or induce the production of inflammatory mediators that, in turn, promote collagen remodeling. Second, the epidermis must be protected from thermal damage. Further studies of optimal treatment parameters, as well as refinement of technology, are needed to attain significant efficacy and consistency with the non-ablative systems. In addition, the mechanisms underlying the clinical improvement observed after non-ablative laser rejuvenation require further investigation. In summary, nonablative laser and light sources have become available as alternatives in rejuvenating photodamaged skin. Although clinical results may be modest compared to traditional resurfacing lasers, these non-ablative systems offer minimal adverse sequelae and, in general, no recovery time when compared with ablative lasers.

References

1   Waldorf WA, Kauvar ANB, Geronemus RG. Skin resurfacing of fine to deep rhytides using a char-free carbon dioxide laser in 47 patients. Dermatol Surg 1995;21:940–6.

2   Lowe NJ, Lask G, Griffin ME. Laser skin resurfacing: pre- and post treatment guidelines. Dermatol Surg 1995;21:1017–19.

3   Lask G, Keller G, Lowe N, Gormley D. Laser skin resurfacing with the Silk Touch flashscanner for facial rhytides. Dermatol Surg 1995;221:1021–4.

4   Lowe NJ, Lask G, Griffin ME, et al. Skin resurfacing with the Ultrapulse carbon dioxide laser: observation on 100 patients. Dermatol Surg 1995;21:1025–9.

5   Ho C, Nguyen Q, Lowe NJ, et al. Laser resurfacing in pigmented skin. Dermatol Surg 1995;21:1035–7.

6   Hruza GJ. Laser skin resurfacing. Arch Dermatol 1996;132:451–5.

7   Fitzpatrick RE Goldman MP, Satur NM, Tope WD. Pulsed carbon dioxide laser resurfacing of photodamaged facial skin. Arch Dermatol 1996;132:395–402.

8   Fitzpatrick RE. Laser resurfacing of rhytides (review). Dermatol Clin 1997;15:431–47.

9   Nanni CA, Alster TS. Complications of carbon dioxide laser resurfacing: an evaluation of 500 patients. Dermatol Surg 1998;24:315–20.

10 Bernstein EF, Chen YQ, Tamai K, et al. Enhanced elastin and fibrillin gene expression in chronically photodamaged skin. J Invest Dermatol 1994;103:182–6.

11 Bernstein EF, Chen YQ, Kopp JB, et al. Long-term sun exposure alters the collagen of the papillary dermis. Comparison of sun-protected and photoaged skin by Northern analysis, immunohistochemical staining, and confocal laser scanning microscopy. J Am Acad Dermatol 1996;34:209–18

12 Fisher GJ, Wang ZQ, Datta SC, et al. Pathophysiology of premature skin aging induced by ultraviolet light. N Engl J Med 1997;337:1419–28.

13 Griffith CEM, Russman AN, Majmudar G, et al. Restoration of collagen formation in photoaged human skin by tretinoin (retinoic acid). N Engl J Med 1993;329:530

14 Ditre CM, Griffin TD, Murphy GF, et al. Effects of alpha-hydroxy acids on photoaged skin: a pilot clinical, histologic, and ultrastructural study. J Am Acad Dermatol 1996;34:187–95.

15 Nelson BR, Metz RD, Majmudar G, et al. A comparison of wire brush and diamond friase superficial dermabrasion for photoaged skin: a clinical, immunology, and biochemical study. J Am Acad Dermatol 1996;34:235–43.

16 Nelson BR, Fader DJ, Gillard M, et al, Pilot histologic and ultrastructural study of the effects of medium-depth chemical facial peels on dermal collagen in patients with actinically damaged skin. J Am Acad Dermatol 1996;32:472–8.

17 Fitzpatrick RE, Tope WD, Goldman MP, Satur NM. Pulsed carbon dioxide laser, trichloroacetic acid, Baker-Gordon phenol, and dermabrasion: a comparative clinical and histologic study of cutaneous resurfacing in a porcine model. Arch Dermatol 1996;132:468–71.

18 Cotton J, Hood AF, Gonin RM, et al. Histologic evaluation of preauricular and postauricular human skin after high energy, short-pulse dioxide laser. Arch Dermatol 1996;132:425–8.

19 Ross EV, Naseef G, Skrobal M, et al. In vivo dermal collagen shrinkage and remodeling following CO_2 laser resurfacing. Lasers Surg Med 1996;18:38.

20 Ross EV, Yashar 55, Naseef GS, et al. A pilot study of in vivo immediate tissue contraction with CO_2 skin laser resurfacing in a live farm pig. Dermatol Surg 1999;25:852–6.

21 Cisneros JL, Rio R, Palou, J. The Q-switched Nd:Yag laser with quadruple frequency. Clinical histological evaluation of facial resurfacing using different wavelengths. Dermatol Surg 1998;24:345–50.

22 Goldberg DJ, Whitworth J. Laser resurfacing with the Q-switched Nd:Yag laser. Dermatol Surg 1997;23:903–7.

23 Goldberg D, Metzler C. Skin resurfacing utilizing a low-fluence Nd:Yag laser. J Cutan Laser Ther 1999;1:23–7.

24 Goldberg DJ, Silapunt S. Q-switched Nd:Yag laser: rhytid improvement by non-ablative remodeling. J Cutan Laser Ther 2000; in press.

25 Lask G, Lee P, Seyfzadeh M, et al. Nonablative laser treatment of facial rhytides. SPIE Proc 1997;2970:338–49.

26 Kelly KM, Nelson JS, Lask GP, et al. Cryogen spray cooling in combination with nonablative laser treatment of facial rhytides. Arch Dermatol 1999;135:691–4.

27 Menaker GM, Wrone DA, Williams RM, Moy RL. Treatment of facial rhytides with a nonablative laser: a clinical and histologic study. Dermatol Surg 1999;25:440–4.

28 Goldberg, DJ. Non-ablative subsurface remodeling: clinical and histologic evaluation of a 1320 nm Nd:Yag laser. J Cutan Laser Ther 1999;1:153–7.

29 Sriprachya-Anunt S, Fitzpatrick RE, Goldman MP. The effect of 1320 nm Nd:Yag laser with dynamic cooling on human skin. Lasers Surg Med 1999;Suppl 11:25.

30 Alster TS. Nonablative cutaneous laser resurfacing: clinical and histologic Is analysis. Lasers Surg Med 1999;Suppl 11:25.

31 Bernstein LJ, Quintana A, Grossman MC, et al. Treatment of striae distensae with a 1320 nm Nd:Yag laser. Lasers Surg Med 1999;Suppl 11:29–30.

32 Weiss RA, Weiss MA, Nestor MS, Turner MS. Nonablative dynamic cryogen spray cooled laser treatment of facial acne scars. Laser Surg Med 2000;Suppl 12:63.

33 Ruiz-Esparza J. Painless nonablative treatment of photoaging with the 1320 nm Nd:Yag laser. Lasers Surg Med 2000;Suppl 11:25.

34 McDaniel DH, Ash K, Zukowski M. Treatment of stretch marks with the 585 nm flashlamp-pumped pulsed dye laser. Dermatol Surg 1994;32:332–7.

35 Alster TS. Treatment of keloid sternotomy scars with 585 nm flashlamp-pumped pulsed dye laser. Lancet 1995;345:1198–200.

36 Alster TS. Improvement of erythematous and hypertrophic scars by the 585 nm flashlamp-pulsed dye laser. Ann Plast Surg, 1994;32:186–90.

37 Alster TS, McMeekin TO. Improvement of facial acne scars by the 585 nm flashlamp-pumped pulsed dye laser. J Am Acad Dermatol 1996;35:79–81.

38 Kilmer SL, Chotzen VA. Pulsed dye laser treatment of rhytids. Lasers Surg Med 1997;Suppl 9:44.

39 Zelickson BD, Kilmer SI, Bernstein E, et al. Pulsed dye laser therapy for sun damaged skin. Lasers Surg Med 1999;25:229–36.

40 Zelickson BD, Kist D. Effect of pulsed dye laser and intense pulsed light source on the dermal extracellular matrix remodeling. Lasers Surg Med 2000;Suppl 12:17.

41 Bjerring P, Clement M, Heickendorff, et al. Selective nonablative wrinkle reduction by laser. J Cutan Laser Ther 2000;2:9–15.

42 Raulin C, Werner S, Hartschuh W, Schonermark MP. Effective treatment of hypertrichosis with pulsed light: a report of two cases. Ann Plast Surg 1997;39:169–73.

43 Raulin C, Goldman MP, Weiss MA, Weiss RA. Treatment of adult port-wine stains using intense pulsed light therapy (PhotoDerm CL): brief initial clinical report. Dermatol Surg 1997;23:594–7.

44 Bitter PJ. Noninvasive rejuvenation of photoaged skin using serial, full-face intense pulsed light treatments. Dermatol Surg 2000;26:835–43.

45 Levy JL. Intense pulsed light treatment for chronic facial erythema of systemic lupus erythematosus: a case report. J Cutan Laser Ther 2000; in press.

46 Bitter P, Goldman M. Nonablative skin rejuvenation using intense pulsed light. Lasers Surg Med 2000;Suppl 12:16.

47 Goldberg DJ, Cutler KB. Non-ablative treatment of rhytides with intense pulsed light. Lasers Surg Med 2000;26:196–200.

48 Goldberg DJ. New collagen formation after dermal remodeling with an intense pulsed light source. J Cutan Laser Ther 2000;2:59–61.

49 Muccini JA Jr, O'Donnell FE Jr, Fuller T, Reinisch L. Laser treatment of solar elastosis with epidermal preservation. Lasers Surg Med 1997;23:121–7.

50 Ross EV, Sajben FP, McKinley JR, et al. Non-ablative skin remodeling: selective dermal heating using an IR laser with surface cooling. Lasers Surg Med 1999;Suppl 11:25–6.

51 Kelley KM, Majaron B, Verkruysse W, Nelson JS. Histologic evaluation of post nonablative resurfacing with the Er:Yag laser in combination with cryogen spray cooling. Lasers Surg Med 2000;Suppl 12:16.

52 Mordon S, Capon A, Levy JL, et al. Nonablative skin remodeling using a 1540 nm laser with contact cooling. Lasers Surg Med. 2000; Suppl 12:18.

COMBINATION TREATMENT (Nicholas J Lowe)

Indications	Potential combination treatments	Chapter reference
Skin laxity	Photoprotection	1
Fine lines	Topical therapy	2,3
	Chemical peels	6,7
Periocular	BTX-A microdermabrasion	8
Perioral	BTX-A following laser resurfacing	10,11
	Dermal fillers	16–18
Neck lines	BTX-A	13–15

13. Botulinum toxin-A development and use for upper facial lines

Jean Carruthers and Alastair Carruthers

INTRODUCTION

The use of botulinum toxin A (BTX-A) for aesthetic purposes began in the glabella where the aesthetic determinant is persistent muscular activity. In the brow, deep glabellar lines and folds are etched by the intellectual characteristics of focus, intensity and determination, yet are perceived by the public at large as the body language for anger, frustration and decompensation. This is particularly true for female subjects. BTX-A gives a safe, effective and localized chemodenervation of the underlying expressive brow musculature and results in an almost immediate softening and relaxation of the folds in question, in both static and dynamic phases of brow activity. The enormous patient acceptance of the glabellar BTX-A effects has led to its use in other upper facial areas such as lateral orbital lines (crow's-feet), horizontal forehead lines, and chemo-brow lift.[1] Cosmetic BTX-A injection is now the second most commonly performed cosmetic procedure in North America.[2]

BTX-A FUNCTION

Botulinum toxin (BTX-A, and also BTX and BoNT-A), manufactured under the trade name Botox® (Allergan Inc, Irvine, CA) is the most powerful neurotoxin known to humans.[3] When initially viewed, it may therefore seem surprising that, in controlled clinical dosing regimen, it has become the most welcome addition to the pharmacologic armamentarium to reduce activity at targeted neuro-muscular junctions. BTX-A blocks the exocytosis of acetyl choline from the presynaptic neurone after it first binds to the neurone membrane. The intracellular effect of the short chain is on oligopeptides necessary for the docking of intracellular acetyl choline vesicles to the neuronal cell membrane prior to their ejection into the myoneural cleft. As the process is enzymatic, even a few molecules will produce this effect and the nanogram-sized doses used provide both clinical safety and efficacy.[4]

The primary effect is one of controlled muscular relaxation that lasts for several months, until existing synapses reactivate or are newly formed.[5]

METHOD OF DILUTION AND INJECTION

Techniques in different clinical settings may vary. The present authors will now describe their own technique and encourage other injecting physicians to find the technique that is most comfortable for them in their own settings.

A dilution of 1 cm³ of sterile saline, without preservative, is used per 100 unit (U) vial of BTX-A. Dilution is performed using 1 cm³ Becton Dickinson tuberculin syringes and an 18–20 gauge needle; a simple hand-held bottle opener is used to remove the metal sleeve from the vial and the grey rubber plug comes out easily with finger manipulation. A 0.3 cm³ Beckton Dickinson 7 mm 30 gauge diabetic syringe/needle is then used to draw up up to 0.3 cm³ (30 U) of BTX-A, taking care to avoid touching the side of the vial and blunting the needle. As many units as are needed for the injection session are drawn up in multiple syringes, planning four to six needle punctures for each since the needle blunts easily.

This technique gives the least volume effect with the greatest accuracy of injection. Most individuals respond within 1–5 days after injection, although in some cases 2 weeks are needed for the full effect to be apparent. IgG neutralizing antibodies have not yet been reported in individuals receiving < 100 U BTX-A per treatment session or in those treated only with current BTX-A.[5]

GLABELLAR FURROWS

The glabella is the most common site for cosmetic injection. The body language 'reading' of glabellar furrows differs in women and men. In men, small to moderate furrows are evidence of an ability to focus, to lead and to be compassionate – all positive attributes. Very deep and long glabellar furrows in men imply failure to cope and to show mastery, the same way even small furrows remove positive projection from the female glabella. Female subjects with glabellar folds are interpreted as having lost inner equanimity and coping skills, to be angry, bitter or chronically disappointed.

The four depressor muscles in the glabella include: (1) corrugator supercilii; (2) orbicularis oculi; (3) procerus; and (4) depressor supercilii. Procerus is injected first because this is the least painful injection site and also one which can be massaged, which immediately gets rid of the discomfort produced by the BTX-A injection. The procerus injection site is just above the imaginary 'X' lines linking the medial brow with the contralateral medial canthus. Typically, 5–10 U of BTX-A are injected at this site (20% of the total glabella dose).

The surface anatomy for the medial corrugator injection is on a line drawn vertically through the medial canthus, intersecting the superior bony orbital margin. Four to 8 U are injected at this site and an additional 3–4 U of BTX-A superior to the first injection point (Figure 13.1), the two injections being 25–30% of the total glabella dose. These sites are not massaged.

The lateral corrugator injection is sited 1 cm above the brow in the mid-pupillary line. Three to

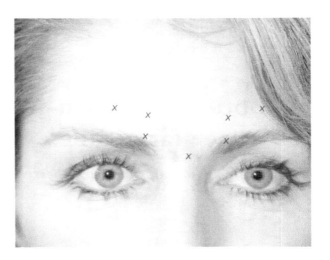

Figure 13.1 *Cutaneous landmarks of the authors' glabellar injection technique.*

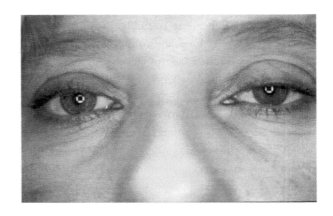

Figure 13.2 *Left upper eyelid ptosis 2 weeks after BTX-A injection.*

5 U of BTX-A are injected (10–15% of the total doses); the site is not massaged in order to avoid channeling BTX-A down through the supraorbital notch (producing eyelid ptosis (Figure 13.2)) or up into frontalis (producing brow ptosis).

A recent multicenter placebo-controlled trial of the treatment of the glabellar area used a uniform dose of 20 U of BTX-A in both women and men in five injection sites somewhat similar to the technique described above.[6] More than 80% of subjects were rated as 'none' or 'mild' at 7–30 days, although all were 'moderate' or 'severe' at the pretreatment visit. A

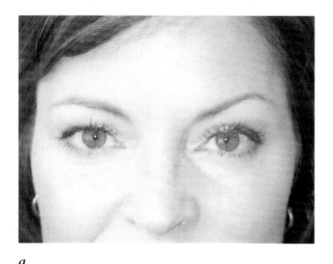

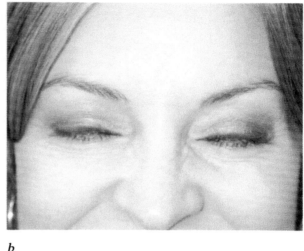

a   *b*

Figure 13.3 *Improved eyebrow symmetry [(A) is pre-treatment, (B) is post treatment] 2 weeks after BTX-A injection.*

similar percentage response was seen in the evaluations at rest, although this was slower in onset, peaking at 30 days instead of 7 days. Interestingly, although the response on maximum frown had declined to 26% at 4 months (probably as a result of low dose), the response at rest hardly declined at all. This finding confirms the present authors' clinical impression that individuals tend to return for retreatment when the dynamic muscular weakness is beginning to wear off but is still present, whereas the smoothing of the brow area is usually still dramatic when compared with pretreatment pictures.

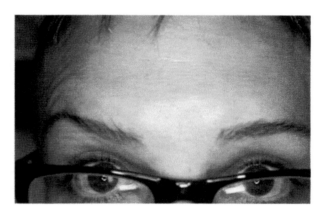

Figure 13.4 *Over-elevation of the lateral right eyebrow following BTX-A injection.*

EYEBROW ELEVATION

Medial and lateral brow ptosis can give unwanted expressions such as anger and ferocity (medial), and anguish and sadness (lateral). The presence of lateral brow ptosis is usually seen after photodamage to the periocular skin when the unopposed action of the vertically oriented of the orbicularis oculi pulls the tail of the brow inferiorly. Injection of 3–5 U of BTX-A into the orbicularis, above the bony orbital margin at the junction with the temporal fusion line, will weaken the depressing action and allow the lateral brow segment to elevate (Figure 13.3).

Post-BTX-A overelevation of the lateral brow can result in a 'Spock' or 'Diablo' effect (Figure 13.4). In other words, untreated frontalis lateral to the treated muscle is overacting to produce this effect. Interestingly, this effect can be desirable in some individuals, although in most it is a problem that requires correction. The aesthetics of the eyebrows, both at rest and on animation, are critical and require great judgement in the use of BTX-A. If the subject wishes the lateral brow to be lower, 1–3 U of BTX-A injected into the frontalis, 1.5 cm above the lateral brow, will drop the tail by 1–3 mm. The effect can be predicted when the individual is asked to voluntarily maximally elevate the brows prior to injection.

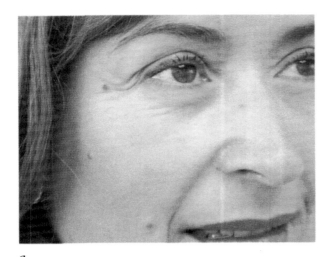
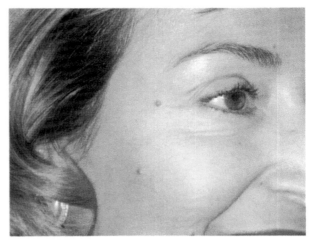

a   b

Figure 13.5 BTX-A induced improvement in the lateral orbital area. (A) is pre-treatment, (B) is post-treatment.

EYEBROW HEIGHT ASYMMETRY

Eighty per cent of adult women have brow height asymmetry, with a vertical discrepancy of 1–3 mm.[7] Until they see their photographs, the individual may be unaware of the pre-existing asymmetry and, furthermore, may feel that the appearance was the result of the BTX-A. Treatment needs to be tailored to administer more BTX-A on the lower side to establish a more symmetric vertical relationship.[8] This manoeuvre is particularly important before upper eyelid blepharoplasty in order that excessive preseptal skin is not removed from the side with the lower brow. BTX-A can also be an important rehearsal to see if a subject requires a surgical brow lift instead of a blepharoplasty.

LATERAL CANTHAL RHYTIDES (CROW'S-FEET)

Crow's-feet are the result of repeated contractions of the vertically oriented fibers of the orbicularis oculi. The lines radiate laterally and superiorly and/or inferiorly from the lateral canthal angle. In youth they only occur in dynamic situations such as smiling or squinting in bright light and they terminate at the lateral bony orbital margin. As time passes they extend over the lateral margin onto the skin of the

cheek and the temple. They are often noted first by friends and colleagues when the face is at rest and the face is viewed obliquely or laterally (Figure 13.5) BTX-A injection will soften and erase these lines. Occasional patients have such long crow's-foot lines that double row of injections is required.[9]

The 'safe zone' for injection is outside the bony margin, in order to avoid diffusion into the extraocular musculature with consequent diplopia, and at least 1 cm above the zygomaticus notch on the lower border of the zygomatic bone, in order to avoid inadvertently treating zygomaticus major and minor which act to elevate the corner of the mouth. The resulting lower facial paresis can last 3–6 months and mimics a Bell's palsy (Figure 13.6).

Before treatment the physician should photograph patients semiprofile when relaxed and in full forced smile. The corner of the mouth should be included in both the before and after photographs to ensure versimilitude. Many individuals that have deep etched crow's-feet at rest also require ablative or nonablative resurfacing procedures and also blepharoplasty. The present authors' believe that BTX-A treatment is a required maintenance therapy for all subjects who have undergone a resurfacing procedure because otherwise the subsequent use of the orbicularis will refold the newly deposited dermal collagen into thicker and more obvious crow's-folds.[10]

SUMMARY

The aesthetic determinant in upper facial aging is persistent muscular action; as a result, BTX-A is the cosmetic treatment of choice for this region. It is useful as both a primary aesthetic enhancement and also as an adjunct to surgical brow lift, blepharoplasty, and ablative and nonablative resurfacing procedures.

For glabellar furrows, horizontal forehead lines, asymmetric eyebrow height, crow's-feet and lateral brow ptosis, BTX-A treatment offers an effective, safe, and affordable intervention with virtually no down time for the subject.[11]

References

1 Carruthers A, Carruthers J. Cosmetic uses of botulinum A exotoxin. In: Klein AW, editor. *Tissue augmentation in clinical practice*. New York: Marcel Dekker; 1998:224–5.

2 Website: American Academy of Cosmetic Surgery. www.cosmeticsurgery.org. November 2000.

3 Carruthers JDA, Carruthers A. Treatment of glabellar frown lines with C botulinum-A exotoxin. J Dermatol Surg Oncol 1992;18:17–21.

4 National Institutes of Health. NIH Consensus Development Conference on Clinical Use of Botulinum A Exotoxin, Bethesda, Maryland, USA. US Dept of Health and Human Services 1990;1–20.

5 Aoki R. Basic science of botulinum toxin type A (Botox). Botulinum Toxin for Experts, Vancouver, October 2000.

6 Standardized photoclassification of static and dynamic glabellar rhytides developed for Phase III FDA trials to establish a cosmetic indication for glabellar Botox chemodenervation, Allergan Pharmaceuticals. Presented as a Poster at the American Academy of Dermatology. Meeting, San Francisco, CA, USA, March 2000.

7 Matarasso A, Terino EO. Forehead brow rhytidoplasty: reassessing the goals. Plastic Reconstr Surg 1994;93:1378.

8 Huilgol S, Carruthers JA, Carruthers JDA. Raising eyebrows with botulinum toxin. Dermatol Surg 1999;25:373–6.

9 Taleppio S. Treatment of large crow's feet. Presented at Botox for the Expert, Vancouver, Canada, October 2000.

10 Carruthers J, Carruthers A. Botulinum toxin and laser resurfacing for lines around the eyes. In: Blitzer A, Binder W, Boyd B, Carruthers A, editors. Management of facial lines and wrinkles. Lippincott Williams and Wilkins; 2000:315–32.

11 Carruthers A Carruthers J. Technique for the cosmetic use of botulinum A exotoxin: Clinical indications and injection. Dermatol Surg 1998;24:1189–94.

COMBINATION TREATMENT (Nicholas J Lowe)

Indications	Potential combination treatments	Chapter reference
Forehead	Photoprotection	2
Glabellar	Topical therapy	3
Periorbital lines	Laser skin resurfacing	10,11
Upper eyelid and	Non-ablative laser rejuvenation	12
brow ptosis	Chemical peels	6,7
	Dermal fillers	16,17
	Periocular surgery	23
	Endoscopic brow lift	24
	Periorbital skin pigmentation	8

14. Botulinum toxin: combination treatments for the face and neck

Nicholas J Lowe

BACKGROUND

The ability of botulinum toxin A (BTX-A) to improve the appearance of facial lines was first reported amongst patients who had been receiving injections for facial dystonias or surgical procedures.[1,2] Since that time there has been very extensive use of this modality of treatment for the relaxation of a wide variety of facial lines and also of ageing lines of the neck. Previously published studies (two double-blind studies) confirm the safety and efficacy of BTX-A in the treatment of upper facial lines.[3,4] Numerous open-label evaluations have also conflrmed the efficacy of this agent.

This chapter will summarize the use of BTX-A on facial lines and its role as a combination treatment in the management of the ageing face. Examples of combinations that may be used with BTX-A are laser resurfacing, non-ablative skin rejuvenation and skin fillers.

INTRODUCTION

Botulisim that causes muscular patalysis as a result of food poisoning was identified in 1897. Alan Scott, an ophthalmologic surgeon in San Francisco, developed the concept of using local injections of BTX-A to selectively inactivate ocular muscles that result in strabismus, whilst looking for a nonsurgical approach to correcting this condition.[5,6]

Subsequently, a wide variety of medical uses[7-16] for BTX-A have been found, treatment of muscle dystonias, strabismus, blethrospasm, muscle spasisity disorders and torticollis, as well as spasisity in Parkinson's disease.[7-11] More recently, BTX-A has been shown to be highly effective as a treatment for hyperactive facial lines of the upper face,[12] forehead, periorbital, paranasal, perioral lower facial and nasolabial regions. In addition, the use of this agent to improve certain features of neck ageing has been proven in clinical observations.

The use of a variety of minimally invasive techniques, e.g. laser skin resurfacing, non-ablative laser rejuvenation and the use of dermal skin fillers, have all been shown to be highly effective in improving the ageing face whilst reducing the need for more invasive surgery. Use of BTX-A prior to these procedures and whilst the improvement effects of these treatments are expected to occur, i.e. over the first 12 months following laser resurfacing and nonablative laser rejuvenation, helps to maintain a less mobile dermis, which is felt to produce a more uniform improvement of the areas treated.

In addition, the adjunctive use of BTX-A to deep glabellar folds and deep perioral rhytides in combination with Dermol fillers also appears to extend the life of temporary fillers.

TYPES OF BTX-A

Botox

There are two principal types of BTX-A currently available and most studies reported relate to the use of Botox® (Allergan Inc, Irvine CA).[13] To produce this toxin, cultures of clostridium botulinum are fermented and the culture undergoes autolysis, releasing BTX complexes that are then harvested by centrifugation and acidification. The reluctant crude toxin is subsequently monitored for contaminatiom, potency and protein content, and the amount of toxin is diluted using a human serum albumin containing dilutant added to the storage vials, which are then subsequently freeze-dried and sealed. Sample vials are checked for integrity, sterility, moisture content and potency. The quantity of active toxin of Botox is defined as 1 unit (U), being the lethal dose of toxin causing death in 50% (LD50) of a group of Swiss Webster female mice. It is interesting to note that the mouse assay, which is at present the standard of measuring potency of commercially available toxin, is a relatively recent development. The original assay utilized by Scott et al. was that of LD50 in the monkey,[5,6] in whom the lethal dose range is apparently less narrow than that in mice.

Lethal doses in humans are not known precisely for the purified toxin but have been estimated from a variety of published clinical catastrophes. The dose of ingested toxin would need to be 10,000–1 million times the parental dose. It has been estimated that an adult male weighing c. 100 kg would succumb to a dose of toxin 3500 times that needed to cause paralysis and death in mice, i.e. 3500 U of Botox. Other data from Scott's studies suggest that a 70 kg human would require a dose of for c. 2800 U for an LD50 dose.[5,6] In other words, there is a wide safety margin on the amount of Botox used for therapeutic purposes, e.g. for facial expression lines, a maximum of 60 U per treatment session is typical.

The procedure of purification of the human serum albumin is felt to be such that it will not allow transfer of communicable diseases.

Dysport

The European BTX-A is called Dysport. It was originally produced by Porton Products in the UK and was licensed for distribution by the Department of Health and Social Security by Speywood. The preparation has been used successfully for blepharospasm torticollis. It is difficult to calculate the direct relationship between Botox and Speywood Ltd who acquired Speywood in 1998, and it is now distributed by Ispen; however, it is suggested that the Dysport unit is less potent than the Botox one.[13,14]

However there are few published guidelines or standards for converting between the two products. Dysport is available in larger number of units per vial (500 U per vial). The present author has extensive experience of the use of Botox in the USA and of both Botox and Dysport in the UK. Table 14.1 lists some of the features of the two commercial preparations and Table 14.2 lists some of the doses of Botox and Dysport used by the present author.

Table 14.1 Details of Botox and Dysport

	Botox	Dysport
Source	Allergan USA Irvine, CA Allergani UK Buckinghamshire, UK (manufactured Ireland since 1997) Tel: (800) 347-4500	Ipsen Ltd (France) (manufactured UK)
Availability	100 U per vial	500 U per vial
Storage	−5°C	Room temperature
Suggested dilutant	Non-preserved saline	Non-preserved saline
Present author's dilution	2.5 cm³ of saline per vial	2.5 cm³ per vial

Table 14.2 The present author's dose range (1 unit Botox equivalent to 5 units Dysport)

	Botox	Dysport
Corrugator muscle	8 U per corrugator	40 U per corrugator
Lateral orbicularis oculi	4.8 U	20–40 U per site
Horizontal forehead lines (usually a maximum of six sites)	4 u per site	20 U per site

The amounts may be decreased or increased depending on several factors, such as patient age, intensity of muscle activity and past responses to botulinum toxin.

Table 14.3 Duration of efficacy of Botox when diluted with unpreserved saline and stored at 4°C

Time stored (days)	Activity (%)
1	90–100
3	70–80
7	40–50
14	Minimal

Efficacy determined by the ability of the Botox solution to reduce upper facial expression lines ≥75% 2 weeks following injection compared with freshly mixed Botox.

COMPARISON OF THE POTENCY OF BOTOX AND DYSPORT

Dilution guidelines

The present author feels that one unit of Botox has an approximately equivalent potency to 4 U of Dysport. Based on these variations and the difference in units per vial available of Botox (100 U) and Dysport (500 U), the conversion factor should be approximately a dilution 2 cm^3 of saline for Botox giving a dilution of 5 U per 0.1 cm^3. A dilution of 2.5 cm^3 of per Dysport gives an approximately equivalent potency of 20 U per 0.1 cm^3.

> Botox: 100 U per vial diluted by 2.5 cm^3 = 4 U per 0.1 cm^3
> Dysport: 500 U per vial diluted with 2.5 cm^3 of saline = 20=U per 0.1 cm^3.

Average units used for treatment

> 0.2 cm^3 Botox (8 U) per corrugator muscle;
> 0.2 cm^2 Dysport (40 U) per corrugator muscle;

0.1 cm^3 (4 U Botox, 20 U of Dysport) to the procerus muscle;
0.1–0.15 cm^2 (8 U Botox, 40 U Dysport) to each crow's-feet area.

Type B botulinum toxin (BTX-B)

In January 2001, BTX-B was approved for cervical dystonia. This toxin was developed by Elan Pharmaceuticals; its name in the USA is Myobloc and in Europe, Neuro Bloc®. To date, no studies comparing BTX-A with BTX-B have been reported but they are currently underway. One theoretical conversion of relative potency is 1 U of Botox to 50 U of Myobloc.

One application of BTX-B may be its use with patients who have developed blocking antibodies to BTX-A. However, this problem is very rare; in fact, with the latest Botox formulations, which contain minimal quantities of protein, there have been no reports of the formation of blocking antibodies (R Aoki, pers comm). Dose ranging studies with BTX-B are currently underway. It does reduce facial lines, but recent studies suggest shorter effect than with BTX-A.

COMBINATION TREATMENT WITH BTX-A

Laser skin resurfacing

There are two types of ablative resurfacing lasers. The CO_2 laser has a wavelength of 10,600 nm and produces up to 100 μm of heat damage per pass depending on the settings of the laser. For resurfacing, the CO_2 laser is usually used in either an ultra-pulse mode (e.g. Coherent UltraPulse) or a continuous-wave mode with a computerized flash scanning device (Sharplan Esc).

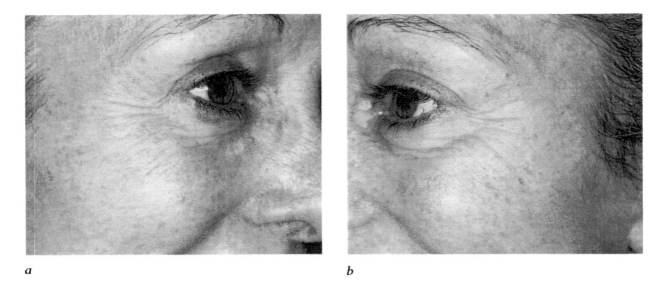

a　　　　　　　　　　　　　　　　　　　　*b*

Figure 14.1 *View of patient before treatment for dynamic rhytides and photoageing.*

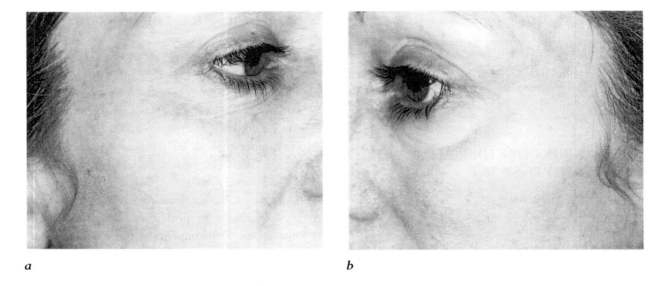

a　　　　　　　　　　　　　　　　　　　　*b*

Figure 14.2 *Same patient 6 months after BTX-A treatment to the periorbital skin and ultrapulsed CO_2 laser resurfacing of the face.*

The other main skin resurfacing laser is the Er:YAG laser that has a wavelength of 2940 nm and generally produces less thermal injury per pass than the CO_2 laser. It also has much more efficient water absorption than the CO_2 laser but has the disadvantage that most Er:YAG do not coagulate bleeding vessels, so the deeper the skin resurfacing the more bleeding is present, which can obscure the resurfucing field. Because the Er:YAG laser is much more efficiently absorbed by the tissue water content than the CO_2 laser there is the possibility of performing much deeper skin destruction.

Following both types of laser resurfacing there is felt to be an initial epidermal wound repair followed by new collagen and connective tissue formation. The maximum improvement from this new tissue formation can take up to 12 months.[15] One of the main problems with laser resurfacing is that dynamic rhytides will return unless they are controlled. This has led to the use of BTX-A as both a pretreatment and

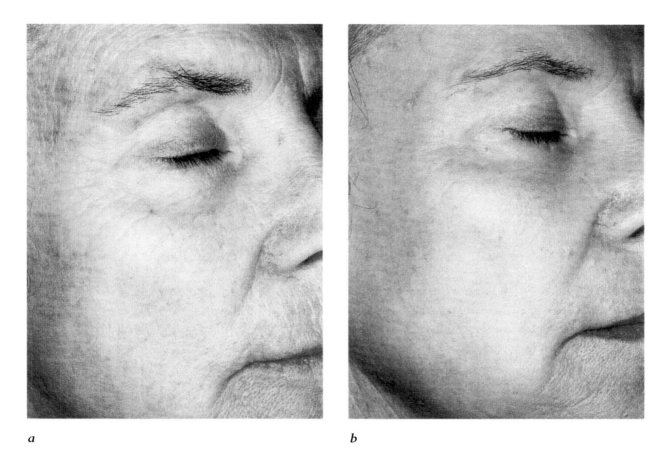

Figure 14.3 *View of patient (A) before treatment and (B) after treatment with BTX-A to the periorbital skin and UltraPulse CO_2 laser resurfacing of the face.*

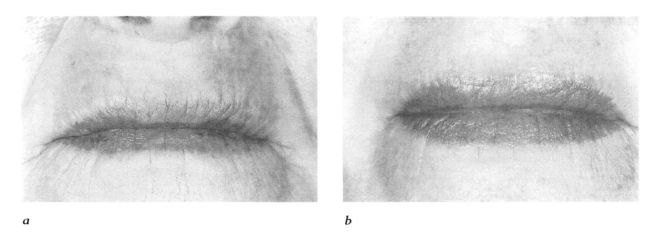

Figure 14.4 *View of patient (A) before treatment and (B) after treatment with BTX-A, insertion of SoftForm implants and CO_2 laser resurfacing of the lips.*

follow-up treatment to be used with laser skin resurfacing. The theory is that if the skin surface is rested as far as possible by muscle denervation with the BTX-A injections, then the subsequent long-term reduction of rhytides by the laser will be more successful than if the dynamic rhytides are not controlled.

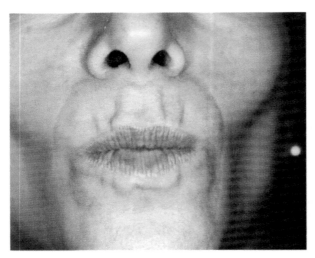
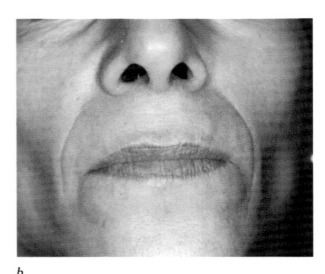

a   *b*

Figure 14.5 *View of patient with severe upper lip rhytides (caused by action of obicularis oris) (A) before treatment at maximum muscle pursing and (B) at rest. Additional treatment would include lip filler and laser rejuvenation.*

Lower face and neck lines

These are covered more fully in Chapter 15. Candidate sites for BTX-A are:

- Perioral lines. The mucosal surface of the lips is anaesthetized with 30% Benzocaine gel and inject through the mucosa (between 4–8 units per lip).
- Marionette lines (downturning of the lateral lips). Here the lower lateral depressor angular oris muscles is injected (usually 4 units per side).
- Platysmal bands (usually 8–12 units per band).

Treatment of these areas of the lower face can then be successfully combined with laser resurfacing, non-ablative laser, chemical peels, dermal fillers, lip implant and topical therapy.

The present author's technique for combining BTX-A with laser resurfacing is as follows:

(1) pretreat with BTX-A, ideally at least 2 weeks prior to laser skin resurfacing;
(2) post-laser treatment, BTX-A should be injected before the muscle activity causes a return of dynamic rhytides, this is usually 3 months after the first injection;

(3) for ongoing treatment with the non-ablative lasers (e.g. CoolTouch), repeat BTX-A injections three to four times over a 1 year period, thus allowing more efficient, smoother dermal connective tissue remodelling (studies are currently in progress to prove this theory);
(4) for selected patients with neck ageing, a combination of BTX-A with cool touch, vascular (for poikiloderma) or superficial resurfacing lasers can be very successful; however, excessive quantities of BTX-A should be avoided on the neck because of deeper effects on pharyngeal and laryngeal muscles.

References

1 Carruthers JD, Carruthers JA. Treatment of glabellar frown lines with C. botulinum A exotoxin. J Dermatol Surg Oncol 1992;18:17–21.

2 Carruthers A, Carruthers J. Cosmetic uses of Botulinum A exotoxin. In Klein AW (ed.) Tissue augmentation in clinical practice. Marcel Dekker New York. 1998. 224–5.

3 Keen M, Blitzer A, Aviv J, et al. Botulinum toxin

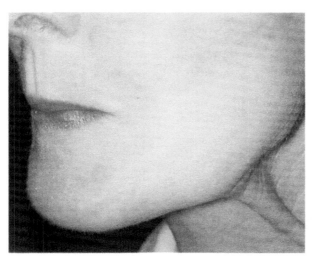
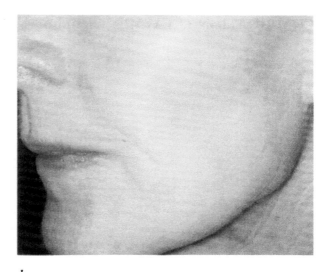

a   b

Figure 14.6 *View of patient with severe neck platysmal muscle banding (A) before treatment and (B) after treatment with BTZ-a. Patient is now a candidate for chemical peels and topical therapy (retinoids) to the neck.*

A for hyperkinetic facial lines: results of a double blind placebo-controlled study. Plast Reconstr Surg 1994;94:94–9.

4 Lowe NJ, Maxwell A, Harper H. Botulinum A exotoxin for glabellar folds: a double blind, placebo controlled study with an electromyo graphic injection technique. J Am Acad Dermatol 1996;35:569–72.

5 Scott AB, Rosenbaum A, Collins CC. Pharmacologic weakening of extraocular muscles. Invest Opthalmol 1973;12:924–7.

6 Scott AB. Botulinum toxin injection into extra ocular muscles as an alternative to strabismus surgery. Opthahmol 1980;87:1044–9.

7 Dutton JJ, Buckley EG. Long term results and complications of botulinum A toxin in the treatment of bleparospasm. Opthalmo 1988;95:1529–34.

8 Gelb DJ, Lowenstein DH, Aminoff MJ. Controlled trial of botulinum toxin injection in the treatment of spasmodic toricollis. Neurol 1989;39:80–4.

9 Savino PJ, Sergott RC, Bosely TM, Schatz NJ. Hemifacial spasm treated with botullnum A toxin injection. Arch Opthalmol 1985;103:1305–6.

10 Kalra HK, Magoon EH. Side effects of the use of botulinum A toxin for the treatment of benign essential belparospasm and hemi-faical spasm. Opthal Surg 1990;21:335–8.

11 Borodic GE, Cheney M, McKenna M. Contralateral injections of botulinum A toxin for the treatment of hemifacial spasm to achieve increased facial symmetry. Plast Reconstr Surg 1992;90:972–9.

12 Lowe NJ, Carruthers JD, Carruthers JA, et al. Scientific Presentation at the European Academy of Dermatology. October 2000.

13 Whurr R. Movement disorders (abstract). 1995;May 10:387.

14 Sampaio C. Movement disorders (abstract). 1995;May 10:387.

15 Lowe NJ, Lask G, Griffin ME, Lowe PL. Skin resurfacing with ultrapulsed carbon dioxide laser: observation on 100 patients. Dermatol Surg 1995;21:1025–9.

16 Carruthers JD, Carruthers JA, Lowe NJ, et al. Scientific Presentation at the American Academy of Dermatology. March 2000.

COMBINATION TREATMENT (Nicholas J Lowe)

Indications	Potential combination treatments	Chapter reference
Forehead	Photoprotection	1
Glabellar	Topical therapy	2
Periorbital	Glycolic acid peels	6
Perioral	Combination peels	7
Lower face	Laser skin resurfacing	10,11
Neck lines	Non-ablative laser rejuvenation	12
Brow and	Chemical peels	7
upper eyelid	Dermal fillers	17,18
ptosis	Endoscopic brow lift	24
	Periorbital skin surgery	8
	Neck rejuvenation	25

ADDITIONAL PHOTOGRAPHIC EXAMPLES OF BTX-A THERAPY

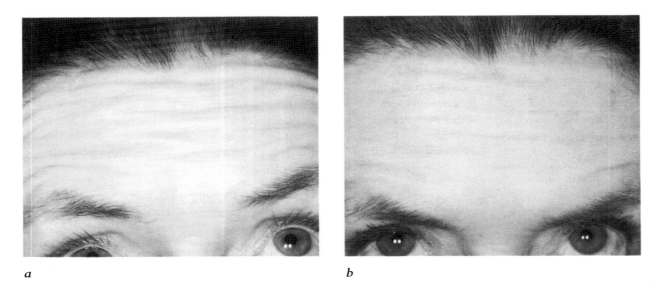

a   *b*

Figure 14.7 *(A) Before treatment with BTX-A. (B) After treatment. Total of 20 units to the forehead.*

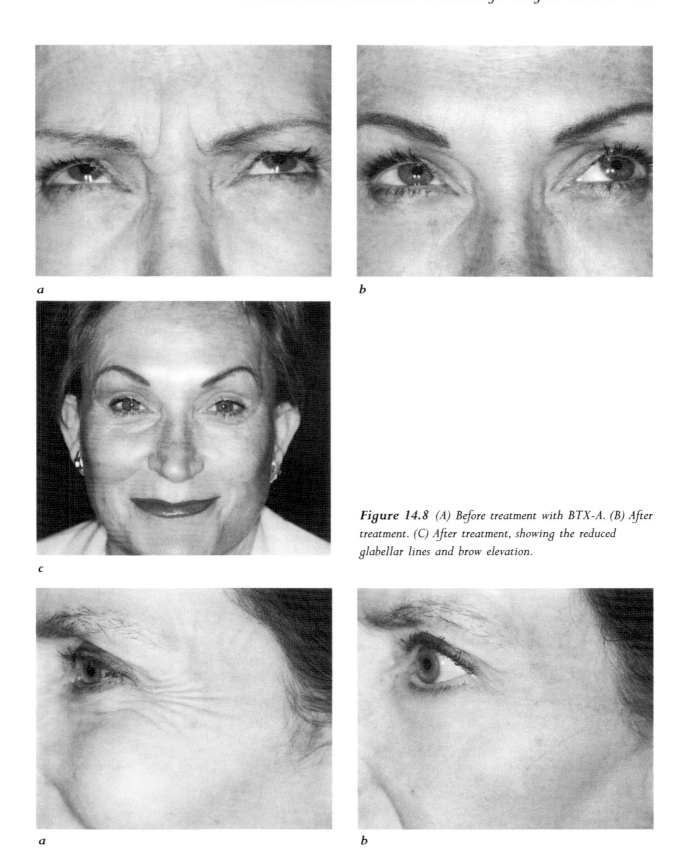

Figure 14.8 *(A) Before treatment with BTX-A. (B) After treatment. (C) After treatment, showing the reduced glabellar lines and brow elevation.*

Figure 14.9 *(A) Before treatment with BTX-A. (B) After treatment. Note the widening of the palpebral angle with larger eye shape.*

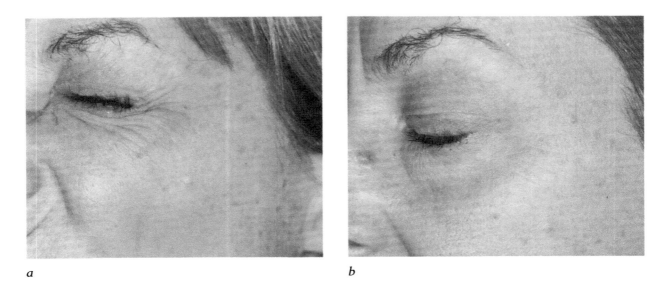

a   b

Figure 14.10 (A) Before treatment. (B) After treatment.

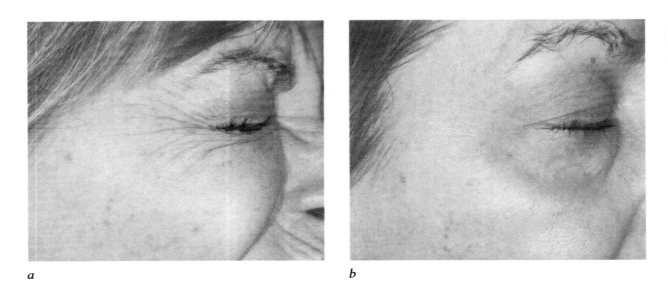

a   b

Figure 14.11 (A) Before treatment. (B) After treatment.

Figures 14.10 and 14.11 Both periorbital areas can now be treated with laser resurfacing or non-ablative laser while maintaining reduced crow's feet.

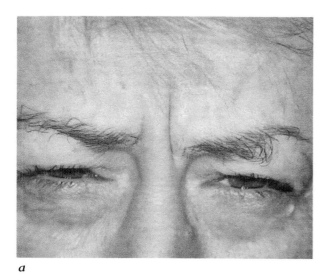

a

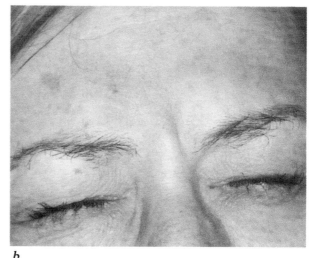

b

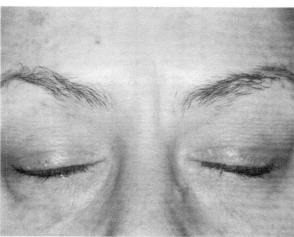

c

Figure 14.12 *(A) Before any BTX-A. (B) Before 2nd BTX-A. (C) Two weeks after 2nd BTX-A. Note the increasing effect with increasing numbers of BTX-A treatment sessions.*

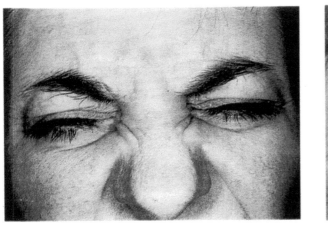
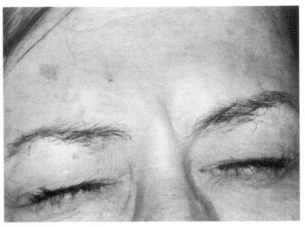

a   b

Figure 14.13 *Prominent procerus action before treatment (A) and after 20 units of BTX-A 12 to procerus, 8 to medial lower corrugator (B).*

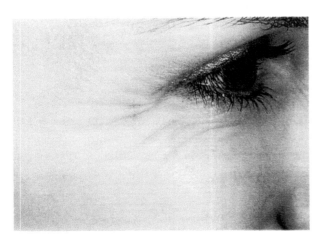
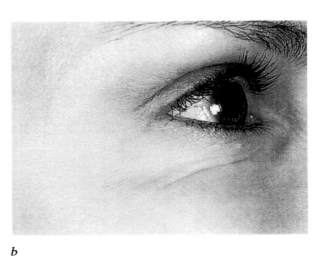

a   b

Figure 14.14 *Crow's feet before BTX-A injection (A) and after 8 units of BTX-A to lateral obicularis oculis muscle (B). Patient needs 2 units of infraorbital BTX-A.*

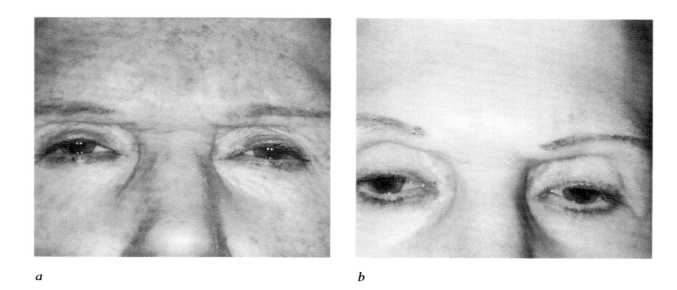

a　　　　　　　　　　　　　　　　　　b

Figure 14.15 *(A) Before BTX to procerus and corrugator followed by full face superficial ultrapulsed carbon dioxide laser resurfacing (B). (See also chapter 11).*

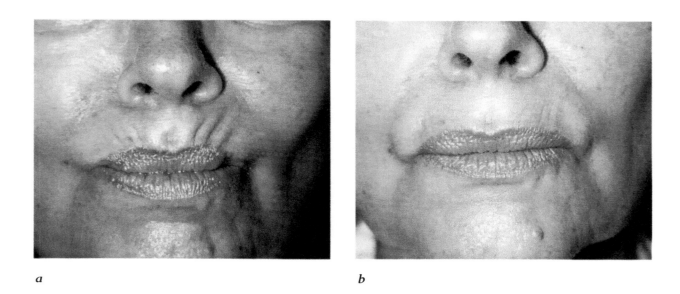

a　　　　　　　　　　　　　　　　　　b

Figure 14.16 *Perioral rhytides before (A) and after (B) BTX-A to upper lip. 2 units into each of four sites into upper lip (total 8 units). Note the 'lengthening' of upper lip plus markedly reduced rhytides. (Both photos taken at lip pursing action).*

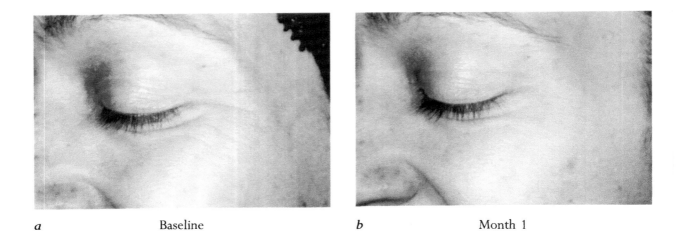

a	Baseline	*b*	Month 1

Figure 14.17 *Crow's feet (A). After BTX-A treatment (B).*

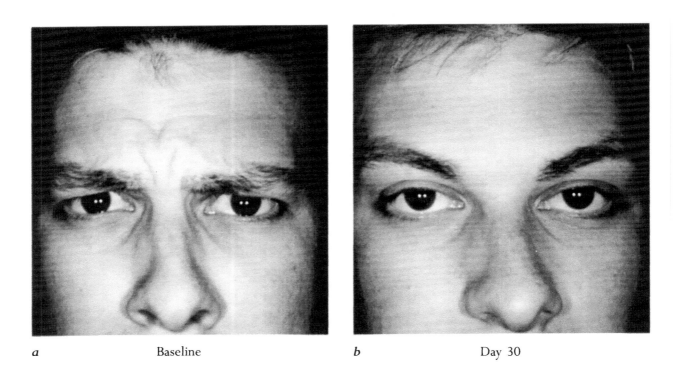

a	Baseline	*b*	Day 30

Figure 14.18 *Pre and post Botox. Note brow elevation and reduced glabellar lines.*

15. Botulinum neurotoxin A for the management of lower facial lines and platysmal bands

Andrew Blitzer

Facial lines and wrinkles have a multifactorial etiology including sun exposure, loss of dermal elastic fibers, skin atrophy, and excessive muscle activity. Hyperfunctional facial lines are caused by skin pleating when there are contracting underlying muscles.

Botulinum toxin injections have been found to weaken muscles, thereby decreasing hyperfunction. Botulinum toxin has been used very successfully for many years in patients with hemifacial spasm, facial tics, or facial dystonia. Patients receiving unilateral injections for these conditions often return asking for injection of the contralateral side to produce a more youthful appearance.[1,2] Over the last decade, much has been written about the use of botulinum toxin for the management of glabellar lines, horizontal forehead lines and crow's feet. With experience, many other facial areas have now been managed with toxin.[3-6]

The materials necessary for botulinum toxin treatments of lower facial lines are botulinum toxin, a standard freezer, non-preserved sterile saline, tuberculin syringes, a small EMG machine, hollow-bore coated 30-gauge monopolar EMG needles, alcohol swabs, and gauze. The author has been using Botox® (Allergan Inc, Irvine, CA). A standard vial contains 100 mouse units (U) of toxin. The toxin is shipped from the manufacturer on dry ice and should be stored in a freezer at −20°C. The frozen, lyophylized toxin is reconstituted with non-preserved sterile saline. The author typically dilutes the toxin to doses giving a volume of 0.1 ml. To minimize the diffusion to adjacent muscles, 4 ml of saline is added as standard to a vial of toxin, making the dose 25 U/ml, or 2.5 U/0.1 ml. In some patients a larger dose is needed and, to prevent excess volume, a more concentrated solution is made by adding 2 ml of saline to a bottle making 50 U/ml, or 5 U/0.1 ml.[5]

Patients who are being considered for lower facial line botulinum toxin therapy are first evaluated with a thorough review of their medical history, medications, and prior plastic surgery. Although there is a paucity of data, patients who are pregnant or lactating should not be injected. Although patients with pre-existing disorders of the neuromuscular junctions have been treated, it is suggested that one proceeds with caution in patients who have Eaton–Lambert syndrome, myasthenia gravis, and motor neurone diseases. It is contraindicated to use botulinum toxin in patients receiving aminoglycoside antibiotics since there may be a synergistic effect of the aminoglycoside and the toxin.

A detailed analysis of the patient's facial lines and skin condition needs to be performed to allow for the optimum treatment and treatment sequence. The hyperfunctional muscle lines are best treated with botulinum toxin injections. Changes in skin are best treated with chemical peels or laser resurfacing. Persistent lines may be treated with injectable filler substances such as collagen. Often, the patient's facial-line therapy requires a combination of these techniques.

Standardized photographs are taken of the patient's face at rest and with activity. The patient's lines, skin condition, any scars and/or asymmetry are noted on the chart. An informed consent is obtained for each patient. This unit's consent form states that the Food and Drugs Administration has approved Botox as safe and effective therapy for blepharospasm, strabismus and hemifacial spasm 'on-label'; cosmetic uses are 'off-label'.

The patient's face is marked for the areas of maximum muscle pull that are causing the bothersome hyperfunctional lines. The points to be injected are drawn or photographed for future reference. The skin area can then be iced or treated with entectic mixture of local anesthetic (EMLA) to decrease the discomfort associated with skin penetration by the needle. Botulinum toxin is then drawn up in a tuberculin syringe with a hollow-bore, coated monopolar EMG needle (Figure 15.1). This needle is connected to the EMG machine, and ground and reference leads placed on the face or in the supra-clavicular area (Figure 15.2). The needle is inserted into the overlying skin at about a 30° angle, thereby impaling the previously marked muscle for injection. The patient is then instructed to accentuate the specific facial expression that produces the unwanted line. If the needle is in an active part of the muscle, a loud burst of activity will be heard on the speaker of the EMG machine. If a distant signal is obtained (low frequency, dull sound), the needle should be moved until it is in a maximal position, before the toxin is injected. This technique is repeated at each area marked for injection. After injection, the patient is asked not to rub or massage the injected area to avoid excess diffusion to adjacent muscles which might cause excessive weakness of these muscles.

Patients who have excessive lip pursing usually have hyperactive mentalis and orbicularis oris muscles. This can occur in patients who have a prognathic jaw or chin implant producing abnormal lip postures and a 'peau d'orange' skin appearance or a 'popply chin'. Small amounts of Botox (2.5–5 U in each mentalis muscle) may be used to compensate for this muscle overactivity and improve chin appearance (Figure 15.3). The injection is given no higher than the half-way point between the vermillion border of the lower lip and the inferior edge of the mentum, and 0.5–1 cm medial to the oral commissure. If the injection is given too high, it will excessively weaken the orbicularis oris, causing a decreased ability to pucker the lips and may cause drooling while drinking fluids. It may also change speech by interfering with plosive and fricative speech elements. The EMG technique is utilized, and the patient asked to pucker their lips. When the needle is in a very active place within the muscle, the toxin is injected.[5,7]

'Marionette' lines are usually the result of hyper-activity of the depressor anguli oris muscle at its connection to the edge of the orbicularis oris muscle.

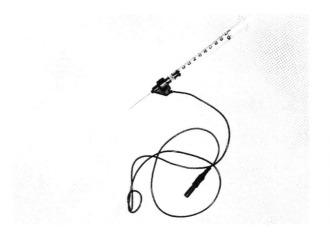

Figure 15.1 *A tuberculin syringe attached to a 30-gauge, hollow-bore, coated monopolar electrode with wire for electrical connection (Medtronics/XOMED).*

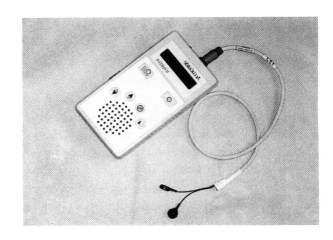

Figure 15.2 *A battery powered EMG machine used for accurate placement of toxin into muscle for facial injections (AccuGuide™–Medtronics/XOMED).*

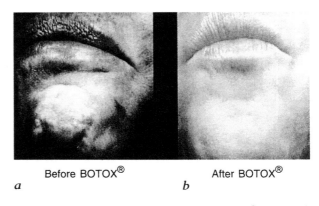

Before BOTOX®   After BOTOX®

a   b

Figure 15.3 *A patient with a 'popply chin' before (A) and after (B) toxin injection (courtesy of Dr Jean Carruthers).*

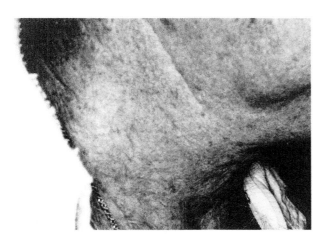

Figure 15.4 *A patient with excess fat in the submental region.*

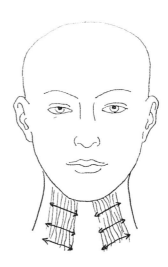

Figure 15.6 *A diagram of injection sites within the platysma muscle.*

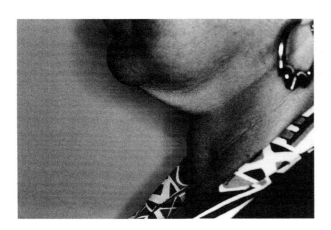

Figure 15.5 *A patient with excess skin in the submental region.*

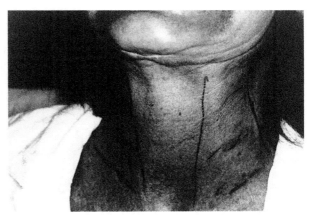

Figure 15.7 *Marking of the platysma muscle and the injection sites on the neck of a patient bothered by platysmal bands.*

A weakening of the depressor anguli oris may decrease or eliminate the lines. Carruthers and Carruthers have described a technique for best managing these lines.[7] In this technique, a point is drawn 7–10 mm lateral to the oral commissure and 8–10 mm inferior to this point: this inferior–lateral point should be in the depressor muscle. A dose of 2–4 U botulinum toxin is injected in 0.1 ml. An excessive dose or volume of injection may cause a weakening of the orbicularis oris producing a change in the ability to pucker the lips causing drooling and/or a change in speech. In some cases a combination of injectable filler and botulinum toxin yields the best results.

Patients who have prominent platysmal bands before or after facelift procedures may also benefit from injections of botulinum toxin, but without the submental incision commonly used for muscle plication. Injection of botulinum toxin will not remove excess fat or skin in the submental area (Figures 15.4 and 15.5) but it will relax the platysma to decrease or eliminate unsightly platysmal bands. The anterior and posterior edge of the platysma is marked on the patient's neck. Horizontal parallel lines are drawn beginning about 2 cm below the inferior border of the mandible, and are repeated every 1.5–2 cm until the end of the platysma banding. Generally, this produces three or four injection sites per

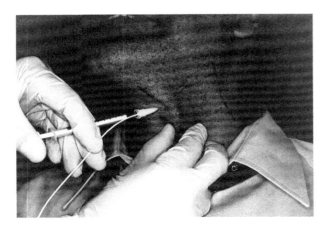

Figure 15.8 Injections of toxin being given with EMG control into the platysmal bands.

side (Figures 15.6 and 15.7). Injection of the bands is performed with a hollow-bore 1½ inch, 27-gauge coated monopolar EMG needle. The needle is passed through the skin at the anterior edge of the platysma and, under EMG guidance, is continued perpendicularly through the muscle fibers. The patient can activate the platysma by depressing their lower lip. The needle may be adjusted so as to remain in the active portion of the muscle. Once the muscle is entered under EMG control, injection of botulinum toxin is given throughout the muscle pass on withdrawal of the needle (Figure 15.8). Each needle pass is injected with 2.5–5.0 U. The dose range is 7.5–20 U per side in the author's series. Other authors report similar results using larger doses without EMG guidance.[8,9] Matarasso et al. reported a

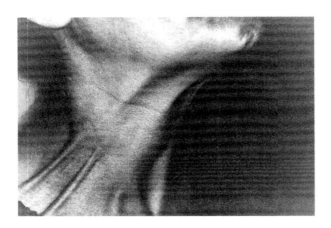

Figure 15.9 A pre-injection lateral oblique photograph showing platysmal bands.

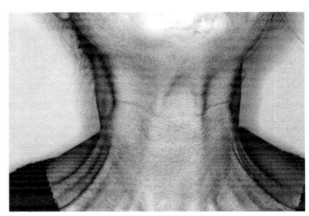

Figure 15.11 A pre-injection anterior photograph showing platysmal bands.

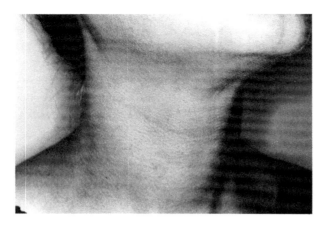

Figure 15.10 A 1-week post-injection lateral oblique photograph showing a marked reduction of platysmal bands.

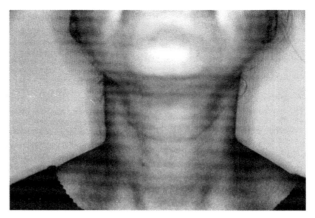

Figure 15.12 A 1-week post-injection anterior photograph showing a marked reduction of platysmal bands.

large series in which patients received 30–250 U; they had an 18% failure rate.[10] The potential complications associated with platysmal band injections from diffusion of toxin to adjacent muscles include dysphagia, related to weakness of the sternohyoid muscles, which decreases laryngeal elevation on swallowing thus making that process more difficult. In addition, if the toxin is injected adjacent to the cricothyroid muscle, weakness may ensue causing changes in vocal pitch. This may be very noticeable in singers.

After the injections are complete, patients are asked to return to the office after 2 weeks to re-evaluate the effect of the toxin. New photographs are taken (Figures 15.9 to 15.12). If the hyperfunctional lines are still bothersome to the patient, additional toxin is injected into the remaining hyperactive portion of the muscle. The dose and the location of the additional toxin is related to the areas of maximal persistent activity. If there is still a minor crease in the skin, but no underlying muscle activity, injections of a filler material can be given to smooth the contour of the skin. After adequate relaxation of the skin, the actinic lines can also be treated using lasers. The author prefers the erbium:YAG laser to remove thinned, elastic wrinkled skin. By pretreating with botulinum toxin, the hyperfunctional lines are diminished or removed, and the new dermal collagen and elastic fibers that form will not be in the functional crease. This produces a better and longer lasting result.[11]

When the muscles are adequately weakened and a pleasing facial skin contour is achieved, the patient is instructed to return to the office if the lines become prominent again; in general, this is about 4–6 months after treatment. In some patients, who have been treated a number of times, the botulinum toxin effect seems to last longer, probably related to behavior modification. These patients have been conditioned to avoid certain undesirable facial gestures thereby avoiding excess pleating of facial skin.

Complications of botulinum toxin injections may lead to mild bruising or local pain related to the injection needle. There also may be weakness of adjacent muscles related to diffusion of the toxin. The amount of diffusion and weakness is technique and dose related. To minimize this possibility, the author uses EMG guidance and small volumes of injected fluid to allow the injection to be placed in the most active area of the muscle with minimum diffusion. If local adjacent muscle weakness occurs, it will disappear with time. The author has not found any long-term hazards or complications of botulinum toxin use. Some patients receiving large doses (300 U or more, such as for torticollis) have developed antibodies to the toxin. These antibodies block the effect of the toxin, making the patient resistant to further therapy. These antibodies have not produced hypersensitivity or anaphylaxis.

Overall, botulinum toxin injections for the management of hyperfunctional lower facial lines has been found to be extremely safe and useful, alone or in combination with other modalities. Patient satisfaction has been very high.

References

1. Blitzer A, Brin MF, Keen MS, Aviv JS. Botulinum toxin for the treatment of hyperfunctional lines of the face. Arch Otolaryngol Head Neck Surg 1993; 119:1018–23.

2. Keen MS, Blitzer A, Aviv JS, et al. Botulinum toxin A for hyperkinetic facial lines: results of a double-blind placebo controlled study. Plast Reconstr Surg 1994;94:94–9.

3. Blitzer A, Binder W, Aviv J, Keen M, Brin M. The management of hyperfunctional facial lines with botulinum toxin: a collaborative study of 210 injection sites in 162 patients. Arch Otolaryngol Head Neck Surg 1997;123:389–92.

4. Carruthers A, Carruthers J. Cosmetic uses of Botulinum toxin. In: Coleman WP, Hanke CW, Alt TH, et al., editors. Cosmetic surgery of the skin: principles and techniques. St Louis: Mosby;1997:231–5.

5. Blitzer A, Binder WJ, Brin MF. Botulinum toxin injections for facial lines and wrinkles. In: Blitzer A, Binder WJ, Boyd JB, Carruthers A, editors. Management of facial lines and wrinkles. Philadelphia: Lippincott William & Wilkins;1999:303–15.

6. Binder WJ, Blitzer A, Brin MF. Treatment of hyperfunctional lines of the face with botulin toxin A. Dermatol Surg 1998;24:1198–205.

7. Carruthers A, Carruthers J. Clinical indications and injection technique for the cosmetic use of botulinum A exotoxin. Dermatol Surg 1998;24: 1189–94.

8. Fulton JE. Botulinum toxin: the Newport Beach experience. Dermatol Surg 1998;24:1219–24.

9. Kane MA. Nonsurgical treatment of platysmal bands with injection of botulinum toxin A. Plast Reconstr Surg 1999;103:656–65.

10. Matarasso A, Matarasso SL, Brandt FS, Bellman B. Botulinum A exotoxin for the management of platysma bands. Plast Reconstr Surg 103:645–52.

11. Carruthers J, Carruthers A. Botulinum toxin and laser resurfacing for lines around the eyes. In: Blitzer A, Binder WJ, Boyd JB, Carruthers A, editors. Management of facial lines and wrinkles. Philadelphia: Lippincott William & Wilkins;1999:315–32.

COMBINATION TREATMENT (Nicholas J Lowe)

Indications	Potential combination treatments	Chapter reference
Forehead	Photoprotection	1
Glabellar	Topical therapy	2
Periorbital	Glycolic acid peels	6
Perioral	Combination peels	7
Lower face	Laser skin resurfacing	10,11
Neck lines	Non-ablative laser rejuvenation	12
Brow and	Chemical peels	7
upper eyelid	Dermal fillers	17,18
ptosis	Endoscopic brow lift	24
	Periorbital skin surgery	8
	Neck rejuvenation	25

16. Temporary dermal fillers – European experiences

Nicholas J Lowe

INTRODUCTION

Over the last 5 years an increasing variety of dermal fillers have been approved for use in Europe and several other countries around the world except for the USA. Most of these consist of various types of hyaluronic acid. These have been used to inject arthritic joints for several years.[1] More recently intradermal filler use has increased, and there are now other fillers in use such as polymerized lactic acid. Many of these newer fillers have had little clinical evaluation and safety testing.[2] Two of the hyaluronic acid fillers – Hylaform and Restylane – have recently been given Food and Drug Administration (FDA) approval for clinical testing in the USA. This chapter addresses the use of these currently non-USA approved dermal fillers; it is hoped that Hylaform and Restylane will be approved in the near future.

A filler that, by definition, produces no risk of allergy is autologous fat filler,[3] which is covered fully in chapter 17.

IDEAL PROPERTIES OF THE IDEAL TEMPORARY FILLER SUBSTANCE

- Non-allergenic
- Nonmigratory
- Wide margin of safety
- Long-lasting effect
- Corrects with a single treatment
- Injectable through a small-gauge needle
- Not detectable once in place

Unfortunately, currently no dermal filler exists that satisfies all of these criteria but it is suggested that some of the newer, longer-lasting hyaluronic acid fillers, such as Perlane, come close. The details of bovine collagen fillers will be covered in chapter 17. These are still the predominantly used temporary dermal fillers in the USA.

SPECIFIC HYALURONIC ACID FILLERS

There are two main types of hyaluronic filler that have been used widely in Europe since 1996, Hylaform™ (Genzyme, Innamed Santa Barbara CA) and Restylane™ (Q-Med Esthetics, Uppsala, Sweden).

Hylaform

Hylaform is a hyaluronic acid extract derived from rooster cones, a variant of this has been used extensively for injection of arthritic joints to provide an artificial sinovial fluid.[1] The Hylaform range has recently been expanded to include original Hylaform, Hylaform Fine and Hylaform Plus. Limited clinical data is needed on Hylaform.[4,5]

Restylane and Perlane

These are microbiologically engineered hyaluronic acid products that are produced by Q-Med Esthetics, Uppsala, Sweden.

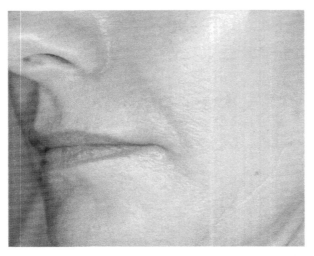

a

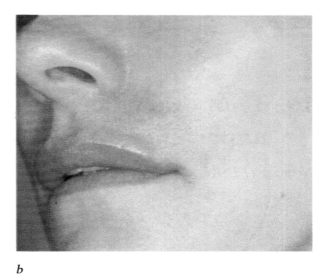

b

Figure 16.1 (A) Before Perlane to upper lip. (B) After Perlane to the nasolabial fold and upper lip.

Restylane is available in three different thicknesses, or viscosities. Restylane Fine is particularly useful for injections of the glabeller area and, if desired the periorbital area. In addition, Restylane Fine can be used as a layer on top of normal Restylane or Perlane. The Restylane 'Fine' line is approximately equivalent in use and persistence, to Zyderm[®] 1 collagen.

Normal Restylane[6] is approximately equivalent to Zyderm 2 in duration and viscosity, and is also very similar in duration and viscosity to Hylaform. The present author has had extensive experience with Hylaform and Restylane since 1996[5] and finds that the average duration of effect for lip augmentation is 3–4 months and for the nasolabial folds is between 9 and 12 months, i.e. very similar to Zyplast[®] collagen.[7]

Perlane is a more viscous version of normal Restylane and has some major advantages when used as filler for the lower face. It has much greater persistence of effect and, in a series of open observations, the present author has found that Perlane lasts up to 9 months or longer as a lip augmenting injection and up to 18 months as filler for the nasolabial folds.

Perlane has become the present author's most used temporary filler for the lower face and Restylane Fine filler of choice for the upper face. Hylaform is a very useful alternative to these should that be the patient's or physician's preference (Figure 16.1).[4–7]

Established hyaluronic acid fillers

- Hylaform
- Hylaform Fine
- Hylaform Plus
- Restylane
- Restylane Fine
- Perlane

INJECTION TECHNIQUE (Figures 16.2 and 16.3)

These agents are injected using a 30-gauge needle: the present author uses a 30-gauge needle other than for Perlane where better results are obtained with the 26 gauge needle supplied. The area has to be anaesthetized with either topical aesthetic creams, ice, injections of local anaesthetics or regional nerve blocks. As yet, none of these hyaluronic acid fillers contain any local anaesthetic.

Pain management: Hyaluronic acid fillers

For optimal patient satisfaction, follow these pain management tips:
- Use anaesthetic cream before the procedure
- Use ice before and during procedure
- Some patients need a dental block with lidocaine.

Inject with tunnelling and retrograde injection technique

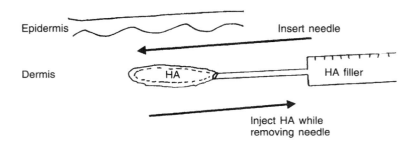

Figure 16.2 HA fillers.

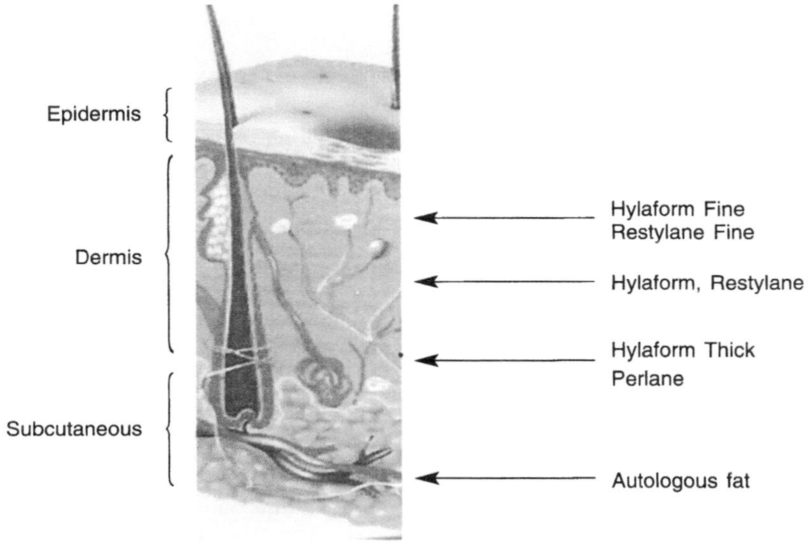

Figure 16.3 Sites for injecting HA fillers.

The 30 gauge needle is passed superficially in the high subdermal plane and, as the needle is slowly removed, the implant is injected into the tunnel created by the needle For Hylaform and Restylane. This gives far fewer injection sites than were previously described for Zyderm and Zyplast collagen technique.

For Perlane and Thick Hylaform a 26 gauge needle is similarly used but in the deeper dermis.

Proper injection

- Use at room temperature, not chilled
- For best results, inject the hyaluronic acid gel slowly
- The 'tunnel' or 'threading' technique is best used
- After injection, massage skin until the material conforms to surrounding contours
- Consider layering a further layer of Hylaform or Restylane over Perlane or Hylaform Thick for further refinement.

Proper technique for fine lines and wrinkles, superficial scars

- Inject material into the papillary dermis
- Insert needle to create a high dermal tunnel
- Inject the hyaluronic acid while withdrawing needle
- Particular care should be taken to avoid overcorrection in thin-skinned areas, e.g. around the eyes and mouth, where any degree of overcorrection is readily visible

---

Proper technique for deeper lines, wrinkles and scars

- Inject material in the mid-dermis (reticular layer)
- Follow, if needed, by a more superficial injection in the papillary level

Reactions to HA fillers		
Timescale	**Reaction**	**Intervention**
Immediate (transient – days)	• Hematoma • Erythema	• None necessary • Camouflage makeup

Delayed
(6–8 weeks)
(rare, 3 / < 700 1996–1999)
(fewer recent reactions seen since 1999)
	• Nodular inflammatory
	• Possibly more severe
	  with Hylaform
	• May last months
		• Intralesional
		  corticosteroid
		• Patience by patient
		  and physician

ADVERSE REACTIONS

Initially, it was hoped that the hyaluronic acid fillers would produce no delayed allergic reactions, but there is a small risk of delayed allergic reactions. There has

now been one case report[8] and a study of over 700 patients injected since 1996 with both Hylaform and Restylane.[5] Of these 100-plus patients, three developed nodular delayed reactions to both Hylaform and Restylane (Figures 16.4 to 16.8). These reactions occurred characteristically 6–8 weeks after injection. It was decided to perform intradermal skin testing on those patients with these reactions, eliciting a similar nodular skin reaction 6–8 weeks after the injection in all but one patient. Subsequently, there have been referrals of three other patients who developed these delayed adverse nodular reactions to both Restylane and Hylaform. Again, all but one of these patients showed positive results to the forearm challenge test (Figures 16.5 and 16.9).[2] (See Table 16.1.)

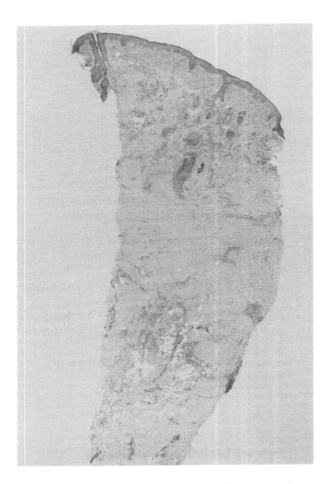

Figure 16.4 *Skin biopsy through a module on the face, which developed due to a delayed allergic reaction to Hylaform. A deep predominantly lymphohistiocystic and plasma cell infiltrate can be seen.*

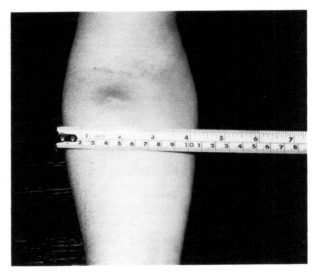

Figure 16.5 *The intradermal forearm challenge test: the positive nodule observed here developed 6 weeks after injection.*

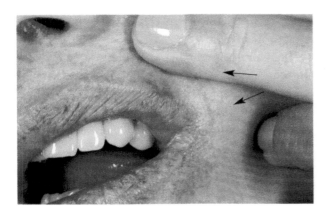

Figure 16.6 *A mild local delayed (6 weeks) reaction to Restylane.*

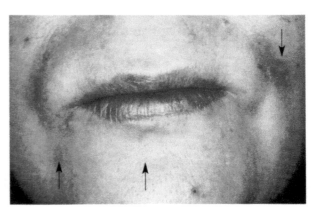

Figure 16.7 *An adverse reaction to Restylane, showing erythematous nodules that developed 6 weeks after injection.*

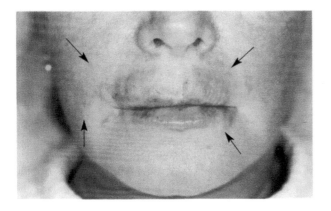

Figure 16.8 *An adverse reaction to Hylaform, showing widespread nodular inflammable reactions that started 8 weeks after injection.*

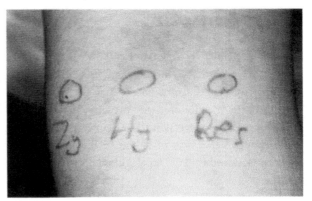

Figure 16.9 *Intradermal skin testing occsionally useful for HA fillers.*

Table 16.1 *Patients developing delayed skin reactions to hyaluronic acid fillers*

Patient*	Hylaform	Reaction sites	Severity	Onset post injection (weeks)	Time to clear	Therapy required	Skin test
1	Hylaform	Lips, glabellar	Severe	10	20 weeks	Yes	+ + to Hylaform, + to Restylane
2	Restylane	Lips, nasolabial	Moderate	7	16 weeks	Yes	– to Hylaform + to Restylane
3	Restylane	Lips	Mild	5	4 weeks	No	Negative to both Hylaform and Restylane
4	Hylaform	Lips, nasolabial	Severe, abscess, nodules	8	20 weeks	Yes	+ + + to Hylaform, – to Restylane
5	Hylaform	Lips, nasolabial	Severe, nodules	8	14 months	Yes	+ + to Hylaform, – to Restylane
6	Restylane	Nasolabial	Mild	5	8 weeks	No	Declined testing

* Patients 1–3 were author's patients (three out of 709 patients); patients 4–6 were referred patients.

Some problems with temporary fillers

- Zyderm/Zyplast
  3–4% delayed allergy skin testing required[9–12]
- Hylaform/Restylane
  Very rare delayed reactions
- Resoplast
  Skin testing required
- Alloderm, Cymera*, Dermologen*, Fascian[13]
  Human-derived tissues – possible viral, prior transmission

*Recently withdrawn in USA

PRETREATMENT SKIN TESTING IN HYALURONIC ACID

Due to the incidence of delayed reactions estimated as being of in the order of three out of 700-plus patients, at present it would seem unnecessary to recommend skin testing. Anecdotally, the present author began performing prospective skin testing on several hundred patients but in the light of failing to find any positive patient reaction this has been abandoned in his practice.

OTHER TEMPORARY FILLERS

Other temporary fillers include AcHyal, an hyaluronic acid filler manufactured by Tedec-Meiji Farma, Madrid. The present author has found this filler to be less as persistent than the Hylaform Restylane and Perlane fillers, and so has largely abandoned using this particular product. However, more controlled studies are needed.

In Europe, another recently promoted filler is New-Fill®. This is polymerized lactic acid filler that is manufactured by Biotech, Luxemburg. Some users suggestions that excellent results can be obtained. Current recommendations for this product are to inject on multiple occasions for optimum persistence.

Recent temporary fillers

- AcHyal
- New-Fill

Recent experiences with New-Fill show that with repeat injections there is a reasonably persistent

filling. It is suggested that this may be due to new collagen formation.

Therefore, in summary numerous temporary fillers are available in Europe, Canada and Australia, and in other countries such as South America and the Far East. The extensively used, tested fillers recommended are Hylaform, Restylane Fine, Restylane and Perlane.

A selection of available temporary filling substances in Europe (2002)

- Biodegradable/transient

Zyderm/Zyplast	Dermal graft
Resoplast	Fat
Alloderm	Fascian
Hylaform gel	Cymetra
Restylane	New-Fill
Perlane	Permaco
AcHyal	Plasmager
Hylan Roman gel	Reviderm intra

Perlane has become the present author's filler of preference for the lower face because of its much longer duration and also because of the relatively small risk of delayed allergic reactions.

Temporary problems that can occur with Hylaform, Restylane and Perlane include a transient erythema at the injected site, bruising, swelling, pain and nodularity if it is not injected with a smooth

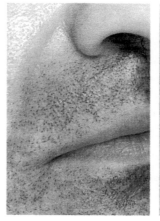 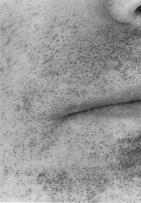

a   *b*

Figure 16.10 *(A) Deep nasolabial fold before treatment; (B) the same patient after injection of 1 cm³ of Hylaform.*

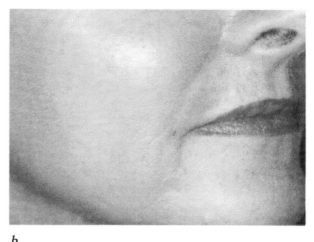
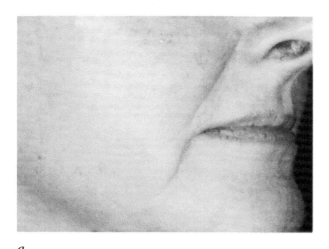

a   b

Figure 16.11 *Prominent nasolabial folds before (A) and after (B) Perlane injections. One syringe (0.7 cm³) to each nasolabial fold*

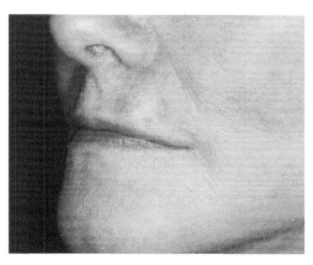
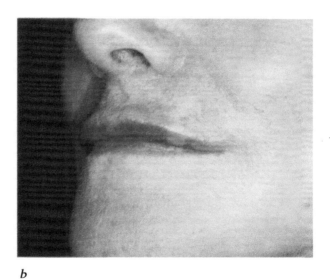

a   b

Figure 16.12 *(A) A thin upper lip before treatment; (B) the same patient after injection of one syringe (0.7cm³) of Perlane.*

technique. In fact, all of these fillers can be moulded between the finger and thumb for several days following injection if there is any lumpiness or nodule formation in the early stages following injection.

These fillers may also be combined with other approaches for the ageing face. These include the use of botulinum toxin A (BTX) together with fine Restylane, for deep glabellar folds, BTX A for perioral rhytides and BTX A together with Perlane or Hylaform for lip augmentation. In addition, careful placement of very small amounts of BTX A under

EMG guidance in the mid-face muscles zygomatic can also be used to reduce the depth of the nasolabial folds, which also results in the effects of injected Hylaform and Perlane lasting longer in these areas.

In most countries these fillers are listed as medical devices and can be released to the public and medical profession with little investigation. However, the present author suggests that further studies into the safety of the fillers and into their duration is required before approval.[2]

Combination approach for fillers

- Combination therapy examples:

  Fillers plus botulinum toxin
  Resurfacing plus fillers
  Non-ablative laser plus fillers

Autologous fat fillers

General
- Safe
- Effective
- Microlipoinjection, fresh or frozen
- Easily harvested
- No significant morbidity or complications
- Beware upper face – fat emboli and blindness reported.

Microlipoinjection: general

Microlipoinjection – syringe harvest method
- Low pressure harvest
- Harvest fresh with local anaesthesia
- Bank frozen (under controlled, labelled conditions at –40°C dedicated freezer)

Microlipoinjection: complications

- Hematoma
- Fat necrosis (too much injected)
- Infection
- Blindness following glabellar injection
- Cyst formation
- Transient correction
- Avoid upper face

In many respects, autologous fat is an ideal filler for most of the lower face, particularly the cheeks and nasolabial folds. Repeat injections of frozen (–40°C) fat is my practice. It is not generally useful for lip augmentation because of swelling, bruising and transient effects.

FUTURE TRENDS IN DERMAL FILLERS

An interesting and potentially exciting new trend is the use of Isolagen® (Isolagen Technologies, Inc., Houston, TX) as an autologous fibroblast derived skin rejuvenation system. Skin biopsies from patients are cultured and freeze-stored in a patented procedure. They can then be reactivated when needed to yield filler substances. Preliminary observations in the USA (Dr William Boss, personal communication) suggest long-term persistence of Isolagen cell implants for facial lines and scars. New studies are about to start in the UK and USA in 2002 with Isolagen.

WHICH PATIENTS BENEFIT FROM FILLERS?

> **Severity grades of nasolabial folds at rest as a guide for fillers**
>
> Grade 1 None
> 2 Minimal
> 3 Mild
> 4 Moderate
> 5 Severe
> 6 Very severe   *Lowe NJ, 2001*

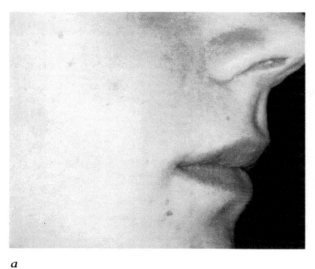
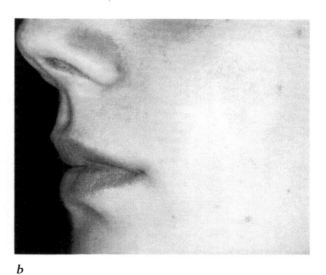

a   *b*

Figure 16.13 *Grade 1. No visible nasolabial folds. No filler required.*

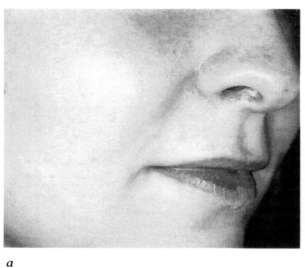
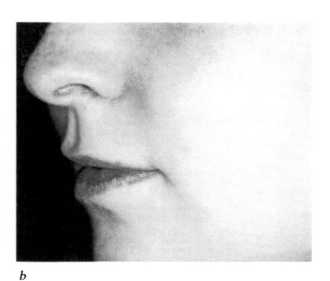

a   *b*

Figure 16.14 *Grade 2. Minimal nasolabial folds. Small amounts of Perlane or Hylaform may be considered, but really not needed.*

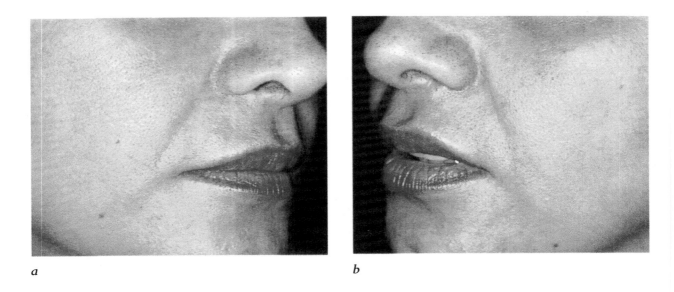

a   b

Figure 16.15 Grade 3. Mild nasolabial folds: patient may be offered Perlane or Hylaform Plus.

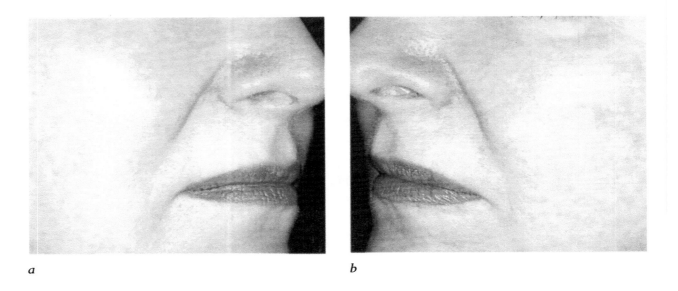

a   b

Figure 16.16 Grade 4. Moderate nasolabial folds. Candidate for Perlane, Hylaform Plus or fat. Could be offered UltraSoft.

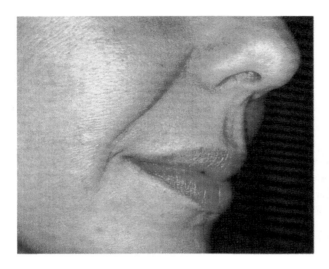 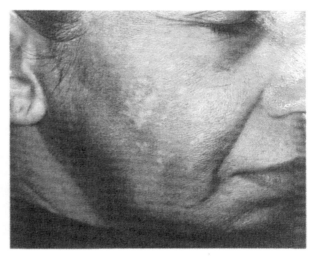

Figure 16.17 Grade 5. Severe nasolabial folds. Candidate for Perlane, Hylaform Plus or fat transfer. Other option UltraSoft implant.

Figure 16.18 Grade 6. Very severe nasolabial folds. Will need large amounts of Perlane, Hylaform Plus or fat. May be offered UltraSoft implant plus above fillers with a second UltraSoft implant later.

References

1 Wright KE, Maurer SG, Di Cesare PE. Viscosupplementation for osteoarthritis. Am J Orthop 2000 Feb;29(2):80–0.

2 Lowe NJ. Editorial: On the need for greater regulation of medical devices. J Cutan Laser Ther 2000;2:1–2.

3 Coleman SR. Facial recontouring with lipostructure. Clin Plast Surg 1997;24:347–67.

4 Piacquadio D, Jarcho M, Goltz R. Evalution of hylan b gel as a soft tissue augmentation implant material. J Am Acad Dermatol 1997;36:544–9.

5 Lowe NJ, Maxwell CA, Lowe PL, et al. Hyaluronic acid skin fillers: adverse reactions and skin testing. J Am Acad Dermatol 2001;45:930–3.

6 Olenius M. The first clinical study using a new biodegradable implant for the treatment of lips, wrinkles, and folds. Aesthetic Plast Surg 1998;22:97–101.

7 Manna F, Detini M, Desideri P, et al. Comparative chemical evaluation of two commercially available derivatives of hyaluronic acid (Hylaform from rooster combs and Restylane from Streptococcus) used for soft tissue augmentation. J Eur Acad Dermatol Venereol 1999;13:183–92.

7 Tromovitch TA, Stegman SJ, Glogau RG. Zyderm collagen: implantation technics J Am Acad Dermatol 1984;10:273–8.

8 Lupton JR, Alster T.S. Cutaneous hypersensitivity reaction to injectable hyaluronic acid gel. Dermatol Surg 2000;26:135–7.

9 Klein AW. In favor of double testing. J Dermatol Surg Oncol 1989;15:263.

10 Hanke CW, Higley HR, Jolivette DM, et al. Abscess formation and local necrosis after treatment with Zyderm or Zyplast collagen implant. J Am Acad Dermatol 1991;25:319–26.

11 Framer FM, Churukium MM. Clinical use of injectable collagen. A three year retrospective review. Arch Otolaryngol 1984;110:93–98.

12 Cooperman LS, Mackinnon V, Bechler G, Pharriss BB. Injectable collagen: a six year clinical investigation. Aesthetic Plast Surg 1985;9:145–151.

13 Fagien S. Facial soft tissue augmentation with injectable autologous and allogeneic human tissue collagen matrix (autologen and dermalogen). Plast Reconstr Surg 2000;105:362–73.

COMBINATION TREATMENT (Nicholas J Lowe)

Indications	Potential combination treatments	Chapter reference
Upper and lower facial lines	BTX-A and B	13,14,15
Lip augmentation	BTX-A and B	14,15
	Laser resurfacing	10,12
Atrophic scar filler	Non-ablative laser	13
	Microdermabrasion	7
	Chemical peels	7
	Photoprotection	1
	Topical therapy	2

17. Temporary dermal fillers – USA experiences

Arnold William Klein

INTRODUCTION

At the turn of the twenty-first century cosmetic enhancement has become an acceptable path for our health-conscious, energetic and fit population, who would prefer the mirror to reflect an image more in tune with how they feel internally. Baby boomers are now reaching the age where their once youthful bodies are starting to show the signs of wear and tear so common in the middle-aged group. Hair is thinning, and wrinkles, stomachs, thighs and love handles are ever more prominent. The leisure time of the 1980s and 1970s, spent in the sun in search of the healthy tan, has taken its toll. People are living longer and obviously want to look good and remove the damage both the sun and time have produced. Naturally, one of the most common reasons for patients to seek cosmetic surgery is for the aging face and the treatment of facial rhytides, the face being the part of the body most seen by others. Next to the hands, the face is typically the most reliable way to determine a person's age.

One of the consequences of time, smoking, the sun and gravity is a loss of dermal collagen in the skin, resulting in wrinkles. These wrinkles tend to appear rather early on facial skin and individuals are inundated with media reports extolling the virtues of creams, injections and surgery to erase these telltale signs of their advancing age. Age-related changes of the lips and mouth include atrophy of both the upper and lower lips, actinic changes of the mucosal surface and vermilion border, and atrophy at the corners of the mouth, causing a downturn of the corners of the

mouth and a resultant aged appearance. Subtle improvements in the lips and their surrounding structures can produce astounding results, rebuilding the perioral structure and regaining a more youthful, rested visage. Another of the earliest signs of aging is an increase in prominence of the nasolabial folds. This, too, is one of the most important areas to be treated with filler substances in order to obtain the aesthetic results sought. But is cosmetic enhancement something new or is it simply something that is now allowed to be uttered publicly?

In reality, the field of soft-tissue augmentation has a long and colorful history, dating back to the late 1800s. Over the years, many implantable substances and devices have been utilized to cosmetically enhance soft-tissue defects and deficiencies. Injectable fat is the oldest material used for tissue augmentation.[1–7] More than 100 years ago, Neuber,[1] in Germany, reported on results from small adipose grafts transplanted for reconstruction of a soft-tissue defect on the face. In the early part of the last century, free-fat grafts were used for tissue augmentation. Subsequently, the use of injectable paraffin became quite popular during the early 1900s. However, it became evident that the injection of paraffin and other oils was associated with a high incidence of undesirable foreign body granuloma formation. In the USA and Europe, the use of paraffin for soft-tissue augmentation was largely abandoned prior to 1920. However, in the Orient, the subcutaneous injection of paraffin was still widely in use well into the 1960s.[8,9]

On the other hand, the injection of some substances, such as pure injectable-grade liquid silicone, while historically extremely useful and beneficial in the skilled hands of certain experienced physicians, has not been approved by the Food and Drug Administration (FDA) and is not available to the practitioner. In fact, in certain states it is illegal.

In the mid-1970s another change occurred. Were there minimally invasive 'minor' procedures and topical agents that could and would produce an improved cosmetic appearance when utilized? The answer was a resounding yes. First, with the introduction of Retin-A, an acidic derivative of vitamin A, it became apparent that there were agents that individuals could use at home to really improve their appearance. Subsequently, bovine collagen became approved as an 'in-and-out' office procedure in the 1980s and minimally invasive cosmetic enhancement began. Indeed, the first injection of collagen into the lip for cosmetic enhancement in 1984 could be described as the shot seen around the world.

Soft-tissue augmentation has become increasingly important as more individuals seek aesthetic improvement without major surgical procedures. Filler substances are indispensable tools to be used when treating the face as stand-alone treatment or in conjunction with laser resurfacing, botulinum toxin and chemical peels. The difficulty comes in choosing the proper treatment techniques and meeting patient expectations. Soft-tissue augmentation has seen a renaissance of interest as an increasing number of patients seek aesthetic improvement without major down time. Why this renewal of interest in filling agents? One huge reason is the availability of Botox® (Allergan, Inc., Irvine, CA), which works superbly in the upper face. Botox has revolutionized many aspects of facial cosmetic surgery and has rapidly become an indispensable tool in the fight against the ravages of time and sun. It is certainly the best advice that can be given to patients now that this terrific treatment is available for the glabellar complex. It not only corrects the problem for the majority of patients but simultaneously also treats the root cause of the rhytide, i.e. the dynamic movement of muscles, usually preventing further progression. This accomplishment of rejuvenating the upper face using Botox has created a need for agents that work equally well in the lower face. Another reason for this renewed interest is the

concept of the three-dimensional face. The youthful face has a much fuller look, not a pulled flat, two-dimensional look. This has become one of the central tenets of the field of soft-tissue augmentation. Filling can augment and even, at times, replace pulling. In addition, subtle lip enhancement is something that is here to stay. In fact, it is the number one indication for injectable fillers.

There are two basic types of wrinkles (rhytides) – dynamic and static.[10] Dynamic rhytides are caused by the action of the muscles and include glabellar, crow's-feet, nasolabial (in part) and forehead wrinkles. Static rhytides are caused by exogenous sources, such as smoking, gravity and sun. Dynamic and static wrinkles can be seen together in areas such as the forehead and cheeks. Dynamic rhytides and others with a combination etiology in the upper one third of the face are normally best treated by botulinum toxin injections.

The choice of an appropriate implant, whether solid or injectable, requires a thorough understanding of the materials available and the etiology of the wrinkle. Fine, superficial rhytides respond best to therapy at the intradermal level. Deeper, more substantial wrinkles typically have a subcutaneous component, with or without a facial muscular element, and are best approached from the subcutaneous space. Often a wrinkle will have both a superficial and deep component, such as the nasolabial fold, and both of these components need to be addressed to obtain optimal results.

Since the earliest experiments with paraffin in 1899, physicians have searched for an ideal bioinjectable material. No matter the origins of implant material, there are important qualities necessary for achieving the goals of a given procedure while minimizing potential adverse effects.[11,12] Though no currently available implant possesses all of these attributes, many options exist that are adequate for a given task, satisfy patients and offer excellent safety profiles. The search for the perfect material to eradicate rhytides, smooth scars and fill traumatic defects continues. New products appear, sometimes with great fanfare, which often fail to fulfill the promise of a better alternative to what is currently in use. There is now a whole host of products and techniques available. What are they and are they of value? Today, physicians have a much larger armamentarium of techniques and material with which to improve facial contours, ameliorate wrinkles and stall the telltale signs of the aging face.

Bovine collagen has become the gold standard of injectable fillers and it is the material against which newer materials are evaluated.[13] Collagen has been used successfully since the early 1980s to fill in the fine lines and wrinkles associated with aging. Collagen is a suspension of bovine collagen fibrils from which the more antigenic end portions of the molecules have been removed.

Fat has been used as an injectable agent since the turn of the twentieth century. Its use was reborn with the advent of liposuction in the 1980s (as an answer to the question of what to do with all the stuff they were sucking out). Fat is used at a much deeper level in the skin than collagen and is applicable for gross correction; it will not correct fine defects. There is a vast difference in results between the use of fresh (recently removed) fat and frozen fat, in that the former provides a much longer duration of correction.

Botox® (Allergan Inc, Irvine, CA) is the new 'magic potion' of cosmetic enhancement. It is a very dilute solution of botulinum A toxin, the same material as that developed for chemical warfare. However, in the dose used for cosmetic procedures there is absolutely no danger to the patient. Botox is used to selectively denervate and relax the muscles in the upper face that cause frown lines, forehead lines and crow's-feet. Over the first few days following its injection, as the muscles relax, the lines 'magically' disappear. When used in the upper face, and in conjunction with collagen in the lower face, remarkable results can be obtained in removing the effects of aging and in providing a more youthful, rested appearance of the face. Botox is the greatest advance in the minimally invasive treatment of the aging face to come along in the last 10 years. It is definitely a home-run in the upper one third of the face and has reawakened interest in other fillers for use in the lower face.[14]

Hyaluronic acid derivatives are products which, in gel form, can be used for soft-tissue augmentation. They have become very popular in Australia, Europe, the UK and Canada, especially for augmentation of the lips. There have been some reports of occasional redness at the injection site. Unfortunately, they are currently not approved for use in the USA.

Manufactured human collagen is a product that is not yet on the market, although an announcement has recently been made of some success in the development of this material. Its use would obviate the need for skin testing such as is done for bovine collagen.

Currently, in the USA, although many materials and substances are available, the most commonly utilized injectable filling agents are autologous fat and Zyderm® or Zyplast® collagen (McGhan Corp, Santa Barbara, CA), with injectable bovine collagen being the single most popular substance used for soft-tissue augmentation.

The duration of correction with any injectable filling substance depends on multiple factors. Implantation technique, the amount implanted, the type of defect and mechanical stresses at the implantation sites all influence persistence of correction.

Natural materials for soft-tissue augmentation include human autografts and allografts, as well as xenografts derived from animals. Autografts are materials harvested from a patient for use only in that individual. There is no risk of rejection and no risk of nosocomial viral or retroviral infection as from human allografts or animal xenografts. Disadvantages include donor site morbidity and limited available quantity, as well as resorption of implanted material. Commonly used autografts include fat and dermis. Semisynthetic implants include human-derived materials, as well as animal-derived materials; the latter category also includes bioengineered molecules that mimic natural ones. With new technological advances, the distinction between these categories is becoming obscured; however, synthetic substances are chemically distinct from those found in human tissue.

Ten years ago, a list of temporary, injectable fillers may have contained five substances but now a veritable cornucopia of agents are available to the practitioner (Table 17.1). Determining the defect will define the substance to be used, e.g. for a very deep defect fat will work but a more superficial defect will require use of Zyderm I or II, and a mid-dermal defect will need a material like Zyplast.

Physicians should counsel patients as to the risks and benefits of injectable substance therapy. Each physician should inform prospective patients about skin testing, the treatment procedure and treatment expectations.

Table 17.1. *Temporary injectable filling agents*

Ac Hyal	Hylaform gel
Arteplast	Hylan Rofilan gel
Autologen	Koken atelocollagen
Botox	Meta-Crill
Cymetra	Newfill
Dermalive	Perlane
Dermalogen	Permacol
Endoplast-50	Profill
Fascian	Recombinant human collagen
Fat	Resoplast
Subcutaneous microlipoinjection	Restylane
Lipocytic dermal augmentation	Restylane-fine
Fibroquel	Reviderm intra
Human placental collagen	Zyderm and Zyplast collagen

ZYDERM AND ZYPLAST COLLAGEN

The normal human dermis is composed of collagen proteins, the most abundant proteins in the human body. Collagen proteins are trimers involving three individual polypeptide chains known as alpha-chains. About 96% of the collagen molecule is helical and these helices are attached to non-helical telopeptides at the amino and carboxy ends. The different types of collagens are each different combinations of alpha-chains. Normal dermal collagen is c. 80% type I collagen and 20% type III collagen. In the human body, similar to secretory proteins, collagen is synthesized in the rough endoplasmic reticulum, modified in the Golgi apparatus and transported to the cell surface where it is secreted as procollagen. The non-helical telopeptide bonds are broken by specific peptidases extracellularly. The collagen molecules then crosslink to form collagen fibrils that then associate to form collagen fibers. Collagen is broken down by specific extracellular collagenases.[8,15]

In 1958, at the Harvard Medical School, Gross and Kirk[16] showed that, under physiologic conditions, a solid gel could be produced by gently warming a solution of collagen to body temperature. In the 1960s, it was found that selective removal of the non-helical amino and carboxy terminal telopeptides significantly reduced the antigenicity of collagen molecules.[17,18] In the early 1970s a team of investigators at Stanford University began work on the development of a clinically useful collagen implant material.[19] This work led Knapp et al.[20] to report on the successful injection of pepsin-solubilized, telopeptide-poor, purified human, rabbit and rat collagen into the subcutaneous tissue of rats. They studied the evolution of the implants over 152 days and reported that the collagen implants remained as a stable graft and were progressively infiltrated by a matrix of viable host connective tissue. The same investigators later conducted an initial trial of human and bovine collagen in 28 human patients, with a 50–85% improvement that was maintained for 3–18 months.[13]

Proceeding from these results, Zyderm collagen was developed by the Collagen Corporation and was tested initially by 14 investigators in 1977–1978. Subsequently, in 1979, the product became widely available to interested physicians in the USA under a Phase III protocol. This was called the Zyderm Clinical Verification Program and had 728 physician participants. In 1980, Stegman and Tromovitch,[21] who were among the initial 14 investigators in the California Cooperative Study Group, reported on the use of Zyderm collagen in the correction of depressed acne and other scars. Subsequently, participants in the full Clinical Verification Program reported on their experience in 5109 patients who underwent testing and subsequent treatment with injectable Zyderm collagen. What became apparent from this study was the superb application this product had for correcting age-related rhytides. Among these 5109 patients, 3.0% developed positive test responses and 1.3% developed transient localized adverse reactions.[22]

In July 1981, after 6.5 years of development, clinical trials and testing, Zyderm Collagen Implant ultimately received FDA approval. This was the first time an injectable xenogenic agent was FDA approved for soft-tissue augmentation. This approval reawakened interest in the entire field of filling agents and, since then, an estimated 1,900,000 individuals worldwide have received injectable collagen implants. Following the approval of the first injectable form, Zyderm I Collagen Implant (ZC-I), the FDA approved two additional formulations, Zyderm II Collagen Implant (ZC-II) and Zyplast Collagen

Implant (ZP). Additionally, a special packaging of ZC-I that contains a 32-gauge needle has been made available (Zyderm I with Fine Gauge Needle; Z-FGN); the barrel of the syringe for this product is specifically suited for use with the supplied 32-gauge, metal-hub needle. Nevertheless, since 32-gauge metal-hub needle are easily affixed to the other ZC-I syringes, some individuals have found this packaging unnecessary.

Zyderm collagen implants ZC-I, ZC-II and ZP are all sterile, purified fibrillar suspensions of bovine dermal collagen. Processing of the material involves purification, pepsin digestion and sterilization. Pepsin digestion removes the more antigenic end portions of the bovine collagen molecule (the telopeptides) without disturbing the natural helical structure. This is critical for the resulting agent to be more immunologically compatible with the human host. Furthermore, the preservation of the helical structure is thought to contribute to substantivity of the product upon implantation. Zyderm collagen implants are all 95–98% type I collagen, with the remainder being type III.[23] The products are suspended in phosphate-buffered physiologic saline containing 0.3% lidocaine. It should be noted that these substances are all taken from the skin of a closed American herd, negating the possibility of contamination with the bovine spongiform encephalopathy virus or prion.[24]

ZC-I, the original material, and ZC-II differ only in concentration: ZC-I is 3.5% by weight bovine collagen whereas ZC-II (introduced in 1983) is 6.5% by weight bovine collagen. ZP, approved in 1985, is the third form of implantable collagen. In ZP, bovine dermal collagen is lightly crosslinked by the addition of 0.0075% glutaraldehyde. Glutaraldehyde crosslinks by producing covalent bridges between 10% of available lysine residues of the bovine collagen molecule. These bridges are intramolecular and intermolecular, as well as between fibrils, resulting in a more robust implant that is essentially an injectable latticework of bovine collagen.[25] As a result of this crosslinkage, ZP is more resistant to proteolytic degradation and less immunogenic.[25,26] Furthermore, the more substantive nature of ZP makes it applicable for deeper contour defects unresponsive to ZC-I or ZC-II.[27,28]

All the products are provided in preloaded syringes that are stored at a low temperature (4°C)

so that the dispersed fibrils remain fluid and small. This allows passage of the products through small-gauge needles. Once implanted, the human body temperature causes the products to undergo consolidation into a solid gel as intermolecular crosslinking occurs in the injected suspension with the generation of a high proportion of larger fibrils.[8] Obviously, Zyplast, which is already chemically crosslinked, probably could not be expected to undergo in vivo crosslinking to the extent of the other products.

Proper patient screening and, especially, skin testing are of the utmost importance in the application of bovine collagen therapy. Individuals who have lidocaine sensitivity, a history of an anaphylactoid event or previous sensitivity to bovine collagen are excluded from testing and treatment. Physicians must counsel patients as to the risks and benefits of injectable collagen therapy. Each physician must inform prospective patients about skin testing, the treatment procedure and treatment expectations. The safety and contraindications of the various injectable collagen formulations have been described elsewhere.[25-28]

Potential allergenicity to injectable collagen is reliably determined by skin testing. Using only one third of the test syringe's contents, the dose is administered in a tuberculin manner in the volar forearm. The site is evaluated at 48–72 hours and again at 4 weeks. A positive skin test is defined as swelling, induration, tenderness or erythema that persists or occurs 6 hours or longer after test implantation. This is a definite contraindication to treatment and patients exhibiting any of these responses are excluded from therapy. A positive skin-test response will be seen in 3.0–3.5% of individuals. Seventy per cent of these reactions will become manifest in 48–72 hours, indicating a pre-existing allergy to bovine collagen.[26,29] Thus, it is imperative to observe the test site at 48–72 hours as well as at the standard 4-week interval. Most authorities now recommend a second test as an additional precaution.[13,30,31] This can be placed in the contralateral forearm or the periphery of the face. It is administered either 2 weeks after the initial test with treatment commencing at 4 weeks after initial testing, or 4 weeks after the initial test with treatment commencing 6 weeks after the first test. The volume utilized for the second test is the same as that used for the first test and, again, skin-test syringes are employed. Since the majority of treatment-associated hypersensitivity reactions occur shortly after the first treatment, double testing greatly reduces the frequency of this most undesirable sequela by changing the first treatment exposure to a second test exposure. Additionally, treatment-associated hypersensitivity reactions that occur after two negative skin tests tend, in general, to be milder, indicating that, possibly, the physician has selected out the most severely allergic individuals. Single retesting of individuals who have not been treated for > 1 year or who were successfully tested or treated elsewhere is strongly recommended. After retesting, a minimum of 2 weeks is recommended for test-site evaluation before commencing treatment.

Injection technique is the single most important factor in the successful application of bovine collagen implants. Tangential halogen lighting is very beneficial because this will often reveal even the subtlest contour defects. Also, magnification greatly increases the precision of injection. The treating physician must remember that the ability to properly implant collagen is an evolutionary process that will improve with experience. Zyderm collagen is implanted in the superficial dermis by serial punctures of the skin with syringes prefilled with the material. With ZC-I, a 30- or 32- gauge needle is used. For extraordinarily fine defects, a 33-gauge needle may be employed. With ZC-II, a 30-gauge needle is necessary in that its viscous nature prevents its use with a 32-gauge needle.

ZC-I is the most versatile of all forms of injectable collagen. It is also the most technique sensitive and the most forgiving. Since it is not crosslinked, it has good flow characteristics. When placed correctly, it will smoothly fill superficial defects. The physician prepares to inject the treatment site by holding it taut between the thumb and forefinger of the non-injecting hand. Next, the needle tip is guided horizontally with the bevel down along the skin surface until it barely penetrates the skin. The hub of the needle is then rocked gently over the thumb of the opposing hand, tenting up the skin with the needle tip and a flow of material is created in the upper dermis as a smooth, yellowish mass that is both wide and flat and not three-dimensional in appearance. With ZC-I, an upper dermal flow is created by applying each subsequent injection at the leading edge of the previously injected volume. This continuous, wide and flat flow

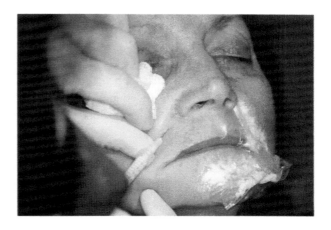

Figure 17.1 *Injection of Zyderm collagen into the nasolabial fold.*

of ZC-I in the upper dermis smoothly augments the applicable soft-tissue defect, thereby providing the most cosmetically pleasing results (Figure 17.1). While persistent beading and overcorrection can be problematic with superficial placement of ZC-II, they are rarely associated with ZC-I therapy.

ZC-II requires greater mechanical force to inject and one must always remember that it undergoes less condensation upon implantation, leaving c. 60% of the injected material at the implantation site, compared to ZC-I, which leaves 30%. As superficial as possible placement of ZC-I and ZC-II is no longer employed, and nor is excessive overcorrection, in that persistent whiteness at the injection site and elevation can be observed with overcorrection.[32,33] However, a slight degree of overcorrection (10–20%) should still be sought when injecting ZC-I and ZC-II. ZC-II is useful for deep acne scars and deep glabellar furrows. Additionally, when certain defects that normally respond to ZC-I are unresponsive, ZC-II can be successfully employed. Techniques for injection with ZC-II are almost identical to those outlined above for ZC-I. While the present author rarely employs ZC-II, some individuals almost certainly find ZC-II a very useful adjunct to soft-tissue augmentation.

ZP is the most robust form of injectable bovine collagen presently approved for use in the USA. Two attributes – the rigid crosslinked structure and the absence of microfibrils – greatly affect the rheology of this product and account for the decreased ability to smoothly flow of this material. The resistance often felt whilst implanting ZP may be explained by these characteristics, as well as possibly the density of the mid-dermal implantation site. In the utilization of ZP, a 30-gauge needle is employed to create a mid-dermal flow of material, again using a serial puncture technique. ZP should be placed neither too superficially nor in the subdermal space. In the former situation it will result in persistent overcorrection with beading, and in the latter one large amounts of material will be required for correction and improvement will be short-lived. With ZP, the syringe is held at a 10–20° angle during the injection process and the material placed slightly deeper than with ZC-I or ZC-II. While implanting ZP the resistance of the dermal matrix is felt against the injecting hand and the plane of the injected site should elevate as the material is being placed. Deliberate overcorrection should be avoided in that the material undergoes little syneresis or condensation upon implantation. It should be noted that some individuals prefer a 90° angle for ZP implantation. If a 90° angle is chosen, only the needle tip should penetrate the skin with numerous serial punctures. While the manufacturer has offered the adjustable depth gauge (ADG) to improve the accuracy of Zyplast implantation, the present author has not found it to increase technical accuracy. Additionally, the practice of molding or massaging ZP after implantation for an improved cosmetic result remains unsubstantiated and could result in the rapid loss of correction as the material is forced into the subdermal space.

The simultaneous use of two products can often provide increased longevity of correction and improved aesthetic results. This is a 'layering' technique, wherein ZC-I or ZC-II is immediately implanted over Zyplast injection sites. Although Botox has become extremely popular for the reduction of wrinkles and lines in the upper third of the face, its application in the lower two thirds is more problematic and collagen implantation is still the treatment of choice. Collagen can also be used in concert with Botox in the upper face to achieve optimal results, e.g. deep glabellar furrows, lower forehead lines and the like.

Full correction can be achieved at one visit if enough material is employed. Correction with all forms of bovine collagen is temporary and requires periodic maintenance at 4- to 12-month intervals.[27]

For all etiologies, 30% of individuals report 18 month longevity of correction, while 70% require touch-up treatments at intervals of 3–12 months. Glabellar frown lines and acne scars appear to retain correction the longest. Indeed, correction with all forms of bovine collagen appears to be lost as the material is displaced in the human from its site of implantation in the dermis into the subcutaneous space.[34] Animal studies using ZC-I and ZP have suggested recipient collagen production after implantation:[35,36] this gradual colonization has been most marked with the use of ZP. In the human, while histologic studies of ZP, as opposed to ZC-I or ZC-II, have revealed some deposition of host collagen, there is no convincing evidence that this deposition contributes to longevity of correction.[37,38] In humans, histologic studies with both ZC-I and ZP have also evidenced excellent biocompatibility with minimal inflammation at sites of implantation.

Indications for ZC-I or ZC-II include horizontal forehead lines, glabellar lines, crow's-feet, nasolabial lines, fine lip lines, marionette lines, shallow acne scars, excisional scars and the like.[27,34–36] Soft, distensible superficial defects and lines are most amenable to ZC-I and ZC-II. Deep nasolabial folds, marionette grooves, deep acne scars and the like respond best to ZP, with or without ZC-I or ZC-II overlay. ZP is also best suited to resurface the vermilion border between the lip and skin for lip enhancement. Additionally, true 'mucosal' injection of ZC-I, ZC-II and ZP is often employed in the lip enhancement process, though the mucosal location is not an FDA-approved site for collagen implantation. ZP is not recommended for use in the glabellar frown lines.[33] Many articles in the literature provide a more detailed discussion of the various indications for ZCI-I, ZCI-II and ZP.[27,33,34]

Adverse treatment responses to injectable collagen can be divided into non-hypersensitive and hypersensitive. Non-hypersensitive reactions include bruising, reactivation of herpetic eruptions and bacterial infection. Additionally, local necrosis due to vascular interruption at the treatment site has been noted with ZP and rarely with ZC-I or ZC-II.[39] In that 56% of these locally necrotic events occur in the glabellar area, physicians are cautioned against using ZP at this site. If, upon injection, a physician notes severe blanching of the area and pain, they should immediately stop injecting because local necrosis has possibly occurred.

The value of massage, warm compresses or nitro-glycerin gel in this situation is, as yet, unsubstantiated. Two reports of partial vision loss after Zyderm collagen therapy have been noted, most likely the result of an occlusive event involving the retinal artery.[40,41] These serious consequences of a cosmetic procedure underscore the need to remember that the dermal site is the proper locale for collagen implantation.

Treatment-associated hypersensitivity reactions to bovine collagen implants are, for the most part, cosmetic and consist of redness and swelling at the treatment site. Rarely, mild systemic symptoms can accompany these reactions. Hypersensitive reactions are almost uniformly associated with anti-Zyderm antibodies,[42,43] which do not cross-react with human collagen.[44,45] 'Cyst–abscess' formation is a rare but severe hypersensitivity response occurring in 4 out of 10 000 treated individuals.[39] Clinically, individuals develop painful, swollen cysts at the sites of treatment. These reactions are usually associated with ZP and rarely ZC-I or ZC-II; 86% of these individuals have associated antibovine antibodies. Incision and drainage, as well as intralesional steroids, have been advocated to manage this most undesirable sequela. This is a long-lasting, severe hypersensitive response that can persist for > 2 years. It should be noted that analysis of extruded material from these abscesses has revealed bovine collagen implant. As to the possibility of bovine collagen inducing connective tissue disease in the human host, retrospective studies, as well as an expert panel convened by the FDA, have found no supporting evidence.[45]

The application of bovine collagen in the circum-oral area is the largest single indication for which these products are used. Thus, an in-depth discussion of the use of bovine collagen as a tool for cosmetic enhancement in this area is warranted. The aging process of the mouth is often associated with the development of circumoral radial grooves, as well as a loss of the three-dimensional aspects of the lips themselves. Therefore, even a small volumetric increase in the size of the lips in selected individuals can produce a most pleasing cosmetic result. Lip augmentation will thus address both the age-related contour loss found in the lips and, by enhancing their size, the radial grooves. Furthermore, lips themselves are the cornerstone of the aesthetic appeal of both the female and male face. Lip enhancement thus

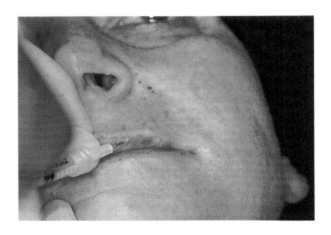

Figure 17.2 *Injection of Zyderm collagen into the lip.*

encompasses both the correctional age-related changes and cosmetic psychosocial improvement. As indicated previously, it should be remembered that, while injection into the glabrous skin surrounding the lips is an FDA-approved indication, mucosal injection is an off-label use (Figure 17.2). One must be sure to counsel the patient regarding the cost as well as the frequent maintenance that is initially required. While various authors have advocated the use of nerve blocks in association with this augmentation, others have unexpectedly found implantation more difficult and the result aesthetically less pleasing when nerve blocks are performed.

A review of the procedure of lip augmentation by six investigators revealed that the best results were achieved by first injecting ZP in the potential space between the lip mucosa and skin (along the vermil-ion border) in the upper and lower lip. This was then followed by ZC-I and ZP directly into the mucosa itself. Remember that the major vascular supply to the lips runs in the mucosa and blind injections of ZP into this area will occasionally result in vascular events, especially after the lips are repeatedly treated. The ideal technique for lip enhancement is variable and is certainly not uniform between physicians or even from patient to patient. Nevertheless, what is outlined below is a basic technique from which the practitioner can individualize. Before the process is begun, both the patient and the physician must be aware that this is a less than painless procedure. First, ZP must be placed in the potential space of the lip.

Initial injection is begun at the right corner of the lower lip. While injecting, the lip is held taut with the thumb of the opposing hand slightly stretching the lip posteriorly from the corner of the mouth. Anterior to the opposing thumb, the potential space at the right corner is entered with ZP, utilizing a 30-gauge needle at an angle of c. 75° from the lip surface with the syringe held parallel to the lower lip. Once the treating physician feels the needle tip drop into the potential space the injection angle is changed to c. 45° from the lip and the flow of material begun across the lower lip in the potential space. If a spot is reached where the material will not easily advance, go to this spot and inject onward from this locale. A smooth yellowish flow of ZP is desired in the potential space and not whitish lumps.

The vermilion potential space of the lower lip should be injected right corner to center and left corner to center. It is very important to place sufficient ZP in the lateral sites of the lower lip in that this will 'lift' the mouth. In the upper lip, the potential space can be entered as in the lower lip, though some individuals prefer to enter the space centrally and inject center to left corner and then center to right corner. This latter approach will preserve the patient's natural cupid's bow. Once outlined, the lip can be further enhanced by placing ZP, ZC-I to ZC-II in the mucosa. All are flowed at this site in a manner similar to that used at other locales. It has been the present author's experience that, after repeated injections, the augmentation process in the lip begins to 'hold', possibly as a result of subtle fibroplasia, and touch-ups are only necessary two or three times a year.

Injectable collagens (ZC-I, ZC-II and ZP) are tools that provide a physician with a manner in which to approach mild contour defects, i.e. defects that signify the aging process or the end result of scarring events. They are a temporary, biocompatible solution to many, but certainly not all, soft-tissue deficiencies. The adverse reaction profile is of an acceptably low level and, indeed, only of local significance. Nevertheless, for both the physician and patient to benefit from these agents, effective reproducible implantation technique(s) must be developed by the treating physician. As the physician's experience with these agents increases, so will their ability to produce aesthetically pleasing results.

BOTULINUM TOXIN
(See also chapters 13–15)

Even though botulinum toxin per se is not a filler, it is impossible to properly discuss rhytide therapy without botulinum toxin as a central component. Botulinum toxin has replaced filler substances as the treatment of choice for crow's-feet, and glabellar and forehead lines. Combining botulinum toxin therapy with resurfacing or filler substances can often dramatically improve efficacy. Predictable and judicious chemical denervation of specific muscles responsible for some rhytides using Botox has become a superb adjunct for the treatment of the aging face.[46,47] Botox is a sterile, vacuum-dried purified form of botulinum A toxin indicated for the treatment of strabismus, blepharospasm and the like.[48] Nevertheless, its off-label use in the treatment of the glabellar frown, horizontal forehead lines, crow's-feet, horizontal neck lines, flaring nostrils and platysmal bands has brought this agent to the attention of the aesthetically oriented physician.[49]

Dynamic rhytides and some with a combination etiology in the upper third of the face are normally best treated by botulinum toxin (Botox) injections. Botox has replaced filler substances as the treatment of choice for crow's-feet, glabellar and forehead lines. While not approved for cosmetic indications, its judicious use has been shown to excellently address certain age-related rhytides. Botox is the greatest advance in the minimally invasive treatment of the aging face to come along in the last 10 years. It is definitely a home-run in the upper third of the face and has reawakened interest in other fillers for use in the lower face.

OTHER INJECTABLE COLLAGEN PRODUCTS

Gamma-irradiated amnion collagen from human placentae has been suggested as an injectable soft-tissue augmentation material and tested in animal studies.[50] This is collagen which is manufactured from human placentae. Placentae are readily available and there have been clinical trials on the material. It was utilized in patients allergic to bovine collagen and produced excellent results. The study was discontinued and the product will probably never come onto the market.

Koken Atelocollagen implant is a 2% monomolecular aqueous solution of collagen of Japanese origin, whereas Zyderm is a suspension containing molecules, fibers and fibrils of collagen. The material is non-fibrillar. Unlike Zyderm, Koken Atelocollagen does not contain lidocaine. It is supplied in cartridges to be injected with a dermal syringe through a 30-gauge needle. The indications, contraindications, testing and injection techniques are the same as those for Zyderm collagen implant. It is manufactured and distributed by the Koken Co. (Japan) but is not available in the USA and so there is no American experience with this product.

Research efforts are currently underway to create a recombinant human collagen. Recombinant human collagen would eliminate the risk of donor viral or prion contamination, eradicate the need for proteolytic cleavage of animal collagen with its attendant degradation and have no potential for allergy. This material will hopefully be available in the near future. Cohesion Technologies (Palo Alto, CA) has recently reported the ability to produce human collagen in the laboratory. This is human collagen that is grown in the cow and separated from the cow's milk. Also, Advanced Tissue Sciences (San Diego, CA) has developed a human collagen that has been bioengineered from a single cell line. This will hopefully be available on the market by early 2002 as Cosmoderm™. Obviously, when this product comes onto the market, it will obviate the allergenicity problems associated with a bovine product.

Resoplast™ (Rofil Medical Internal, Breda, The Netherlands) is bovine monomolecular collagen in solution. Concentrations of 3.5% and 6.5% are available. Indications and techniques of implantation are similar to those for Zyderm collagen and a skin test is provided. It has not been approved for use in the USA.

Fibroquel® (Aspid Division) is an injectable form of porcine collagen described in Brazil.

OTHER AUTOLOGOUS PRODUCTS

Autologen® is true autologous collagen. It is a sterile suspension of intact collagen fibers prepared from the patient's own tissue. Research on the development of Autologen was performed from 1988 to 1994 by Kelman and DeVore;[51] a patent was secured in 1994 and the material was subsequently available on the market. Host skin from a prior procedure is forwarded to Collagenesis for processing into a suspended autologous, fibrillar material, usually of a 3.5% concentration. Three square inches of skin produces 1 cm³ of Autologen at this concentration. The material is returned to the physician in prefilled syringes. It is applicable for fine lines, wrinkles, depressions and lip augmentation. It must be placed as superficially as possible. It has been used in 1100 individuals and they state there is a greater longevity of correction than with bovine collagen because of the impact of the autologous composition. It is manufactured by Collagenesis Inc. (Beverly, MA); however, the company has stopped accepting shipments of new skin for processing and Autologen is presently not available.

Plasmagel is an autologous, blood-derived augmenting material. Ascorbic acid and lidocaine are added to blood plasma. The material is heated to form a gel and then injected. It is applicable for wrinkles, contour defects, acne scars and lip augmentation.[52]

OTHER ALLOGENIC PRODUCTS

These products are not FDA approved. Because they are derived from human tissue, they are not required to undergo the FDA approval process, just as autologous products do not require FDA approval for their use.

Cymetra™ is micronized, cryofractured Alloderm. The material is rehydrated with 1 cm³ of Xylocaine. No allergy prescreening or testing is required according to the manufacture. Donor screening and viral inactivation is performed. The material is obtained from the American Association of Tissue Banks (AATB) guideline-compliant tissue banks. It is implanted with a 26-gauge needle into the subcutaneous space. The treatment area is gently massaged. Clinical studies on 200 patients to date evidenced no allergic or immunologic reactions. Adverse reactions are bruising, redness, swelling and wrinkling of skin. Eye pain with temporary vision loss has been reported. All the adverse reactions are reported as transient and occur at a rate of 2.1%. It is manufactured by Lifecell Corp. (Branchburg, NJ) and distributed by Obagi Medical (Chicago, IL).

Dermalogen™ is human tissue collagen matrix from the dermal layer of donor skin specimens and was introduced in 1998. It is manufactured by the same company that produces Autologen and uses the same technology as that product. It is suspended in a neutral pH buffer and is predominately composed of collagen fibrils, but it contains other matrix proteins such as elastin. Extensive donor screening is undergone, including interviews with next of kin. It is sterilized and undergoes viral inactivation procedures and a prion inactivation step. Of course, HIV and hepatitis tests are performed. The sources of the donor skin are tissue banks accredited by the AATB. Nearly two million tissue and organ transplants have been done without any cases of communicable disease. There has been much discussion about the necessity of skin tests with Dermalogen to which some people have been positive. The incidence of erythema and problems with the skin tests are much less with the present products than with the original formulations. The material is produced in a nominal 3.5% concentration with no local anesthetic added (although the true concentration is c. 5%). A newer 2.8% concentration form of Dermalogen is on the horizon. The company says to use it with Emla or a nerve block: the present author uses it only with Emla. The company states that implantation is associated with new vessel formation and host collagen deposition. Patients have been followed for up to 6 months and some increase of longevity has been reported with Dermalogen compared with bovine collagen, but at 12 months they were equal. It is a useful product for people who are allergic to bovine collagen. Dermalogen is injected somewhere between the level of injection of Zyderm and Zyplast, as superficial as one can get this agent, and is used with a 30-gauge needle. The present author's experience has been that it is very difficult to inject, although the new, lower concentration holds promise of being much more manageable. It is manufactured and distributed by Collagenesis, Inc. (Beverly, MA).

Fascian (Fascia Biomaterials, Beverly Hills, CA), which is preserved, particulate fascia lata, derived from screened human cadavers, has recently become available. The material is freeze-dried and typically pre-irradiated. This injectable form of fascia lata can be injected when soft-tissue augmentation is desired. Historically, preserved fascia grafts have a proven efficacy and an excellent safety record over the past 73 years. In a clinical trial, Burres[53] followed 81 subjects for 6–9 months after implantation without incidence of infection, allergic reaction or acute rejection. Soft-tissue augmentation was evident 3–4 months after grafting, or longer in most cases. Histologic studies have demonstrated that, as in other locations with larger grafts, small pieces of fascia lata implanted intradermally were digested as an extraneous tissue and replaced with native collagen. This later reinvestment of the allograft matrix by the host fibroblast response generated a vascularized sheet of collagen that essentially restores the original elements found in native fascia, and was titled recollagenation. A recent study of samples of commercial sources of human allograft fascia showed that they all contained residual DNA fragments.[54] Injectable material is supplied in particle sizes of < 0.25, < 0.5 or < 2.0 mm. The Fascian particles are hydrated in 3–5 cm of 0.3% lidocaine solution prior to injection. The injected area is pre-undermined with a 20-gauge needle and the material injected into the preformed tunnel with a 16–25-gauge needle, depending on the size of the particles used. According to Burres, histologic studies have demonstrated that, as in other locations with larger grafts, small pieces of fascia lata implanted intradermally were digested as an extraneous tissue and replaced with native collagen.[53]

SUMMARY

As can be seen from the above discussion, there are many injectable substances available for soft-tissue augmentation. Obviously, the techniques and substances for soft-tissue augmentation are increasing at an accelerated rate. This is possibly a result of an understanding on the part of the cosmetically oriented physician that the three-dimensional aspects of the face must be preserved in achieving the best aesthetic result. Although one must be familiar with all of the techniques, materials and options, it is preferable to become very proficient in only two or three different methods so that patients can be given a few options while the physician is experienced in the techniques offered. Really, it is not what is used that is most critical, it is how it is used. A physician should not be a jack of all trades and a master of none. The choice of implant material should be based on the location of the defect, the potential for hypersensitivity reaction, the desire for permanency and the patient's feelings about the need for a 'natural feel' of the implant. There is a whole encyclopedia of substances to choose from to satisfy these criteria. Of course, safety should be the primary concern when using any implant material and, thus, to do no harm. As newer products are developed, the methods of soft-tissue enhancement will continue to change, hopefully bringing improved results to patients.

References

1. Neuber F. Fettransplantation. Chir Kongr Verhandl Dsch Gesellch Chir 1893;22:66.

2. Neuhof H. The transplantation of tissues. New York: Appleton & Company; 1923.

3. Boering G, Huffstadt AJ. The use of derma-fat grafts in the face. Br J Plast Surg 1968;20:172.

4. Stevenson TW. Fat grafts to the face. Plast Reconstr Surg 1949;4:458.

5. Peer LA. The neglected 'free fat graft', its behaviour and clinical use. Am J Surg 1956;92:40.

6. Katocs AS, Largis EE, Allen DO. Perfused fat cells: effects of lipolytic agents. J Biol Chem 1973;248:5089.

7. Gurney CE. Studies on the fate of free transplants of fat. Proc Staff Meet Mayo Clin 1937;12:317.

8. Matton G, Amseeuw A, De Keyser F. The history of biomaterials and the biology of collagen. Aesth Plast Surg 1985;9:133–40.

9. Urback F, Wilne SS, Johnson WC, Davies RE. Generalized paraffinoma (sclerosing lipogranuloma). Arch Dermatol 1971;103:277–85.

10. Kaminer M, Krause M. Filler substances in the treatment of facial aging. Med Surg Dermatol 1998;5:215–21.

11. DeLustro F, Condell RA, Nguyen MA, et al. A comparative study of biologic and immunologic response to medical devices derived from dermal collagen. J Biomed Mat Res 1986;20:109–20.

12. Klein AW, Rish DC. Injectable collagen: an adjunct to facial plastic surgery. Facial Plast Surg 1987;4:87.

13. Knapp TR, Kaplan EN, Daniels JR. Injectable collagen for soft tissue augmentation. Plast Reconstr Surg 1977;60:389.

14. Klein AW. Cosmetic therapy with botulinum toxin. Dermatol Surg 1996;22:757–9.

15. Hollister DW, Byers PH, Holbrook KA. Genetic disorders of collagen metabolism. In: Harris, Hirschorn, editors. Advances in human genetics 12. New York: Plenum Press; 1982:1–86.

16. Gross J, Kirk D. The heat precipitation of collagen from neutral salt solutions: some rate-regulating factors. J Biol Chem 1958;233:355–60.

17. Davidson PF et al. The serologic specificity of tropocollagen telopeptides. J Exp Med 1967;126:331–49.

18. Schmitt FO et al. The antigenicity of tropocollagen. Proc Natl Acad Sci USA 1964;51:493–7.

19. Stegman SJ, Tromovich TA. Injectable collagen. In: Stegman SJ, Tromovich TA, editors. Cosmetic dermatology surgery. Chicago: Yearbook Medical Publishers; 1984:131–49.

20. Knapp TR, Luck E, Daniels JR. Behavior of solubilized collagen as a bioimplant. J Surg Res 1977;23:96–105.

21. Stegman SJ, Tromovitch TA. Implantation of collagen for depressed scars. J Dermatol Surg Oncol 1980;6:450–3.

22. Watson W, Kay RL, Klein, et al. Injectable collagen: a clinical overview. Cutis 1983;31:543–6.

23. Wallace DG, McPherson JJ, Ellingsworth LE, et al. Injectable collagen for tissue augmentation. In: Nimni ME, editor. Collagen, Volume III Biotechnology. Boca Ratan: CRC Press; 1988:117–44.

24. Bulletin Collagen Corporation. Bovine Spongiform Encephalopathy.

25. McPherson JM, Ledger PW, Sawamura S, et al. The preparation and physiochemical characterization of an injectable form of reconstituted, glutaraldehyde crosslinked, bovine corium collagen. J Biomed Mat Res 1986;20: 79.

26. DeLustro F, Smith ST, Sundsmo J, et al. Reaction to injectable collagen in human subjects. J Dermatol Surg Oncol 1988;14(Suppl):49.

27. Klein AW. Indications and implantation techniques for the various formulations of injectable collagen. J Dermatol Surg Oncol 1988;14(Suppl):27–30.

28. Elson ML. Corrections of dermal contour defects with the injectable collagens: choosing and using these materials. Semin Dermatol 1987;6:77.

29. Cooperman LS, Mackinnon V, Bechler G, Pharriss BB. Injectable collagen: a six-year clinical investigation. Aesth Plast Surg 1985;9:145.

30. Klein AW. In favor of double testing. J Dermatol Surg Oncol 1989;15:263.

31. Elson ML. The role of skin testing in the use of collagen injectable materials. J Dermatol Surg Oncol 1989;15:301.

32. Klein AW. Implantation techniclues for injectable collagen: two-and-one half years of personal clinical experience. J Am Acad Dermatol 1983; 9:224.

33. Bailin PL, Bailin MD. Collagen implantation: clinical applications and lesion selection. J Dermatol Surg Oncol 1988;14 (Suppl):49.

34. Stegman SJ, Chus S, Bensch K, Armstrong R. A light and electron microscopic evaluation of Zyderm Collagen and Zyplast implants in aging human facial skin: a pilot study. Arch Dermatol 1987;123:1644.

35. Armstrong R, et al. Injectable collagen for soft tissue augmentation. In: Boretos JW, Eden M, editors. Contemporary clinical applications, new technology and legal aspects. Park Ridge, NJ: Noyes Publications; 1984:528–36.

36. McPherson JM, et al. An examination of the biologic response to injectable, glutaraldehyde cross-linked collagen implants. J Biomed Mat Res 1986;20:93.

37. Kligman AM, Armstrong RC. Histologic response to intradermal Zyderm and Zyplast (glutaraldehyde cross-linked) collagen in humans. J Dermatol Surg Oncol 1986;12:351.

38. Kligman AM, Histologic responses to collagen implants in human volunteers; comparison of Zyderm collagen with Zyplast implant. J Dermatol Surg Oncol 1988;14(Suppl):35.

39. Hanke CW, Hingley HR, Jolivette DM, et al. Abscess formation and local necrosis after treatment with Zyderm or Zyplast collagen implant. J Am Acad Dermatol 1991;25:319–26.

40. DeLustro F, Smith ST, Sundsmo J, et al. Reaction to injectable collagen: results in animal models and clinical use. Plast Reconstr Surg 1987;79:581.

41. McGraw R, et al. Sudden blindness secondary to injection of common drugs in the head and neck, part 1: clinical experiences. Otolaryngology 1978;86:147.

42. McCoy JP, et al. Characterization of the humoral immune response to bovine collagen implants. Arch Dermatol 1985;121:990.

43. Cooperman LS, Michaeli D. The immunogenicity of injectable collagen, part 2: a retrospective review of seventy-two tested and treated patients. J Dermatol Surg Oncol 1984; 10:647.

44. Siegle RJ, McCoy JP, Schade W, et al. Intradermal implantation of bovine collagen: humoral responses associated with clinical reaction. Arch Dermatol 1984;120:183.

45. Klein AW. 'Bonfire of the wrinkles'. J Dermatol Surg Oncol 1991;17:543–4.

46. Blitzer A, Brin MF, et al. Botulinum toxin for the treatment of hyperfunctional lines of the face. Arch Otolaryngol Head Neck Surg 1993; ••:1018–22.

47. Carruthers JDA, Carruthers JA. Treatment of glabellar frown lines with C botulinum – A exotoxin. J Dermatol Surg Oncol 1992;18: 17–21.

48. Jankovic J, Hallet M, editors. Therapy with botulinum toxin. New York: Marcel Dekker; 1994.

49. Carruthers A. Botulinum A exotoxin use in clinical dermatology. J Am Acad Dermatol 1996;34:788–97.

50. Spira M, Liu B, Xu Z et al. Human amnion collagen for soft tissue augmentation – biochemical characterizations and animal observations. J Biomed Mat Res 1994;28: 91–6.

51. Kelman CD, DeVore DP. Human collagen processing and autoimplant use. US Patent No 5,332,802; July 26 1994.

52. Krajcik R, Orentreich DS, Orentreich N. Plasmagel: a novel injectable autologous material for soft tissue augmentation. J Aesthet Acad Dermatol Cosmet Surg 1999;1:109–15.

53. Burres S. Recollagenation of acne scars. Dermatol Surg 1996;22:364–7.

54. Brunk D. DNA material lingers in human allografts. Skin Allergy News Jan 2000;4.

COMBINATION TREATMENT (Nicholas J Lowe)

Indications	Potential combination treatments	Chapter reference
Nasolabial folds	Photoprotection	2
Lip augmentation	Topical therapy	3
Periorbital lines	Glycolic acid	6
Scars	Chemical peels	7
	Laser resurfacing	10,11
	Non-ablative laser	12
	Vascular skin lesions	9
	Pigmentation treatment	8
	Botox	8
	Permanent fillers	19
	Fat transfer	18

18. Liposuction of the neck and microlipoinjection of the face

Richard D Glogau

INTRODUCTION

The human face shows its advancing age in many ways, but one of the subtlest yet demonstrative signs of aging is the redistribution of relative volumes of subcutaneous fat in the face. For example, there is a gradual loss of fat around the mouth and in front of the chin, which taken together with the gravitational effects of the sagging superficial musculo-aponeurotic system (SMAS) gives rise to the deeper and longer nasolabial folds on either side of the mouth. The lips lose their subcutaneous fat, accentuating the vertical rhytids secondary to repetitive motion of the orbicularis oris muscle. There is usually a hollowness that develops in the mid-lower cheek as the fat thins. The round prominence of the malar cheeks gives way to a flattening as the fat both thins and descends caudally with time. There is an increasing depression over the temporal fossae, a deepening of the eye, protuberance of the fat above the globes of the eye, and bulging as the infraorbital fat pushes anteriorly against the orbicularis oculii. And finally, of greatest importance to this discussion, the submental area begins to acquire an increase in fat volume, while the skin overlying the platysma in the neck gradually thins with time.[1–4]

In order to restore the youthful appearance of the face, the surgeon would like to remove fat in some areas and add fat back to others. The seminal work of Illouz,[5–8] Fournier,[9,10] and Fischer[11] introduced liposculpture to modern medicine. But the advance of local anesthetic solutions through Klein's crystallization and refinement of Illouz's original formula brought liposuction to the forefront of cosmetic surgery.[12–14] Liposuction[15–36] and microlipoinjection (or autologous fat grafting)[16,17,24,25,27,28,37–65] are two interrelated techniques in the cosmetic surgery armamentarium that have been used to address the problem of volume contour changes in the aging face.

REMOVING FAT FROM THE SUBMENTAL NECK

When planning liposuction of the face, the surgeon must be cautious about the long-term ramifications of removing fat. Just as there has been movement away from pro forma removal of the infraorbital fat pads in blepharoplasty in favor of repositioning the fat,[66] in the present author's opinion, there is usually little need to apply liposuction to the subcutaneous cheek and nasolabial folds. While buccal fat pad extraction enjoyed a period of popularity,[67–70] in the long term patients are better served by retaining and repositioning the fat in their cheeks to maintain round, youthful contours.

Attempts to minimize the nasolabial folds by flattening the cheek lateral to the fold with liposuction were popular in the early days of liposuction.[16,23,25,26,32,71–73] Now such a procedure is rarely indicated. Instead of diminishing the nasolabial fold, the unintended and unflattering consequence of suctioning lateral to the folds is the loss of the convexity of the cheek, leading to an older, flatter appearance of the cheek.

Facial liposuction, given today's understanding of the importance of volume and contour in the face, is a misnomer. It should more properly be labeled submental liposuction, i.e. it is directed to the neck and submental area where it can be used judiciously in certain patients to sharpen the submental angles. If there is extensive platysmal banding, plication and draping of the muscle via rhytidectomy may yield results superior to submental liposuction alone.[74] Tightening the skin of the neck with shrinkage obtained from applying laser energy to the underside of the neck skin has been proposed as an alternative to traditional rhytidectomy for the neck when excessive skin and prominent muscle banding are noted.[4,75] But many patients who have prominent submental fat benefit from liposuction alone, with accompanying contraction of the overlying skin that follows as a consequence of this procedure.[15,29,31,35,36,72,76–79]

TRANSFERRING FAT BACK INTO THE FACE

Fat harvested expressly for transfer or incidental to body liposuction procedures can be used to inject the nasolabial folds, cheeks, chin, mental creases, lips, and even the temples and forehead. Fat grafting has been in the medical literature for many years, receiving a tremendous awakened interest following the introduction of liposuction surgery in the late 1970s.[5,16,17,21,24,25,27,37–40,42–44,46–51,54–63,80–109] Current anxieties over the sources of soft-tissue augmentation fillers, e.g. cadavers, bovine, porcine, etc., in this era of bovine spongiform encephalopathy and prions may have refocused attention on the utility of using the patient's own tissue for augmentation.[110]

This chapter will focus on the techniques used for liposuction and lipotransfer in the face, with emphasis on variation limitations, as there are as many different methods as there are surgeons.[111] However, some trends emerge that may guide the interested physician to developing their own technique.

SUBMENTAL LIPOSUCTION

Who is a candidate for submental liposuction? Generally, a patient who has acquired familial submental fat who does not have platysmal banding as their major cosmetic complaint, and who has reasonable skin tone, without significant solar elastosis, is a good candidate for submental liposuction. Patients should be in otherwise good health, and have been off aspirin products and anticoagulants for at least 7–10 days prior to surgery. Age is less of a barrier to submental liposuction than is the condition and the quality of the neck skin.

RELATIONSHIP OF THE CHIN TO THE SUBMENTAL ANGLE

If the patient is sitting in neutral upright position gazing straight ahead, a plumb line can be dropped from the upper lip, lightly touching the lower lip and providing a theoretical line which the most anterior point of the chin should just graze (Figure 18.1). If there is substantial distance between the chin and the plumb line, consideration should be given to chin augmentation, a simple procedure that can be undertaken at the same sitting as the submental liposuction (Figure 18.2a and b). Substantial improvement in the side profile can occur without liposuction, purely on the basis of bringing the chin forward to the plumb line with the lips (Figure 18.3a and b). But even without chin augmentation, one can achieve gratifying changes in the profile with liposuction alone (Figure 18.4a and b).

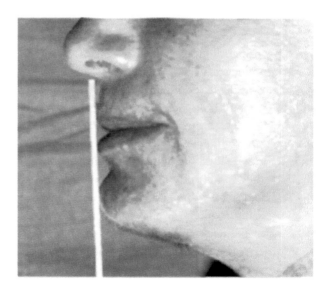

Figure 18.1 *A straight edge laid on the lips should show the chin just touching when viewed in profile. If there is significant distance between the chin and the straight edge, a chin augmentation may be considered.*

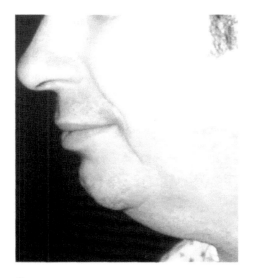
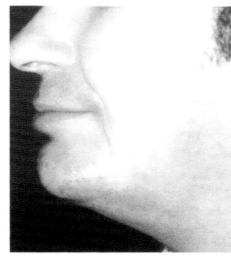

a
b

Figure 18.2
(A) Demonstration of the effect of combining chin augmentation with submental liposuction; (B) six-month follow-up.

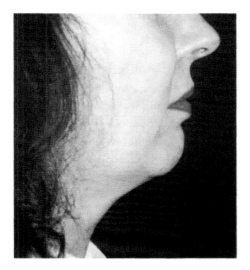
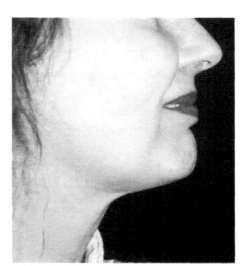

a
b

Figure 18.3
(A) Demonstration of the effect of chin augmentation alone; (B) six-month follow-up.

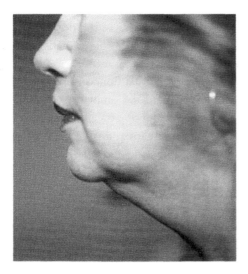
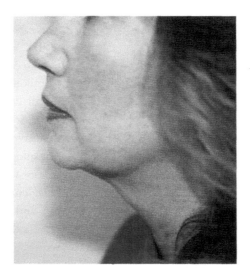

a
b

Figure 18.4
(A) Demonstration of the effect of submental liposuction alone; (B) six-month follow-up.

MARGINAL MANDIBULAR NERVE

When performing submental liposuction, it is important to recognize the location of the marginal mandibular branch of the facial nerve (Figure 18.5).[112] Although using blunt cannulae with the tumescent technique should minimize any trauma to the nerve, it occasionally happens that some minor trauma produces a neuropraxis, where the nerve is weakened slightly. This can interfere with the normal position and functioning of the corners of the mouth. In all cases, the neuropraxis is temporary and spontaneously resolves over several weeks, occasionally months.

ANESTHESIA

The submental area and jowls are easily anesthetized utilizing tumescent anesthesia, utilizing dilute lidocaine 0.05% solution and epinephrine, as described elsewhere.

A total of < 100 cm³ is required to anesthetize the submental fat, anterior upper neck and jowls along the mandibular margin. With such small volumes, machine-assisted infiltration is not required, and all the anesthetic can be placed with a 19-gauge needle through a small wheal of local anesthetic just under the chin in the midline. A small infiltration cannula can then be used to extend the anesthetic solution to the ears along the jaw line in either direction.

INCISION PLACEMENT

Almost all surgeons agree on the location of the primary cannula entry point – in the midline, in a flexural crease just posterior to the chin, usually located in a small crease that appears when the neck flexes forward. A stab incision with a #11 blade provides ready access to a small cannula and heals without a visible scar.

Depending on the presence or absence of jowling and fat alone the jaw line, small stab incisions can be made just behind the earlobes, providing ready access to the area along the jaw line from both sides. These are often quite useful in the more obese patient, where sharpening the contour along the jaw line is desirable. Less commonly, small stabs can be placed behind the angle of the jaw or underneath the jowls themselves. These sites are less desirable because of their higher visibility and should only be used in unusual cases.

CANNULA SELECTION AND TECHNIQUE

The cannula used varies according to the preferences of the surgeon. Many surgeons prefer small-gauge needle cannula, i.e. 12-gauge, or at most a 2 or 3 mm diameter cannula. Flatter spatula-tipped cannulae are useful because they facilitate the blunt dissection of the skin and assist in breaking up attachments of skin underlying fascia. If there is a great deal of loose skin, a rasping cannula may be used to scrape the underside of the skin and stimulate fibrosis and retraction. It is generally said that the skin in this area is forgiving, and one is often encouraged to freely scrape the underside of the skin. However, an undesirable fine wrinkling of the skin can be seen in the long-term follow-up, which can be precipitated by overly aggressive suctioning of the underside of the dermis.

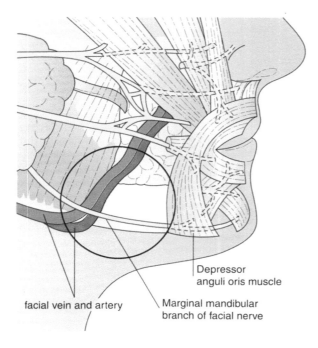

facial vein and artery

Depressor anguli oris muscle

Marginal mandibular branch of facial nerve

Figure 18.5 The location of the marginal branch of the facial nerve as it crosses the mandible, just anterior to the artery which can easily be palpated.

In general, the suctioning is carried out from the chin to the level of the cricothyroid cartilage, and from the ear down to the anterior border of the sternocleidomastoid muscle on the sides. Particular attention is paid to the area of the jowls just under the mandible, taking care to avoid unnecessary trauma to the marginal mandibular nerve. Positioning the patient on their back and asking them to jut their chin forward towards the ceiling will put the neck in high relief. The difference produced by the suctioning becomes immediately evident.

Surprisingly little fat is usually extracted. Even large necks seldom yield > 25–30 cm³ of fat, and many smaller necks give up only enough globules of fat to be seen in the proximal portions of the suction tubing. Following suctioning, the stab incisions may be closed with rapidly absorbable 6-0 gut or something similar. The neck is then supported with either a tape dressing that runs from ear to ear or an elastic compression garment that can be removed for showering and worn at night for a week. Final contour results may not be evident for several months, as fibrosis and retraction follow the usual course in liposuction.

CHIN AUGMENTATION

If the chin profile would benefit, a small chin implant can be placed at this point in the procedure. The extraoral approach may be utilized by widening the stab incision made for the suctioning in the midline below the chin. Techniques for placement vary, but essentially a submuscular pocket is created just anterior to the periosteum, and a soft, silicone implant (modified Beekhuis) can readily be placed to extend the chin in profile. Details for placement of the implant can be obtained from descriptions of the technique in the surgical literature.[1,19,31,70,113]

LIPOTRANSFER

If filling the perioral area, nasolabial folds or premalar cheeks is desired, a ready amount of fat can quickly be harvested from the subcutaneous fat over the upper outer hips, waist or abdomen. The donor site is infiltrated with tumescent anesthetic as if preparing for liposuction. Cortisone and hyaluronidase are omitted from the anesthetic solution if it is to be used for harvesting donor fat. It is necessary to wait 10–15 minutes for the skin to blanch well. Usually, 100 ml of tumescent anesthetic solution is sufficient.

A 10 cm³ syringe with a Luer-lok hub, blunt-tipped 12-gauge needle, is introduced through a small stab incision into the subcutaneous fat. It is easier to extract the fat if the syringe is primed with 1–2 cm³ or normal saline to remove any dead space before introducing the harvesting needle into the fat. By extending the plunger to create a small vacuum, and rapidly moving the needle/syringe up and down along the long axis of the syringe, perpendicular to the skin that is grasped with the non-dominant hand, fat is rapidly aspirated into the syringe.

When the syringe is two thirds full, the needle is removed, and the syringe capped and then allowed to stand for several minutes to permit the fat to float above the infranatant: the infranatant is then discarded. Sterile saline or Ringer's lactate is then drawn into the syringe, the contents are gently agitated and the syringe is again rested, allowing the fat to rise above the infranatant, which is again discarded. This washing procedure is repeated until the infranatant is relatively free of blood. By keeping the entire system within the harvesting syringe, the sterility of the material is maintained. No air or break in the system is allowed.

Using a Luer-lock transfer device, the fat is then placed in a sterile fashion into either 3 or 1 ml syringes for injection. Fresh fat requires a 14-, 16- or 18-gauge needle to inject. With such large needles, it is important to: (1) anesthetize the recipient site with a small wheal of lidocaine 1% with epinephrine to blanch the skin and minimize bleeding; (2) enter the skin with the bevel up and the needle almost parallel to the skin. This avoids 'punching' a small defect in the skin that potentially will heal with a small pit.

INJECTING FAT

Fat can be injected into the face in a variety of places to augment the subcutaneous volume. Most surgeons agree that freshly harvested and immediately injected fat has the best opportunity to correct volume deficits.[43,45,48,65,80] However, fat that is harvested and not immediately used can be frozen for future use as an injectable filler substance. While it is unlikely that such frozen fat achieves the status of a viable graft, there is eventual production of volume probably secondary to resulting fibrosis as a response to the injected fat. For those who are concerned about the nature and safety of allogenic filler materials, frozen fat offers a useful if somewhat cumbersome solution for soft-tissue augmentation.

Typically, the nasolabial folds can be injected by advancing a needle gently from a puncture site lateral to the corner of the mouth, moving the needle just under the skin and advancing the tip towards the nose (Figure 18.6a and b). At the farthest point of advancement of the needle tip, the plunger is aspirated to make sure the tip is not in an intravascular location. The fat is injected slowly as the needle is withdrawn. A similar technique can be used for the pre-malar cheeks and chin (Figure 18.7a and b).

While many surgeons use fat for lip injection,[50,64] the present author has largely avoided the technique. The aversion stems from two factors: (1) the ease of injuring the labial artery; (2) the bulkiness of the fat that precludes any aesthetic shaping of the vermilion border and blunts the Cupid's bow of the lip. Other filler agents are usually preferable from an aesthetic viewpoint.[114]

Injection of fat around the eyes, particularly the glabellar area, has been associated with immediate blindness.[105,115] Injection of fat directly into the upper nasolabial fold has been associated with intravascular injection, stroke and tissue slough.[88,116,117] These areas are best treated only by

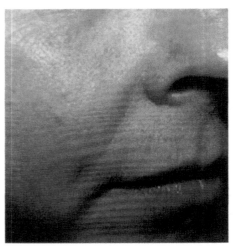

a

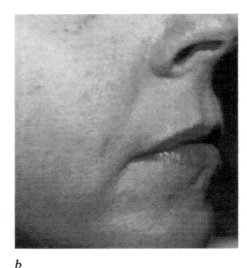

b

Figure 18.6

(A) Demonstration of the effect of microlipoinjection into the nasolabial folds and marionette lines at the corners of the mouth; (B) six-month follow-up.

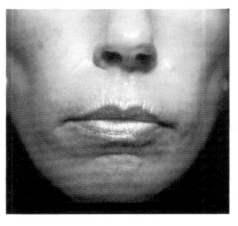

a

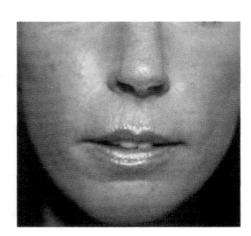

b

Figure 18.7

(A) Demonstration of fat grafting to correct the hollow cheeks; (B) six-month follow-up.

experienced transplanters, utilizing low-flow and low-pressure techniques, because of the high potential morbidity.

As a general safety precaution, using excessive pressure to inject fat is potentially catastrophic because of possible inadvertent intravascular injection. If the syringe becomes jammed, it should be removed and cleared rather than trying to force the fat out under ever greater pressure.

LONG-TERM FOLLOW-UP

The major problem with fat transplantation and injection is its unpredictability.[22,57,58,62,90,91,98] Certainly, when the graft takes, the results can be gratifying;[46,50,53,80,91,118-120] however, more often than not, the material is slowly broken down and absorbed, and repeated injections may be needed. Long-term studies debate the ultimate fate of the fat graft. While fresh fat can often produce dramatic results, it is more reasonable to think of frozen fat as a useful short-term filler. Aesthetically, the appeal of the fat remains – it can provide broad contouring that is soft and natural, which is difficult to achieve by any other means at present. The surgeon can often achieve results that cannot be accomplished with other agents, but it is difficult to reliably promise success with fat grafts.

References

1. Moreno A, Bell W, You Z. Esthetic contour analysis of the submental cervical region: a study based on ideal subjects and surgical patients. J Oral Maxillofac Surg 1994;52:704–13; discussion 713.

2. Renaut A, Orlin W, Ammar A, Pogrel M. Distribution of submental fat in relationship to the platysma muscle. Oral Surg Oral Med Oral Pathol 1994;77:442–5.

3. Kamer F, Lefkoff L. Submental surgery. A graduated approach to the aging neck. Arch Otolaryngol Head Neck Surg 1991;117:40–6.

4. Cook WJ. 'Cook weekend alternative to the facelift'. Liposuction of the face, neck, and jowls with laser dermal resurfacing and platysmal plication. Dermatol Clin 1999;17:773–82.

5. Illouz YG. The fat cell 'graft': a new technique to fill depressions [letter]. Plast Reconstr Surg 1986;78:122–3.

6. Illouz YG. Surgical remodeling of the silhouette by aspiration lipolysis or selective lipectomy. Aesth Plast Surg 1985;9:7–21.

7. Illouz YG. Illouz's technique of body contouring by lipolysis. Clin Plast Surg 1984;11:409–17.

8. Illouz YG. Body contouring by lipolysis: a 5-year experience with over 3000 cases. Plast Reconstr Surg 1983;72:591–7.

9. Fournier PF. Who should do syringe liposculpturing? [editorial]. J Dermatol Surg Oncol 1988;14:1055–6.

10. Fournier PF. Why the syringe and not the suction machine? J Dermatol Surg Oncol 1988;14:1062–71.

11. Fischer G. Liposculpture: the 'correct' history of liposuction. Part I [see comments]. J Dermatol Surg Oncol 1990;16:1087–9.

12. Klein J. The tumescent technique for liposuction surgery. Am J Cosmet Surg 1987;4:263–7.

13. Klein JA. The tumescent technique. Anesthesia and modified liposuction technique. Dermatol Clin 1990;8:425–37.

14. Klein JA. Tumescent technique for regional anesthesia permits lidocaine doses of 35 mg/kg for liposuction. J Dermatol Surg Oncol 1990; 16:248–63.

15. Adamson P, Cormier R, Tropper G, McGraw B. Cervicofacial liposuction: results and controversies [see comments]. J Otolaryngol 1990;19:267–73.

16. Asken S. Facial liposuction and microlipoinjection. J Dermatol Surg Oncol 1988;14:297–305.

17. Asken S. Microliposuction and autologous fat transplantation for aesthetic enhancement of the aging face. J Dermatol Surg Oncol 1990;16: 965–72.

18. Asken S. Perils and pearls of liposuction. Dermatol Clin 1990;8:415–19.

19. Bach D, Newhouse R, Boice G. Simultaneous orthognathic surgery and cervicomental liposuction. Clinical and survey results. Oral Surg Oral Med Oral Pathol 1981;71:262–6.

20. Bisaccia E, Scarborough DA, Swensen RD. Syringe-assisted liposuction: a cosmetic surgeon's office technique. J Dermatol Surg Oncol 1988;14:982–9.

21. Chajchi A, Benzaquen I. Liposuction fat grafts in face wrinkles and hemifacial atrophy. Aesth Plast Surg 1986;10:115–17.

22. Chrisman BB. Liposuction: removal of body and facial fat deposits by subcutaneous suction. Hawaii Med J 1985;44:180, 183–4.

23. Chrisman B. Liposuction with facelift surgery. Dermatol Clin 1990;8:501–22.

24. Coleman WP. The history of liposuction and fat transplantation in America. Dermatol Clin 1999;17:723–7.

25. Collins PC, Field LM, Narins RS. Liposuction surgery and autologous fat transplantation. Clin Dermatol 1992;10:365–72.

26. Daher JC, Cosac OM, Domingues S. Face-lift: the importance of redefining facial contours through facial liposuction. Ann Plast Surg 1988;21:1–10.

27. Field LM. Re: Microliposuction and autologous fat transplantation for aesthetic enhancement of the aging face [letter; comment]. J Dermatol Surg Oncol 1991;17:914–15.

28. Horl HW, Feller AM, Biemer E. Technique for liposuction fat reimplantation and long-term volume evaluation by magnetic resonance imaging. Ann Plast Surg 1991;26:248–58.

29. Jacob C, Berkes B, Kaminer M. Liposuction and surgical recontouring of the neck: a retrospective analysis. Dermatol Surg 2000;26:625–32.

30. Johnson D, Cook WJ. Advanced techniques in liposuction. Semin Cutan Med Surg 1999;18:139–48.

31. Kane N. Cervical liposuction: results and controversies. J Otolaryngol 1991;20:69.

32. Kesselring UK. Facial liposuction. Facial Plast Surg 1986;4:1–4.

33. Kovacs B, Smith R, Cesteleyn L, Claeys T. Submental liposuction in maxillofacial surgery. Acta Stomatol Belg 1992;89:37–45.

34. Mottura A. Liposuction: more curettage than aspiration. Aesth Plast Surg 1991;15:209–14.

35. Samdal F, Amland P, Abyholm F. Syringe-assisted microliposuction for cervical rejuvenation. A five year experience. Scand J Plast Reconstr Surg Hand Surg 1995;29:1–8.

36. Tapia A, Ferreria B, Eng R. Liposuction in cervical rejuvenation. Aesth Plast Surg 1987;11:95–100.

37. Cortese A, Savastano G, Felicetta L. Free fat transplantation for facial tissue augmentation. J Oral Maxillofac Surg 2000;58:164–9; discussion 169–70.

38. Fulton JE, Suarez M, Silverton K, Barnes T. Small volume fat transfer. Dermatol Surg 1998;24:857–65.

39. Schuller-Petrovic S. Improving the aesthetic aspect of soft tissue defects on the face using autologous fat transplantation. Facial Plast Surg 1997;13:119–24.

40. Fournier PF. Facial recontouring with fat grafting. Dermatol Clin 1990;8:523–37.

41. Coleman WP, Alt TH. Dermatologic cosmetic surgery. J Dermatol Surg Oncol 1990;16:170–6.

42. Silkiss RZ, Baylis HI. Autogenous fat grafting by injection. Ophthal Plast Reconstr Surg 1987;3:71–5.

43. Markey AC, Glogau RG. Autologous fat grafting: comparison of techniques. Dermatol Surg 2000;26:1135–9.

44. Glogau RG. Microlipoinjection. Autologous fat grafting. Arch Dermatol 1988;124:1340–3.

45. Donofrio LM. Structural autologous lipoaugmentation: a pan-facial technique. Dermatol Surg 2000;26:1129–34.

46. Berman M. Rejuvenation of the upper eyelid complex with autologous fat transplantation. Dermatol Surg 2000;26:1113–16.

47. Karacalar A, Ozcan M. The superdry technique for lipoplasty of the leg and the no-touch technique for autologous fat transplantation. Plast Reconstr Surg 2000;106:738–40.

48. Lidagoster MI, Cinelli PB, Levee EM, Sian CS. Comparison of autologous fat transfer in fresh, refrigerated, and frozen specimens: an animal model. Ann Plast Surg 2000;44:512–15.

49. Coleman WP. Fat transplantation. Dermatol Clin 1999;17:891–8, viii.

50. Gatti JE. Permanent lip augmentation with serial fat grafting. Ann Plast Surg 1999;42:376–80.

51. Mandrekas AD, Zambacos GJ, Kittas C. Cyst formation after fat injection. Plast Reconstr Surg 1998;102:1708–9.

52. Ersek RA, Change P, Salisbury MA. Lipo layering of autologous fat: an improved technique with promising results. Plast Reconstr Surg 1998;101:820–6.

53. Coleman SR. Facial recontouring with lipostructure. Clin Plast Surg 1997;24:347–67.

54. Nordstrom RE, Wang J, Fan K. 'Spaghetti' fat grafting: a new technique. Plast Reconstr Surg 1997;99:917–18.

55. American Academy of Dermatology. Guidelines of care for soft tissue augmentation: fat transplantation. J Am Acad Dermatol 1996;34:690–4.

56. Matarasso A, Matarasso SL. Autologous fat transplantation. Plast Reconstr Surg 1995;69:933.

57. Niechajev I, Sevcuk O. Long-term results of fat transplantation: clinical and histologic studies. Plast Reconstr Surg 1994;94:496–506.

58. Gormley DR. Autologous fat transplantation: evaluation and interpretation of results. J Dermatol Surg Oncol 1993;19:389–90.

59. Lewis CM. The current status of autologous fat grafting. Aesth Plast Surg 1993;17:109–12.

60. Lam A. Moy R. The potential for fat transplantation. J Dermatol Surg Oncol 1992;18:432–4.

61. Eppley BL, Snyders Jr R, Winkelmann T, Delfino JJ. Autologous facial fat transplantation: improved graft maintenance by microbead bioactivation. J Oral Maxillofac Surg 1992;50:477–82.

62. Pinski KS, Roenigk HH. Autologous fat transplantation. Long-term follow-up. J Dermatol Surg Oncol 1992;18:179–84.

63. Bircoll M. Injectable technique of autologous fat transplantation. Plast Reconstr Surg 1990;85:149.

64. Fulton JE, Rahimi AD, Helton P, et al. Lip rejuvenation. Dermatol Surg 2000;26:470–4; discussion 474–5.

65. Sattler G, Sommer B. Liporecycling: a technique for facial rejuvenation and body contouring. Dermatol Surg 2000;26:1140–4.

66. Hoefflin SM. The youthful face: tight is not right, repositioning is right [letter]. Plast Reconstr Surg 1998;101:1417.

67. Matarasso A. Buccal fat pad excision: aesthetic improvement of the midface. Ann Plast Surg 1991;26:413–18.

68. Guerrerosantos J, Manjarrez-Cortes A. Cheek and neck sculpturing: simultaneous buccal fat pad removal and subcutaneous cheek and neck lipoplasty. Clin Plast Surg 1989;16:343–53.

69. Newman J. Removal of buccal fat pad by liposuction [letter; comment]. Plast Reconstr Surg 1990;86:885–6.

70. Newman J, Dolsky RL, Nguyen A. Facial profileplasty by liposuction extraction. Otolaryngol Head Neck Surg 1985;93:718–31.

71. Stegman SJ. The application of lipo-suction in dermatology. Adv Dermatol 1986;1:211–19.

72. Goodstein WA. Superficial liposculpture of the face and neck. Plast Reconstr Surg 1996;98:988–96; discussion 997–82.

73. Fischer G. Liposculpture. 3. Surgical technique in liposculpture. J Dermatol Surg Oncol 1991;17:964–6.

74. Kamer F, Minoli J. Postoperative platysmal band deformity. A pitfall of submental liposuction. Arch Otolaryngol Head Neck Surg 1993;119:193–6.

75. Cook WJ. Laser neck and jowl liposculpture including platysma laser resurfacing, dermal laser resurfacing, and vaporization of subcutaneous fat [see comments]. Dermatol Surg 1997;23:1143–8.

76. Samdal F. Treatment of the neck in facial rejuvenation surgery using a simplified method of syringe assisted microlipoextraction. Scand J Plast Reconstr Surg Hand Surg 1990;24:253–7.

77. Lake D. Cosmetic surgery of the neck as an office procedure. J Dermatol Surg 1976;2:397–9.

78. Lambros VC. Fat contouring in the face and neck. Clin Plast Surg 1992;19:401–14.

79. Guerrerosantos J. Liposuction in the cheek, chin, and neck: a clinical study. Facial Plast Surg 1986;4:25–34.

80. Sommer B, Sattler G. Current concepts of fat survival: histology of aspirated adipose tissue and review of the literature. Dermatol Surg 2000;26:1159–66.

81. Reiche-Fischel O, Wolford LM, Pitta M. Facial contour reconstruction using an autologous free fat graft: a case report with 18-year follow-up. J Oral Maxillofac Surg 2000;58:103–6.

82. Nishimura T, Hashimoto H, Nakanishi I, Furukawa M. Microvascular angiogenesis and apoptosis in the survival of free fat grafts. Laryngoscope 2000;110:1333–8.

83. Latoni JD, Marshall DM, Wolde SA. Overgrowth of fat autotransplanted for correction of localized steroid-induced atrophy. Plast Reconstr Surg 2000;106:1566–9.

84. Lapiere JC, Aasi S, Cook B, Montalvo A. Successful correction of depressed scars of the forehead secondary to trauma and morphea en coup de sabre by en bloc autologous dermal fat graft. Dermatol Surg 2000;26:793–7.

85. Erol OO. Facial autologous soft-tissue contouring by adjunction of tissue cocktail injection (micrograft and minigraft mixture of dermis, fascia, and fat). Plast Reconstr Surg 2000;106:1375–87; discussion 1388.

86. Sataloff RT, Hawkshaw M, Shaw A. Autologous fat injection: the intraoperative endpoint. Ear Nose Throat J 1999;78:534.

87. Har-Shai Y, Lindenbaum ES, Gamliel-Lazarovich A, et al. An integrated approach for increasing the survival of autologous fat grafts in the treatment of contour defects. Plast Reconstr Surg 1999;104:945–54.

88. Feinendegen DL, Baumgartner RW, Vuadens P, et al. Autologous fat injection for soft tissue augmentation in the face: a safe procedure? Aesth Plast Surg 1998;22:163–7.

89. Fagrell D, Enestrom S, Berggren A, Kniola B. Fat cylinder transplantation: an experimental comparative study of three different kinds of fat transplants. Plast Reconstr Surg 1996;98:90–6; discussion 97–8.

90. Chajchir A. Fat injection: long-term follow-up. Aesth Plast Surg 1996;20:291–6.

91. Coleman SR. Long-term survival of fat transplants: controlled demonstrations. Aesth Plast Surg 1995;19:421–5.

92. Viterbo F, Marques M, Valente M. Fat-tissue injection versus graft: experimental study in rabbits. Ann Plast Surg 1994;33:1184–92.

93. Moscona R, Shoshani O, Lichtig H, Karnieli E. Viability of adipose tissue injected and treated by different methods: an experimental study in the rat. Ann Plast Surg 1994;33:500–6.

94. Marques A, Brenda E, Saldiva PH, et al. Autologous fat grafts: a quantitative and morphometric study in rabbits. Scand J Plast Reconstr Surg Hand Surg 1994;28:241–7.

95. Samdal F, Skolleborg KC, Berthelsen B. The effect of preoperative needle abrasion of the recipient site on survival of autologous free fat grafts in rats. Scand J Plast Reconstr Surg Hand Surg 1992;26:33–6.

96. Hambley RM, Carruthers JA. Microlipoinjection for the elevation of depressed full thickness skin grafts on the nose. J Dermatol Surg Oncol 1992;18:963–8.

97. Lewis CM. Transplantation of autologous fat. Plast Reconstr Surg 1991;88:1110–11.

98. Ersek RA. Transplantation of purified autologous fat: a 3-year follow-up is disappointing [see comments]. Plast Reconstr Surg 1991;87:219–27.

99. Ellenbogen R. Autologous fat injection. Plast Reconstr Surg 1991;88:543–4.

100. Fournier PF. Reduction syringe liposculpturing. Dermatol Clin 1990;8:539–51.

101. Chajchir A, Benzaquen I, Wexler E, Arellano A. Fat injection. Aesth Plast Surg 1990;14:127–36.

102. Bartynski K, Marion MS, Wang TD. Histopathologic evaluation of adipose autografts in a rabbit ear model. Otolaryngol Head Neck Surg 1990;102:314–21.

103. Stephenson KL. Passot and fat grafts. Plast Reconstr Surg 1989;84:700–1.

104. Moscona R, Ullman Y, Har-Shai Y, Hirshowitz B. Free-fat injections for the correction of hemifacial atrophy. Plast Reconstr Surg 1989; 84:501–7; discussion 508–9.

105. Dreizen NG, Framm L. Sudden unilateral visual loss after autologous fat injection into the glabellar area. Am J Ophthalmol 1989;107: 85–7.

106. Chajchir A, Benzaquen I. Fat-grafting injection for soft-tissue augmentation. Plast Reconstr Surg 1989;84:921–34; discussion 935.

107. Illouz YG. Present results of fat injection. Aesth Plast Surg 1988;12:175–81.

108. Ellenbogen R. Free autogenous pearl fat grafts in the face – a preliminary report of a rediscovered technique. Ann Plast Surg 1986; 16:179–94.

109. Meade CJ, Ashwell M. Site differences in fat cell size – a transplantation study. Proc Nutr Soc 1979;38:62A.

110. Underwood A, Rogers A, Murr A, et al. Cannibals to cows: the path of a deadly disease. Newsweek 2001;137:53–61.

111. Stegman SJ. Technique variations in liposuction surgery. Dermatol Clin 1990;8:457–61.

112. Liebman EP, Webster RC, Gaul JR, Griffin T. The marginal mandibular nerve in rhytidectomy and liposuction surgery. Arch Otolaryngol Head Neck Surg 1988;114:179–81.

113. Newman J, Dolsky RL, Mai ST. Submental liposuction extraction with hard chin augmentation. Arch Otolaryngol 1984;110: 454–7.

114. Klein A, Elson M. The history of substances for soft tissue augmentation. Dermatol Surg 2000; 26:1096–105.

115. Teimourian B. Blindess following fat injections [letter]. Plast Reconstr Surg 1988;82:361.

116. Feinendegen D, Baumgartner R, Schroth G, et al. Middle cerebral artery occlusion and ocular fat embolism after autologous fat injection in the face [letter]. J Neurol 1998;245:53–4.

117. Egido J, Arroyo R, Marcos A, Jimenez-Alfaro I. Middle cerebral artery embolism and unilateral visual loss after autologous fat injection into the glabellar area [letter]. Stroke 1993;24:615–16.

118. Hanke C. Fat transplantation: indications, techniques, results. Dermatol Surg 2000;26: 1106.

119. Fournier P. Fat grafting: my technique. Dermatol Surg 2000;26:1117–28.

120. Pinski K, Coleman WR. Microlipoinjection and autologous collagen. Dermatol Clin 1995;13: 339–51.

COMBINATION TREATMENT (Nicholas J Lowe)

Indications	Potential combination treatments	Chapter reference
Nasolabial folds	Photoprotection	2
Lip augmentation±	Topical agents	3,4
Hollow cheeks	Glycolic acid peels	6
Atrophic acne scars	Chemical peels	7
Facial deformity e.g. hemifacial atrophy	Laser skin resurfacing	10,11
	Botox	13–15
	Temporary fillers	16,17
	Permanent fillers	19
	Ocular plastic procedures	23
	Surgical procedures	24

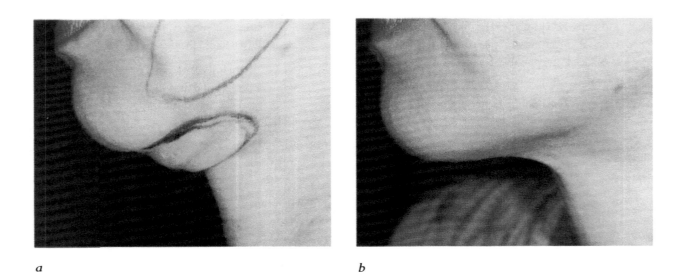

a   b

Figure 18.8
Liposuction of the chin using tumescent anaesthesia and microcanular. Provided by NJ Lowe.

19. Dermal fillers: permanent injectable and implant devices

Nicholas J Lowe

INTRODUCTION

Permanent fillers have a long history of use in correcting some of the features of facial ageing, particularly those associated with signs of the lower face. The ideal skin filler would consist of an inert substance that would be readily implanted, produce no local tissue reactions, have a natural feel, and would be readily removable should the patient's desire or facial contour change.

Numerous permanent fillers have been used over the years and are listed in Table 19.1 Some of these fillers have, unfortunately, become the subject of controversy and have been banned by a number of national regulatory authorities, e.g. the use of silicone as a dermal filler, and Arteplast, Evolution.

Table 19.1 Some permanent injectable skin fillers (non-biodegradable)

- Artecoll[1]
- Bioplastique[2]
- Dermalive
- Silicone[3]
- Porfill
- Metacrill

Other more recent trends have included the use of modified forms of e-PETE or Gore-Tex®,[4] e.g. SoftForm™[5] or UltraSoft™ manufactured to give hollow, softer feeling tubular implants (Tables 19.2–19.4).

Table 19.2 Properties of Gore-Tex

• Features	• Side-effects
Strands	Wrong placement
Oral contour	Extrusion
Circular contour	Hardening
Sometimes difficult to remove	Contraction
	Pyogenic granulomas

Table 19.3 Properties of SoftForm

• Features	• Side-effects
Hollow tubular design	Wrong placement
Placement is critical	Extrusion
Good stability in nasolabial folds	Hardening
Less stable in lips	Contraction
Designed to be removed	Pyogenic granulomas

Most recently Ultrasoft has been developed as a softer, more pliable type of SoftForm. Studies with this material are underway.

Table 19.4 Properties of UltraSoft

• Features	• Side-effects
Hollow tubular design	To be determined
2.5 times softer than SoftForm	
Less contractions anticipated	

This chapter provides information about the use of SoftForm based on a group of 250 patients over the last 3 years.

Table 19.5 Properties and problems of silicone injections

- **Summary**
  Developed in the 1930s
  Different viscocities
  Medical-grade liquid silicones used for tissue
  augmentation since 1965
  Filtered 350 centistokes
  Many patients treated over the past 20 years
  Dermatological and podiatric uses
- **Problems**
  Migration
  Cellulitis
  Not covered by malpractice insurance in the USA
  Overcorrection and nodule formation

INJECTABLE PERMANENT FILLERS

A list of some of these types of injectable permanent fillers is provided in Table 19.1. A variety of important features is to be found with these different fillers.

One particular problem associated with these injectable fillers is that once injected they cannot be removed. Therefore, if a defect has been overcorrected this problem will remain.

Some of the fillers have been associated with a variety of other problems, e.g. Artecoll® can give persistent nodular reactions in the lips and nasolabial folds (Lowe NJ, pers obs). These can be difficult or impossible to treat and will sometimes require excision or overfilling with other fillers such as fat or hyaluronic acids (see Chapters 16 and 17) to correct some of the nodularity (Table 19.5).

Silicone skin-filling injections are now rarely used in the USA except by a small number of experts who feel that, correctly injected, they still have benefits (D Duffy, pers comm). To avoid overcorrection a 'microdroplet' method is generally recommended.

Table 19.6 Potential side-effects of injectable fillers

- **Artecoll** (methacrylate and collagen)
  Delayed allergy
  Nodules
  Overcorrection
- **Arteplast** (no longer used)
- **Dermalive** (methacrylate and hyaluronic acid)
  Similar to Artecoll

The present author's use of these permanent filler injections is limited to depressed atrophic scars using Artecoll or Dermalive. To avoid overcorrection, the injection is administered using a constant in–out movement of the needle under the defect and, if necessary, the process will be repeated some weeks later.

STRUCTURE OF SOFTFORM AND ULTRASOFT – DETAILS OF THE DEVICE

SoftForm is an extruded form of e-PETE, which is the substance comprising Gore-Tex. It was developed with a facial plastic surgeon in San Francisco, the goal being to develop a usable, safe, predictable, implantable device that could also be removed if so required. These goals have been partially met, as will now be described.

The implants are a tubular type of modified Gore-Tex[5] that comes as a presterilized package complete with a pointed trocar and covering sleeve that protects the SoftForm material. Different sizes of SoftForm are available, and are summarized in Table 19.7. The section is based on experience with a group of over 100 patients treated with SoftForm over the last 3 years.

Table 19.7 SoftForm features / *UltraSoft features*

SoftForm features	UltraSoft features

- **Sizes (diameter in mm)**
  2.4 (rarely used)
  3.2
  4.0
	- **Tubular**
	  4.0 mm

	- **Slotted** 4.0 mm

- **Pretreatment for lip implants**
  Acylovir po + po antibiotics
	- **Tubular**
	  4.8 mm

- **For nasolabial folds** Antibiotics po	Different lengths are now available.

It is the present author's preference to predominantly use the 4 mm diameter implant. Occasionally, for nasolabial folds that do not require major correction or for lips that require little correction, the 3.2 mm diameter device is used; however, use of the 2.4 mm diameter device has virtually stopped. Typically, the length of the implant utilized is 50 or 70 mm for the nasolabial folds, and 90 mm for the upper and lower lip implants.

NASOLABIAL IMPLANTATION OF SOFTFORM

It is most important to follow a systematic technique in both selecting patients as well as planning for the implant prior to the start of any procedure. Patients must be fully informed of the potential problems of the implant and the present author utilizes a comprehensive information consent form for this purpose (see Appendix, p.X). In this consent form, patients are informed that the implants may migrate, that small residual scars from the nasolabial implants may be noted and that the implants may, at times, be palpable, particularly if they are placed too superficially. If the implant migrates to a high subdermal level then the occurrence of reactions such as pyagenic granulomas may also occur.

An ideal patient has a deep but well-defined nasolabial fold. Generally the broader the nasolabial folds the poorer the response to SoftForm implants. However, SoftForm implants may be used in these broader nasolabial folds as a basis for further less permanent fillers such as the hyaluronic acid fillers, e.g. Zyplast collagen, or fat transfer. This combination of treatment often leads to greater persistence of the temporary implant. Slotted (oval shaped) UltraSoft is useful for broader nasolabial folds.

Selection of patients

A summary of suitable patients is given in Table 19.8. Well-defined nasolabial folds are required, as is a lack of history of previous problems. Great care must be taken when treating patients who have had other permanent injected implants such as Artecoll or silicone, as the placing of the tubular implant can occasionally lead to accentuation of nodules caused by the previous implants: it may be necessary to refuse to treat such patients. One day prior to the procedure patients are put on a systemic antibiotic that is usually one of the cephalosporens e.g. Keflex 250 mg twice daily or erythromycin 250 mg twice daily.

On the day of the procedure the patient is examined in an upright sitting position. The positions of the implants are marked onto the patients nasolabial folds. The line of implantation is slightly medial to the nasolabial fold and the implant is directed upwards from the lower injection site towards the lateral part

Table 19.8 Patient selection for undergoing nasolabial implantation with Softform — UltraSoft

- Aware these are permanent implants
- No abnormal bleeding risk
- Willing to stop aspirin and NSAID temporarily
- Aware of the possibility of implant replacement

of the ala nasae. Just prior to reaching the ala nasae, the trocar and implant are angled slightly laterally to then appear through the excision site.

It is essential that these markings are made accurately before any local anaesthesia is given to the patient, as occasionally this may distort the facial contours and incorrect placement of the implant may ensue.

Local anaesthesia

Local anaesthesia is routinely used prior to the placement of the implant. The present author's favoured technique involves the use of 2% Xylocaine with epinephrine. A dental mandibular nerve is conducted by initially anaesthetizing the mucosa at the base at the upper canine teeth with 30% benzaciane gel c. 2–3 cm^3 of the Xylocaine with epinephrine is then injected using a 30-gauge half or one inch needle. The patient is then left for this dental nerve block to take effect. Subsequently, injections will be made at the upper and lower ends of the implant site where the incision and excision openings will be made. In this way it is possible to achieve complete anaesthesia of the area.

Insertion of implants (see Figure 19.1)

Incisions are made using a nokor 16-gauge needle (Beckton Dickinson nokor needle), which has the advantage of being a miniature scalpel that leaves a smaller scar than is achievable with most other scalpel blades. Entry with the nokor needle is made at an angle and, in most cases, lower incision point is made at a slightly different level to the corresponding incision point on the contralateral side; this is done so that should there be any marks the non-symmetric incision points will look less obvious. The area is cleansed with sterile fluid such as Betadine or Hibiclens. The device with the trocar is then inserted

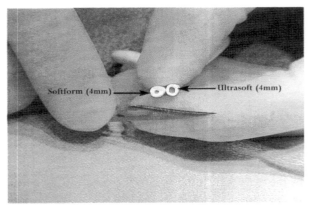
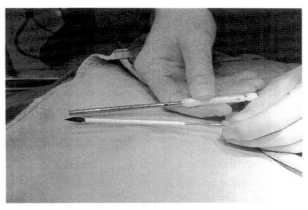

a *b*

Figure 19.1 *(A) Tubular UltraSoft and SoftForm implants. (B) SoftForm/UltraSoft tubular implants and trocar. Courtesy of Tissue Technologies and Dr C Maas.*

through the lower incision point and, by palpation from within the mouth and from outside the cheek, the placement of the trocar in the subdermal plane is ensured.

The implant is then inserted under the line drawn on the patient. Depending on the nature of the subdermal tissue, it is sometimes necessary to insert the trocar using a twisting motion to ease implantation. The implant is inserted slightly medial to the nasolabial fold, towards the alae nasea. Subsequently, just prior to reaching the alae nasea, the trocar is angled slightly laterally and then emerges through the exit incision. The safety hold on the trocar is then released and, by shielding and holding the end of the trocar to prevent rapid expulsion, the tubular cover over the implant is then withdrawn, taking great care to concertina the skin so that the implant is visible at either end of the insertion openings. The tissue is then stretched and gently draped over the implant. The patient opening their mouth widely often assists this. The present author then prefers to leave the implant in place untrimmed whilst the procedure is repeated on the other nasolabial fold.

Following insertion of both implants, the positions are checked for depth as well as correct location just medial to the nasolabial folds. The implants are trimmed transversely across the incision sites so that when their skin tissue is stretched slightly the implant will fall into the incision and excision openings. Once this is performed the ideal is not to be able to see the

implant, i.e. the implant should fall down below the dermis that then fully covers the implant. The present author uses colourless 6.0 Ethilon sutures to close the openings on the face, usually inserting two or three closely placed sutures per incision. The systemic antibiotics are then continued for 7 days following the placement of the implant and the sutures are removed on the sixth or seventh day.

LIP AUGMENTATION USING SOFTFORM AND ULTRASOFT IMPLANTS

This can be a highly successful procedure to give permanent correction for the thinning lip and thin lips with multiple vertical rhytides; it can also be successfully combined with laser skin resurfacing to give a significant rejuvenation of the atrophic upper lip, particularly where multiple rhytides are appearing.

As for nasolabial fold candidates careful patient selection is critical for permanent lip augmentation with SoftForm or UltraSoft implants. In patients with severe lower facial ageing loss of subcutaneous fat may mean undergoing other procedures, including fat transfer and laser resurfacing, either instead of or in addition to SoftForm or UltraSoft implantation.

The present author has experienced a higher incidence of problems with implant migration in older patients, possibly due to less dense subcutaneous tissue that may lead to greater implant migration.

Specific techniques of lip implantation

In the present author's opinion the optimum technique that gives patients the most satisfactory results is to use a single implant technique for both upper and lower lips. This is not the technique that was originally utilized for the upper lip by Mass et al.[1] Initially, they used double-implant technique, which unfortunately left many patients with a gap between the two implants in the mid-line of the upper lip. This became particularly evident when there was any contraction of the implant, which inevitably occurs, albeit to variable degrees in different patients. In addition, it was very difficult to disguise the implant exit incisions in the middle of the upper lip.

Implants in the upper lip

The patient is carefully selected and will be given an informed consent form to read, preferably weeks ahead of the procedure. One day prior to starting the procedure the patient is placed cephalosporin antibiotics, e.g. Keflex 250 mg daily or erythromycin 250 mg daily (as for nasolabial fold implantation). In addition, for the lips the patient is given Acyclovir 400 mg po twice daily. This is because it is often not possible to obtain an accurate history of herpes simplex virus infections and the present author feels that it is better to cover all patients for the possibility of infection.

On the day of the procedure the patient is examined seated vertically and photographs are taken from all angles. The patient is then marked as regards the insertion and exit incisions- these are placed at the angles of the mouth posterior to the border of the lip, thereby ensuring that the incisions are not visible. With the gentian violet marker the intended lip line and shape is drawn onto the patient.

Local anaesthesia

The same technique is employed as described for nasolabial implantation above, with one additional injection: after the full effects of the dental block are observed, usually after 10–15 minutes, a further injection through the benzocaine gel is placed into the medial portion of the upper lip to ensure full anaesthesia.

INSERTION OF THE IMPLANT

The insertion may start either from the left or right, depending on the preferences of the surgeon. The insertion and exit incisions are again made using a 16-gauge nokor needle. A pretunnelling technique will be used if the 4 mm implant is to be employed as it eases insertion of the implant. The implant is placed in the subdermal plane following its placement though the insertion incision. The implant is then angled towards the Cupid's bow on the side of the insertion. If the patient desires to retain or to have a Cupid's bow resulting from the implant then, at the lateral side of the Cupid's bow, the direction of the insertion of trocar is changed to point downwards, then laterally, then upwards and then downwards again towards the exit incision.

Some patients prefer a lip enhancement without an obvious cupid's bow, in which case the insertion is made without the change in direction of the trocar. After the trocar has been passed through the lip successfully and then through the exit incision, the lip is gently concertinaed over the metal trocar, the safety device released, the metal sleeve removed and, while holding one end of the implant gently, the trocar is removed. The implant is centralized and the lip is gradually and gently stretched over the implant, taking care not to stretch the implant itself.

Finally, the implant is trimmed transversely across the ends of the implant at the correct length so that when allowed to retract into the lip no visible implant is seen at the insertion and exit incisions. Black 60 Ethilon sutures may be used – the sutures should not be visible as they are hidden by the angle of the lips. These sutures usually stay for between 5 and 6 days.

LOWER LIP AUGMENTATION WITH SOFTFORM AND ULTRASOFT IMPLANTS

A very similar procedure is followed to that described for the upper lip with the exception that there is a steady placement of the implant along the lower lip line between the insertion and the exit incisions without any need for movement of change of direction of the implant.

The local anaesthesia for the lower lip implant is usually most effectively performed using a mental block of 2% Xylocaine with epinephrine; once that has taken effect then 30% benzocaine gel is placed inside the lower lip and further injections are performed to ensure that the lip is fully anaesthetized.

It is rare for the present author to place upper and lower implants at the same session, as the implant in the upper lip can often change the exact placement requirements for the lower lip implant and may also influence the decision of the size of lower lip implant, i.e. whether the patient will have a better balance with a 4 mm diameter implant or 3.2 mm diameter implant.

Patient advice to be followed after recieving a SoftForm implant is given in Table 19.9.

Table 19.9 *Post-SoftForm implant instructions*

For optimal results following a SoftForm implant procedure follow these guidelines.

Do:
- apply a small amount of antibiotic ointment two to three times a day
- apply ice to the implantation area for 24–48 hours to reduce swelling and discomfort
- keep sutures clean and dry

Do not:
- manipulate, move or push on the implant
- pick at the stiches or area surrounding the incisions
- apply make-up or lipstick until sutures are removed
- make exaggerated or excessive lip or facial movements for 2 weeks following surgery, including:
  eating hard to eat items, e.g. apples,
  excessive talking/laughing,
  excessive kissing

Call the surgeon's office if you experience:
- drainage or pus from the incision site
- redness lasting longer than 10 days
- appearance of a lump or pimple-like bump
- excessive pain lasting more than 4 days

REMOVAL TECHNIQUES

It is essential that patients be counselled that the removal of an implant is occasionally necessary usually due to implant migration, the presence of incomplete extrusion of the implant, pyogenic granuloma and changes to the lower face e.g. further thinning that results in palpability of the implant. The present author has not seen any cases of postimplant infection but this would be another indication for removal. One of the present author's patients was struck on the lip post-SoftForm by a golf ball! This resulted in extrusion and replacement.

Removal has been practical in all of the cases where it has been required, sometimes up to 2 years after implantation. The technique of removal is to anaesthetize the area as described above. A small incision is made over one of the ends of the implant (the nasal end is usually chosen for nasolabial folds in order to minimize any scarring).

An incision is made with a number 11 scalpel blade, followed by the smallest incision possible, followed by blunt scissor dissection utilizing ocular magnification. It is then possible to identify the end of the implant. This is grasped with a mosquito surgical clamp and, by gentle and variable traction, the implant is removed intact. Some of the implants that have been removed have been sent for histological examination, which has shown an ingrowth of tissue into the lumen of the implant and also some cross-growth of tissue through the material of the implant (Figure 19.8). However, in the present author's experience this has not resulted in difficulties in implant removal.

After implant removal the patient can be offered further implantation. However, it is advised that the patient allows the tissue reaction to resolve after removal of the implant and a period of several months re-evaluation of the need for further implantation can be undertaken.

SUMMARY COMMENTS ON SOFTFORM AND ULTRASOFT

These dermal implants have become a useful part of the present author's practice for lower facial rejuvenation but only in selected patients. It has been found that lip implantation has a higher rate of complications (about 10–15%) than nasolabial fold implantation (about 5%). Lip implantation problems include seromas, pyogenic granulomas; extrusion and migration of the implant. All of these seem to be independent of the care of implantation technique. However, fewer problems have been seen with a single 4 mm thick 90 mm lip implant than the original double-implant technique.

Combining lip implantation prior to laser skin resurfacing has proved particularly useful. This has lead to good results in many patients as a result of the implant enhancing the volume of the atrophic lip and acting as a preventative structure for the development recurring rhytides.

The implants are certainly not for all patients. Patients who are concerned about the occasional need for implant removal are clearly not candidates.

It has also been noted that in some patients where the implants have been removed several months to 2 years after implantation that there has been some continued improvement in either the atrophic lips or the nasolabial folds. It is presumed that this is a result of the hollow implant encouraging the growth of tissue (presumably fibroblast derived) into the area, resulting in formation of new subdermal tissue.

CONCLUSIONS

SoftForm and UltraSoft implants have proved to be a useful treatment for lower facial ageing. Careful patient selection and attention to implantation technique is essential. Patients need to be fully informed as to the potential problems and of the need for possible implant removal. Other non-removal injectable permanent fillers are useful in some situations, but patients must be warned of irreversible complications.

References

1. Lemperle G, Hazan-Gauthier N, Lemperle M. PMMA microspheres (Artecoll) for skin and soft-tissue augmentation. Part II: Clinical investigations. Plast Reconstr Surg 1995;96:627–34.

2. Ersek RA, Beisang AA 3rd. Bioplastique: a new textured copolymer microparticle promises permanence in soft-tissue augmentation. Plast Reconstr Surg 1991;87:693–702.

3. Simons G, Mazaleyrat P, Masurel T. Utilization of injectable microimplants in aesthetic facial surgery. Aesthetic Plast Surg 1992;16:77–82.

4. Cisneros JL, Singla R. Intradermal augmentation with expanded polytetrafluoroethylene (Gore-Tex) for facial lines and wrinkles. J Dermatol Surg Oncol 1993;19:539–42.

5. Maas CS, Eriksson T, McCalmont T et al. Evaluation of expanded polytetrafluoroethylene as a soft-tissue filling substance: an analysis of design-related implant behavior using the porcine skin model. Plast Reconstr Surg 1998;101:1307–14.

COMBINATION TREATMENT (Nicholas J Lowe)

Indications	Potential combination treatments	Chapter reference
Nasolabial fold	Laser resurfacing	10,11
	Non-ablative laser rejuvenation	12
	Chemical peels	6,7
Lip augmentation	Topical therapy	2
	Photoprotection	1

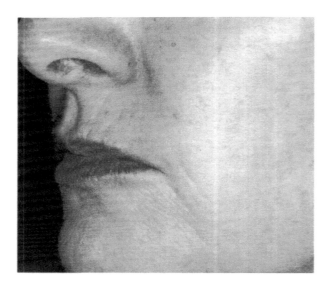

a Pre-implant

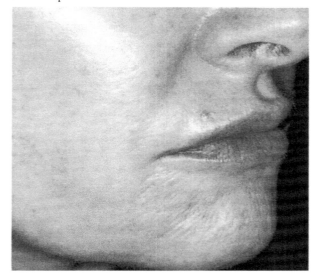

b Pre-implant

c Post-implant

d Post-implant

Figure 19.2 *SoftForm upper lip 4.0 mm × 90 mm.*

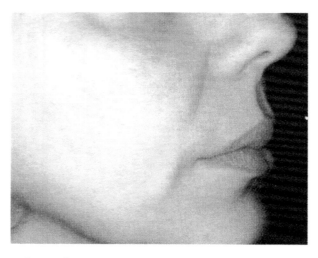 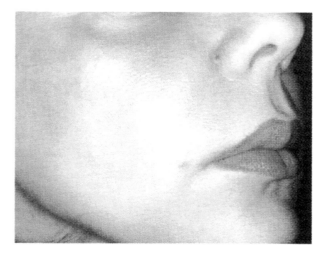

a Pre-implant   *b* Post-implant

Figure 19.3 *SoftForm nasolabial fold 3.2 mm × 7.0 mm.*

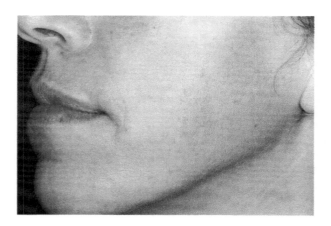 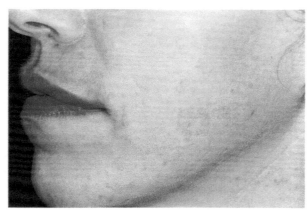

a Pre-implant   *b* Post-implant

Figure 19.4 *Pre and post SoftForm implant to upper lip. A single 4.2 mm × 90 mm was used with change of direction at the mid lip to preserve the 'Cupid's Bow'.*

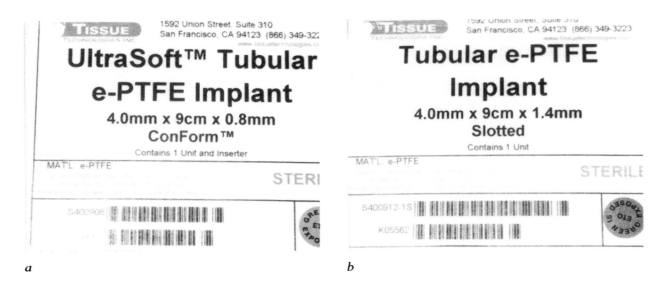

a   *b*

Figure 19.5 *There are now two different types of UltraSoft – a tubular version for lips (a) and a slotted version for nasolabial folds (b).*

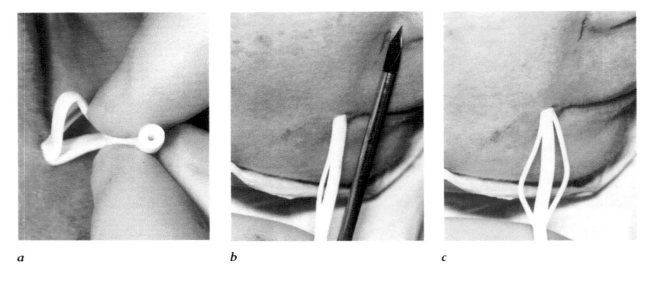

a   *b*   *c*

Figure 19.6 *Slotted UltraSoft showing tubular ends (a) and introducer trocar (b) with a patient who is having the slotted implant to her nasolabial folds (c).*

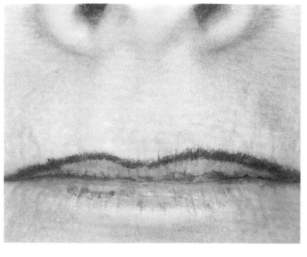

a

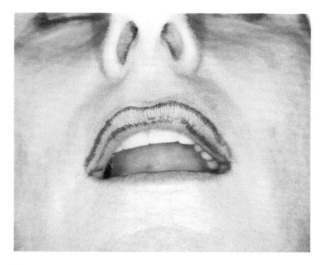

b

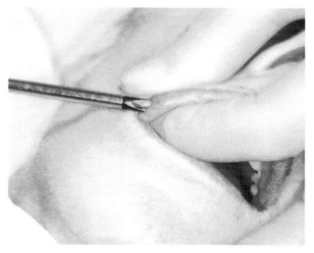

c

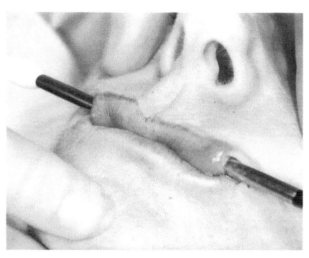

d

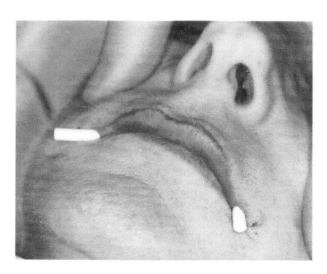

e

Figure 19.7 *(a) Before Ultrasoft implant to upper lip. See markings in gentian violet. Also note right side upper lip smaller than left. She will also have a full face ultra-pulsed carbon dioxide laser skin resurfacing. (b) Placement markings plus planned incision marks at angles of lips before Ultrasoft. (c) Ultrasoft 4 mm × 90 mm tubular implant. Trocar beimg inserted after 2% Xylocaine – Elpinephrine (Adrenaline) nerve block plus local infiltration. (d) Implant trocar in place through upper lip. (e) Trocar removed, Ultrasoft implant about to be trimmed.*

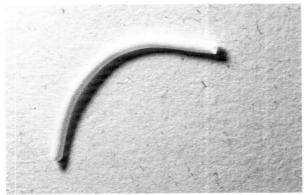

a

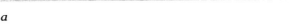

b

Figure 19.8 (a) An example of a 3.2 mm SoftForm implant prior to use. (b and c) A cross section of a SoftForm implant removed after 18 months from a patient's upper lip to replace 2 implants with 1. See the capsule formation and some fibroblast growth through the implant.

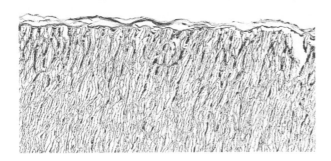

c

20. Objective measurement of lips augmented with SoftForm using three-dimensional laser surface scanning

Brian Coghlan, Beverly Westwood and Sue Nicholl

INTRODUCTION

Surgical improvement of the features of the lips may include augmentation to give a fuller and more sensuous appearance, resurfacing to reduce rhytides and permanent tattooing to accentuate the vermillion border. Advancement and filling is effective in rejuvenation of the senile lip and in cosmetic augmentation. A variety of autogenous, homogeneous and alloplastic materials, and different surgical implantation techniques have been used in an attempt to achieve this.[1–7] Implantation of crystal silicone, polyacrylamide hydrogel,[4] polytef (Gore-Tex®),[1,2,7] including expanded polytetrafluoroethylene,[4] bovine collagen, autologous fat,[8] and dermis fat graft have all been evaluated with mixed success.[4] No single material has yet been found to achieve a soft and long-lasting effect. Gore-Tex, an alloplastic material, is an expanded fibrillated polytetrafluoroethylene polymer. It was established safe as a vascular graft many years ago. It has been claimed that the Gore-Tex implant does not produce a big enough change in the appearance of the lip,[7] although others have found it safe, simple and effective.[2] Bovine collagen does not provide permanent results. Homogeneous materials such as Zyderm® (McGhan Corp, Santa Barbara, CA) usually undergo significant resorption within months. Autogenous tissue grafts and flaps can give unpredictable results and donor morbidity. Alloplastic materials usually result in complications, including immunological reactions, rigidity of the material and extrusion.

Patients presenting for lip augmentation procedures frequently have requests for different cosmetic outcomes. These can be placed in three groups:

(1) More mucosal show of the lip 'pout'
(2) Enhanced Cupid's-bow definition of the upper lip
(3) More clearly defined vermilion/skin junction.

The ideal lip augmentation procedure should result in a soft, predictable and permanent change without visible scarring. It is difficult for the surgeon to describe the outcomes of various procedures and there are no published reports on the amount of augmentation achieved by implants of different sizes. Managing the patient's expectations is a key element in their overall satisfaction with the procedure.

All of our patients presenting for lip augmentation procedures are routinely photographed using digital technology. Selected patients also have their lips scanned using three-dimensional (3D) laser-imaging technology, an established technique in maxillo-facial surgery.[9,10] The patients are scanned immediately before the implantation procedure and 3 months following the procedure. All of the patients who have SoftForm implants to their lips are asked to complete a questionnaire. A series of 10 consecutive patients who have had 3D laser scanning, observations from these scans and a summary of the patients' questionnaires is presented in this chapter.

During the past year, one of the present authors has implanted a total of 121 pieces of SoftForm™ (Biomatrix Inc, Ridgefield, NJ). These were placed at lip, nasolabial crease and glabellar sites. Patients who have had implants in their lips in conjunction with other procedures such as rhytidectomy or rhinoplasty are not included in this series as the impact of the additional procedures might influence the outcome, as the overall appearance of the face will have changed.

SoftForm has already been evaluated clinically and found to have the unique advantage of forming a well-accentuated Cupid's bow.[4] In this study, the SoftForm tubes were still palpable 3 months after implantation.

METHODS AND MATERIALS

Patients were selected based upon their desire for upper and lower lip augmentation, wishing for more volume of the lower lip and more definition of the Cupid's bow of the upper lip. Patients taking aspirin, or those with a local skin condition or a sensitivity to Gore-Tex were not included (manufacturers' precautions). Prior to surgery, all patients were counselled about the procedure. They were provided with literature about SoftForm and, having read it and received answers to any questions, they signed consent for the procedure. Patients who had previously had collagen injections to the lips were considered suitable for the procedure, provided that more than 3 months had elapsed since the last injections and that no residual collagen could be felt on medical examination. All patients were photographed with their lips relaxed but not smiling. They attended the Department of Medical Physics and Bioengineering, University College London Hospital (UCLH), where they were prepared for the 3D laser surface scanning. The hair was held back with a band and the patients were seated in the scanning chair. The subjects were all scanned on the optical surface scanner.[9,10] This uses a low-powered infrared laser beam, which is rotated typically through 250°, fanned vertically onto the face. The scan takes about 15 seconds during which time the patient needs to keep still. Profiles are collected and converted into 3D coordinates of points lying on the surface of the face. The precision is more than 0.5 mm.

The scans from before and after the implant were loaded into the UCLH 3D surface registration package. The two scans were registered by moving each image into the same 3D space and observing the difference between the surfaces. This is represented as a colour-coded image of differences in millimetres. The maximum change over the region of the implant was measured for each subject (see Figure 20.5).

The patients were marked whilst upright, detailing the red/white mucocutaneous junction of the upper and lower lips. All patients received prophylaxis with oral antibiotics and those with a history of herpes simplex infection also received an oral antiviral agent.

Patients were positioned on the operating table with their back 45° to the vertical. A mixture of lignocaine with adrenaline and marcaine were infiltrated into an infraorbital and mental nerve block, as well as small blebs of local anaesthetic at the intended entry and exit sites on the lips. The skin was prepared, the face draped and the entry points were defined using a number 15 scalpel blade. Two pieces of 3.2 mm SoftForm were tunnelled (using the introducer) into the upper lip so that the central part of the cylinder augmented the mucocutaneous junction (the alternative technique using a single implant across the top lip was not used as it is best for upper lip volume augmentation and not Cupid's bow definition). The introducer was advanced as far as the philtral colunm and then withdrawn to exit through the marked point. The cannula was removed, as well as the trocar, the edges of the implant were trimmed to a 45° angle and the central part of the cylinder was opened using the tip of the trocar. It was positioned so that the medial end was placed up into the base of the philtral colunm and the lateral end was buried well into the orbicularis muscle. Closure was with two 6/0 Prolene sutures at each entry site. The lower lip had a single piece of 2.4 mm SoftForm tunnelled along the mucocutaneous junction and a similar closure technique was used.

The patients were sat upright afterwards with swabs soaked in iced water against the lips. They were encouraged to remain upright for the rest of the day and to sleep propped up on pillows in order to minimize swelling. Follow-up was arranged for 7 days later when the sutures were removed. The patients were given a questionnaire to complete immediately prior to the procedure and at the 3-month follow-up visit (a copy is attached in the Appendix). The questionnaire was designed to be as minimally suggestive as possible; consequently, patients were asked to use their own words to describe their feelings and appearance, and were also required to complete a visual analogue scale rating their personal appearance.

RESULTS

In this case series 10 patients had a total of 30 pieces of SoftForm implanted, 20 into the top lip and 10 into the bottom lip. Using 3.2 mm implants only in the top lip, an average augmentation of 1.99 mm was achieved (standard deviation (SD), 0.85 mm; range, 1.1–3.9 mm. For the lower lip, using 2.4 mm implants, an average augmentation of 2.48 mm was achieved (SD, 1.31 mm; range, 0.7–5.0 mm).

APPEARANCE OF LIPS BEFORE SOFTFORM

The 10 patients in this series were asked what words they would use to describe their lips prior to having SoftForm implants; the results are presented in Figure 20.1.

It is noted from Figure 20.1 that only one patient described her lips as looking normal before surgery; the majority felt that their lips were thin (seven out of 10) and either flat or lacking definition (six out of 10).

Subjective feelings about lips before augmentation

The patients in the series were asked to describe their feelings about their lips prior to the augmentation procedure; the results are presented in Figure 20.2.

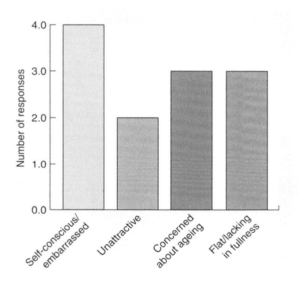

Figure 20.2 Feeling about lips before SoftForm.

Expected outcome versus actual outcome

The patients in the series were asked to describe both their expected and actual outcomes of lip augmentation; the results are presented in Figure 20.3.

It is interesting to note that whilst the pre-implant expectations focused on the anticipated physical aspects of the implants the vast majority of actual outcomes focused upon the positive psychological effects.

Appearance rating

The patients in the series, were asked to complete a 10 cm visual analogue scale to indicate how they

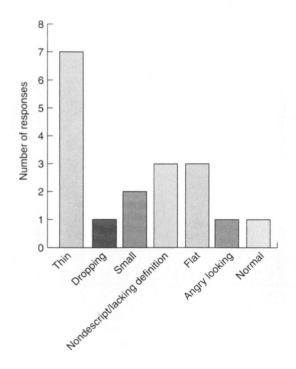

Figure 20.1 Appearance of lips before SoftForm.

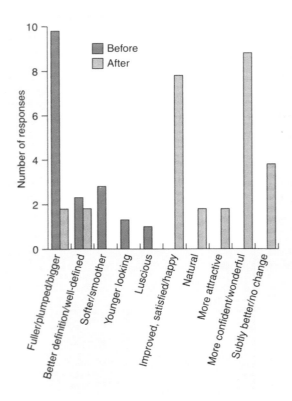

Figure 20.3 *Expectations versus outcomes.*

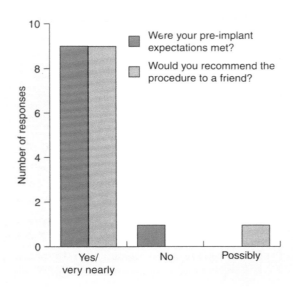

Figure 20.4 *Pre-implant expectations.*

rated their appearance following surgery. The left-hand side of the line represented 'worse than previously' and the right-hand side 'better than previously'. The average mark was 7.34 cm, indicating that appearance was considered to have improved following implantation. This number was derived from nine responses as one patient did not complete this evaluation. The range of scores obtained varied from 4.9 cm from the least satisfied patient to 9.7 cm from the most satisfied patient.

Pre-implant expectations

The patients in the series were asked whether their pre-implant expectations were met and whether they would recommend the procedure to a friend; the results are presented in Figure 20.4.

In all but one case (nine out of 10) the pre-implant expectations were met and the same number of nine out of 10) would definitely recommend the procedure to a friend.

Laser measurement

The 3D laser scanner was used to measure the augmentation in the lips. All post-implant scans were taken 3 months after the implants had been inserted. The pre- and post-implant scans were superimposed and the difference in size was calculated by computer programme; the results are presented in Figure 20.5.

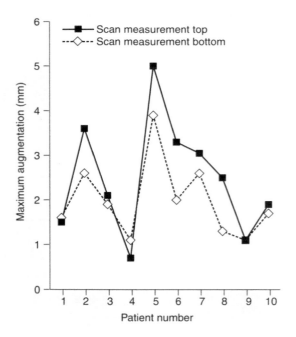

Figure 20.5 *Augmentation of the lips.*

The procedure

The patients in the series were asked to describe their lip augmentation procedure; the results are presented in Figure 20.6.

With respect to the procedure itself, the majority of responses indicated that it was uncomfortable and some rated it as frightening or traumatic. None of these patients received any sedation with the local anaesthetic.

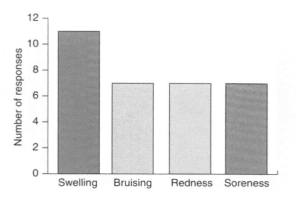

Figure 20.7 *Adverse experience.*

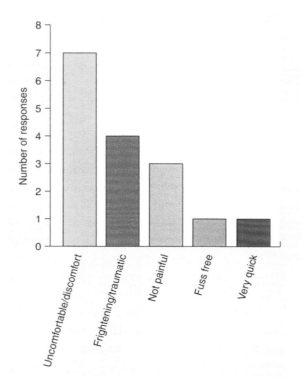

Figure 20.6 *Words used to describe the lip augmentation procedure.*

Adverse experiences

All of the patients in the series experienced some of the symptoms of swelling, bruising, redness and soreness following the procedures; the results from the questionnaire are presented in Figure 20.7.

Patients were recommended to ice the lips and to take non-aspirin, non-NSAID analgesics. One patient had an infection 5 days after the procedure, which the present authors believe was because her anaesthetist husband removed the sutures 2 days early to save her return visit at 7 days. Subsequently, one of the

wounds broke down and the implant protruded through it: an infection ensued which was treated with antibiotics and resolved satisfactorily. The patient's husband resutured the wound and the implant did not need to be removed. No other adverse device experiences were reported and 6 months post-procedure all implants are still in situ.

Effects of the procedure on daily life

The patients in the series were asked to describe the effect of lip augmentation on their daily lives; the results are presented in Figure 20.8.

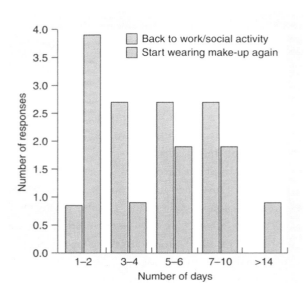

Figure 20.8 *Effects of the procedure on daily life.*

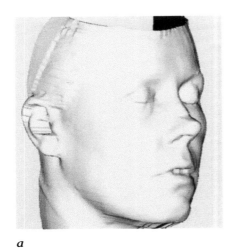
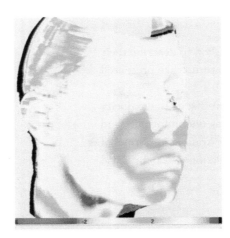

a   *b*

Figure 20.9 (a) Preoperative 3D laser scan, (b) Post SoftForm image superimposed on preoperative image. Warm colours are advancements, measured in millimetres.

The results show that procedure itself did not keep the patients out of action for very long. The majority returned to work or social activity and began wearing make-up again within 6 days.

3D images of a patient before and after surgery

3D images of a patients before and after lip augmentation are presented in Figure 20.9.

DISCUSSION

When offering a patient a choice of materials for lip augmentation it is clearly important to be able to provide a reasonable estimate of the degree of augmentation the procedure is likely to achieve, and to match this to expectations and aesthetic requirements. Although other techniques based on photography and computer imaging have been developed, none is totally satisfactory in providing the patient with an accurate and quantitative impression of how the end result might appear.

Patients chose to have their lips augmented with SoftForm because they understood it to be safe and to provide a long-lasting result. On the whole, their expectations of the procedure were modest and the quantitative results demonstrate that they are happier with a smaller lip projection than the surgeon might have expected.[5] Only one patient described her lips as looking normal prior to the procedure. The other words used were flat, thin, lacking definition – at face value, fairly innocuous descriptions. It is only when these words are juxtaposed to the words used in answer to the question, 'what words would you use to describe your feelings about your lips prior to your implants?', that the negative connotations become apparent. The words such as 'self-conscious', 'embarrassed', 'unattractive' and 'concerned about ageing' imply that all of the women (10 out of 10) in this series expected to become more attractive following the SoftForm implants. It was perceived that the consequent increase in lip volume would make the difference. However, when asked what words they would use to describe what they expected their lips to look like, there was no stated expectation of heightened attractiveness or enhanced self-esteem. Examples were better definition, younger looking, luscious, softer. Words used to describe the actual outcome confirmed the improvement of self image, e.g. more attractive, more confident, wonderful, improved. The visual analogue scale (VAS) scores confirmed this perceived enhancement of appearance, even though only nine responses were given and the score includes the response from the least satisfied patient.

All but one of the patients had their pre-implant expectations met and would definitely recommend the procedure to a friend. This is interesting, as there is no direct correlation between the degree of augmentation and the degree of satisfaction in appearance. Indeed, the least satisfied patient showed almost the average augmentation for both top and bottom lips and this was the only patient who had undergone previous lip augmentation surgery with collagen injections.

The maximum augmentation measured is consistent with that obtained using other augmentation techniques and methods of measurement.[6,7] The explanation for a mean 2.0 mm anterior augmentation for a 3.2 mm diameter implant in the upper lip may be due to the adaptation of the soft tissues of the upper lip preventing a full augmentation with the implant compressing the local lip anatomy. The lower lip augmentation of 2.5 mm with a 2.4 mm implant could be from eversion of the lower lip due to the implant placement in the musculocutaneous junction. The 3D surface laser-scanning method relies on the subjects achieving the same facial expression between the two scans. Any alteration in the facial musculature, such as frowning or smiling or other unexpressed tension, could impact upon the measurements. Whilst every effort was made to attain this, there were some quite noticeable differences in some subjects such as lengthening of the jaw, lips further apart, smiling or frowning slightly. Smiling would spread the lips and appear to reduce the thickness of the lips and hence mask the measurable difference. This inevitably reduces the reliability of the measurement technique but is equally a limitation of the other techniques that have been referenced in this paper. Some compensation for the differences could be made by the use of registration points, local to the lips but unaffected by the procedure, to match the pre- and postprocedure scans. At this stage in the development of the scanning technique, it was felt that volume measurements of the lips could not be derived from the data with sufficient accuracy or robustness.

All of the patients found the procedure to be uncomfortable and some rated it as frightening or traumatic, despite the fact that eight out of 10 of the patients rated the pre-implant counselling as good or excellent. This highlights just how important it is to prepare the patients for the procedure and suggests that the clinic staff might underestimate the impact of the procedure in their explanations. None of the patients commented that the procedure itself was actually painful. The use of sedation techniques in addition to the local anaesthetic blocks might be appropriate for some patients.

Statement of sponsorship: Collagen UK Ltd kindly donated the SoftForm implants and also paid for the laser scanning.

Note: all patients signed two consent forms; one for the implant procedure and one for publication of photographs or laser/digital images.

References

1 Linder RM. Permanent lip augmentation employing polytetrafluoroethylene grafts. Plast Reconstr Surg 1992;90:1083–90.

2 Conrad K, MacDonald MR. Wide polytef (Gore-Tex) implants in lip augmentation and nasolabial groove correction. Arch Otolaryngol Head Neck Surg 1996;122:664–70.

3 Hubmer MG, Hoffman C, Popper H, Scharnagl E. Expanded polytetrafluoroethylene threads for lip augmentation induce foreign body granulomatous reaction. Plast Reconstr Surg 1999;103:1277–9.

4 Niechajev I. Lip enhancement: surgical alternatives and histological aspects. Plast Reconstr Surg 2000;105:1173–83.

5 Maloney BP. Cosmetic surrgery of the lips. Facial Plast Surg 1966;12:265–79.

6 Castor SA, Wyatt CT, Papay FA. Lip augmentation with AlloDerm acellular allogenic dermal graft and Fat Autograft: a comparison with autologous fat injection alone. Aesth Plas Surg 1999;23:218–23.

7 Wang J, Fan J, Nordstrom REA. Evaluation of augmentation with Gore-Tex facial implant. Aesth Plast Surg 1997;21:433–6.

8 Fulton JE, Rahimi ADA, Helton P, et al. Lip rejuvenation. Dermatol Surg 26;5:470–5.

9 Linney AD, Campos J,. Richards R. Non-contact anthropometry using projected laser line distortion: three dimensionalg graphic visualisation and applications. Optics Lasers in Eng 1997;28:137–55.

10. Moss JP, Linney AD Grindrod SR, Mosse CA. A laser scanning system for the measurement of facial surface morphology. Optics Lasers in Eng 1989;10:179–90.

21. Hair transplantation techniques

Dow B Stough and Jeffrey M Whitworth

BACKGROUND

The field of hair restoration is an exciting and dynamic specialty in contemporary medicine, although the general public is largely unaware of the results possible with the refined techniques now available – advanced technologies are enabling surgeons to achieve better results than ever before. The field of hair restoration includes both medical and surgical modalities, and this chapter will attempt to clarify the salient aspects of the hair restoration process. Pretreatment, treatment, and posttreatment considerations will be discussed.

CONSULTATION

Individuals considering hair restoration surgery should expect to meet with a physician to discuss their hair loss history, and their surgical and medical options. In the consultation a plan for hair restoration is sought and received. This process is crucial for both patient and physician, an outcome that is satisfactory to both parties hangs in the balance of a successful consultation. This is the time when a patient's preconceived notions and desires, perhaps fraught with emotion, are modified by a physician's knowledge. The doctor will express concerns about patient expectations and gauge what can feasibly be obtained (Figure 21.1). Often, the patient and doctor begin from two divergent perspectives and by the end of the consultative phase have a common understanding, a common goal, and a well-defined plan for achieving this end. If the

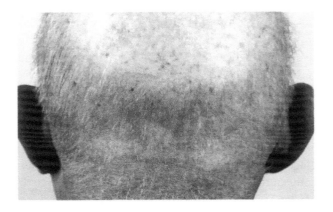

Figure 21.1 *Many males who experience severe alopecia in their early teens and twenties will progress to a Norwood VII stage alopecia. With proper planning and execution, these individuals can be transplanted at an early age without fear of decline in the cosmesis of the transplant.*

physician's explanations and understanding appear inadequate, the patient should seek consultation with another surgeon. Likewise, the physician should proceed with caution if the patient cannot grasp explanations of the proposed treatment plan, its risks and benefits.

THE PHYSICIAN'S ROLE

A patient visiting for consultation should receive frank, open, and honest communication regarding their hair loss. The patient should gain a clear under-standing of the short- and long-term treatment plan along with potential complications.

Patient history

During the consultation, the physician will inquire about the patient's ultimate goal, previous hair trans-plants or scalp surgeries, and medical history. The physician should specifically ask what is most impor-tant to the patient; the simple question, 'What is your goal?', is most helpful. This consideration is of criti-cal significance in the authors' preoperative evalua-tions as it is the basis from which patient expectations can be synchronized with surgical and medical capabilities. A history of previous hair transplants or scalp surgeries, both of which factor into preopera-tive planning from the standpoint of scalp elasticity, recipient site creation, and donor strip harvesting, is imperative. A medical history should include questions regarding previous bleeding problems, medication ingestion and medication allergies, as well as a history of herbal and vitamin intakes (garlic, gingko biloba and vitamin E all have the potential to contribute to intra-operative and postoperative bleeding). Preoperative evaluation may also include assessing the need for preoperative antibiotics in select cases; the present authors do not recommend preoperative antibiotics on a routine basis.

CANDIDACY

Useful criteria for assessing an individual's predica-tion as a candidate for hair transplantation include the degree of baldness, caliber of the hair shaft, skin to hair color match, donor hair volume, donor hair density and patient expectations.[1,2]

Pattern of baldness

Individuals with androgenetic alopecia who possess primarily anterior baldness are more suitable candi-dates for hair restoration than those with excessive loss in the vertex. This is because transplantation limited only to the anterior scalp utilizes less donor hair. A complete restoration of the vertex area is potentially problematic. This can result in isolation of

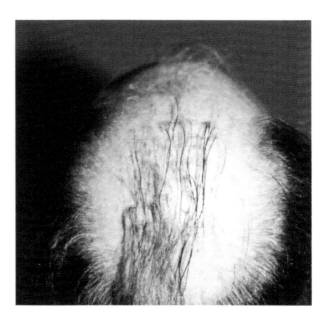

Figure 21.2 *A 55-year-old male who received standard 4mm punch autografts in his twenties. The progression of baldness has created a halo of alopecia surrounding the grafts. Such progression of baldness is predictable and limits attempts at a complete restoration in the vertex area.*

transplanted hair in an unnatural pattern referred to as a donut or halo deformity (Figure 21.2). Although additional transplants can be performed in the vertex, an insufficient donor supply to continue supporting the earlier transplant often exists, result-ing in an increasing prominence of this 'halo'. Patients desiring transplantation of their vertex are routinely refused by the present authors, although rare excep-tions are noted.

Unlike vertex alopecia, frontal alopecia lends itself to a definable and attainable goal of facial framing. This framing shortens the face and serves to draw the attention of the observing eye away from the upper forehead to the mid-face, especially the eyes. Thus, in transplanting a bald individual, the scalp becomes a 'nonissue' by redirection of attention to the central one-third of the face as opposed to the scalp. Facial framing imparts a reminiscence of a younger self to the patient when examining his reflec-tion. For these reasons, the presence of an isolated frontal forelock or complete anterior alopecia makes one a stronger candidate for hair restoration than one with the presence of isolated vertex balding. Most men seeking consultation for hair restoration have a combination of frontal and vertex balding. The greater the component of frontal baldness, the stronger the surgical candidate.

Occipital hair density

Patients with high donor hair density yield a greater number of grafts per unit area of scalp. This large donor supply is most advantageous. Men require 13–15 hairs per 4 mm field as a minimum to be considered for transplants. In terms of follicular

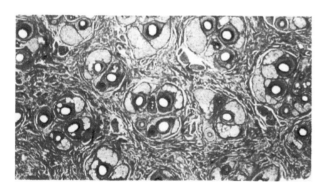

Figure 21.3 *A close-up of the donor area depicting varying numbers of hairs within a follicular unit grouping. In this photograph, one, two and three follicular units are easily identified. (Courtesy of Dr Francisco Jimenez.)*

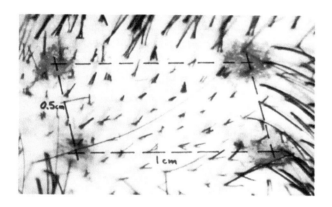

Figure 21.4 *The histology of follicular unit groups at the level of the mid-dermis demonstrating the close association between the sebaceous gland and the hair follicles. Each follicular unit group is enveloped by blue stroma which corresponds to peri-follicular collagen. A follicular unit group may contain one to five hairs. (Courtesy of Dr David Whiting.)*

units, at least 8–10 follicular units per 4 mm field must be observed in the donor area (Figures 21.3 and 21.4).

Caliber

Hair transplant surgeons generally speak of hair caliber or volume when discussing hair shaft width. Larger width (> 80 μm) hair is of higher cosmetic value than fine hair.[3] Patients possessing fine hair (< 80 μm), are destined to have a sparse quality to their transplant, even with dense transplantation of grafts in the recipient area. Persons with curlier hair are better candidates for hair transplantation because the curly hair imparts an illusion of density.

Skin to hair color match

The color of hair relative to the color of skin is important. People with a hair color that closely matches their skin color have a lower contrast of transplanted hair against the background of scalp skin. These individuals have optimal short- and long-term results because of a decreased prominence of the follicular unit as it exits the scalp. This is the concept behind scalp camouflaging products that reduce the contrast of hair color to skin color. Patients having light hair color and fair skin are better candidates than those with dark hair color and fair skin.

Patient expectations

The final consideration in assessing a person's candidacy for hair restoration surgery is the individual's expectations. If a patient approaches with unrealistic expectations or desires, and these desires are unable to be modified through careful consultation, this person is a poor candidate for hair transplantation.

Men in their late teens and early twenties with the beginnings of frontotemporal recessions often desire restoration of their hairline to its original juvenile location. Such cases are problematic. These young men presently maintain enough hair for facial framing and will receive limited aesthetic benefit from surgery. Another consideration when planning a hair restoration procedure is that due to the progression of male pattern baldness, patients can be left with an unnatural zone of baldness between transplanted hair and further recessions. If a transplant is placed low at an early age it may eventually appear unnatural. Individuals that obtain a restoration of their original low-lying hairline often seek corrective surgery in the future.

FEMALE PATTERN ALOPECIA

Women with female pattern alopecia experience hair loss in a different pattern than males, thus the above discussion of the presence or absence of frontal baldness does not typically apply to women. Patterns of female loss do bear their own considerations in assessing any given woman's quality as a candidate for hair restoration.

Usually, in female hair loss the most anterior segment of the frontal hairline is maintained to a greater extent than the scalp posterior to it. In its mildest form, it may be noticeable only as a slight expansion of the parted hair. In its most severe form, female alopecia may occur as diffuse, severe thinning of hair in all areas of the scalp (diffuse unpatterned alopecia).[2] Women from either extreme are poor surgical candidates.

Those with mild female pattern alopecia are poor surgical candidates due to their total hair volume being such that appreciable differences in pretransplanted scalp versus post-transplanted scalp are not obvious. Those with diffuse unpatterned alopecia are poor surgical candidates for the obvious reason that the entire scalp is suffering hair loss, thus, the donor area is of limited value as it is just as susceptible to loss as hair elsewhere on the scalp. Women who are the best patients for hair transplantation are those with high density donor hair and extensive hair loss or thinning of the frontal scalp. A frontal thinning pattern of < 10–13 (follicular units per cm^2) is required to proceed with a recommendation of hair transplantation in individuals experiencing female pattern alopecia. These patients will receive the greatest cosmetic benefit.

MEDICAL TREATMENT/THERAPY

Currently, there are only two medically proven treatments for hair loss; one being minoxidil and the other finasteride. Minoxidil exerts its effects on the cells of the hair follicle, although its precise mechanism of action in androgenic alopecia and female pattern alopecia is not known.[5] Common side-effects of topical minoxidil include unwanted facial hair growth (especially disconcerting to women) and skin irritation or localized skin allergy to a component of the minoxidil solution. Rarely, patients may complain of headaches or chest pain.

The oral medication indicated for use in the treatment of male pattern baldness only is finasteride in a 1 mg per day dose. At this time, side-effects include changes in sexual function that manifest in men as decreased libido, ejaculatory dysfunction or erectile dysfunction. It should be noted that the incidence of these side-effects is only slightly higher than the placebo, and less than 2% overall. Gynecomastia is also a side-effect infrequently reported with finasteride administration. While the incidence of all adverse effects are low, anecdotal, nonstatistical reports among transplant surgeons reflect a somewhat higher incidence of decreased libido and gynecomastia than well-documented studies by the pharmaceutical house. The value of these reports cannot be assessed. Finasteride is not indicated for the treatment of female pattern alopecia due to the potential for birth defects in the form of feminization of a male fetus. For this reason, women of reproductive potential should neither ingest nor handle finasteride.

The advantages of medications are well established: both minoxidil and finasteride are likely to slow or halt hair loss in a given individual. Once stabilization of the bald scalp is achieved, the area requiring a transplant is also stabilized and subsequently less donor hair will need to be harvested. This theoretical scenario is one reason hair transplant surgeons have embraced finasteride. A select few individuals will experience impressive regrowth with minoxidil, finasteride or both. These lucky patients have the capability of achieving the most complete and natural hair restoration possible. The downside for those who experience regrowth with the use of medications is that continuous administration is necessary to maintain a clinical response. One would expect loss of hairs regrown or maintained by either minoxidil or finasteride upon discontinuation of either treatment.

HAIR RESTORATION SURGERY

Donor strip harvesting

Most surgeons favor taking a single, elliptical donor strip that may range in width from 6 mm to 1.2 cm. There are c. 1000 follicular units in a 20 cm long by 6 mm wide strip of tissue. An 11 cm long by 1 cm width strip of tissue will yield similar results in those with adequate density.

Prior to surgery, 15 cm³ of 0.5% lidocaine with 1:200,000 epinephrine is administered to the donor area. Immediately before excising the area, 20 cm³ of saline solution is injected to create dermal turgor, 3 cm³ syringes are used to administer this saline. Planck's law dictates that the pressure generated in a small syringe is much greater than that in a larger syringe. Syringes larger than 3 cm³ cannot achieve firm tumescence of the occipital area, which is necessary to minimize donor strip transection (Figure 21.5).

Using an elliptical harvest with a double blade, one limits the surface area of the scalp that is cut blindly. This allows the donor strip harvest to be performed with limited transection of donor hair.[7] The blade is held parallel to the patients hair follicle, though not perpendicular to the skin in order to avert hair shaft transection. The scalpel blade is inserted approximately 5 mm into the scalp, enough to reach a depth of 1–2 mm below the terminus of the hair follicles. The strip is then tapered into an elliptical

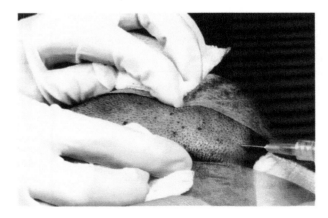

Figure 21.5 *Super tumescence of the occipital area is achieved with 3 cm³ syringes and saline injected into the mid-dermal plain. Rock-hard tumescence minimizes hair shaft transection.*

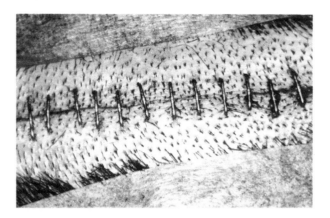

Figure 21.6 *Closure of the donor area with staples.*

pattern and cut from the base using sharp scissors: hemostasis is obtained. The present authors prefer wound closure with surgical staples (Figure 21.6).

Graft creation

Once the donor tissue is harvested, the strip is placed in a Petri dish containing chilled isotonic saline. The techniques used for subsectioning the donor strip are accomplished with great precision using a range of methods. At one extreme, automated graft sectioning can be achieved using donor tissue which has been harvested with a multibladed knife. These thin strips of tissue are laid across 1–2 mm wide spaced, parallel blades of an automated graft cutter. By applying pressure, a number of micro- or minigrafts are created. At the other extreme, the elliptical donor tissue is taken and dissected with a number 10 surgical blade using backlighting and microscopic magnification. In the former method, transection of hair follicles will be at a maximum; in the latter method, transection of hair follicles will be at a minimum. The aesthetic benefits of hairs in a nontransected state is currently controversial; however, purists of follicular unit transplantation advocate the use of microscopes for creation of follicular unit grafts.[3] Though there is evidence that transected hair will grow, the quality of any given hair involves its cross-sectional area and transected hairs have demonstrated diameter of growth less than that of their parent hair.[3] In between the aforementioned examples, one might find a surgeon who uses backlighting with no magnification;

Table 21.1 *A comparison of follicular unit techniques*

Technique	Advantages	Disadvantages
Simultaneous needle stick and graft placement	Microscopic dissection limits follicular transsection The physician is free to engage in other activities after the donor strip is harvested	Microscopic dissection contributes to slower procedure times Microscopic dissection requires training and time for technicians to become proficient
Simultaneous blade slit and graft placement	Very fast implantation phase and total time Physician control of graft position and spacing Larger slits accept chubbier grafts, that require less tissue trimming. (This may translate to a higher quality of transplanted hair)	Insertion requires a two-person team, one person must be a physician
Separated needle stick and graft placement	Microscopic dissection limits follicular transsection The physician is free to engage in other activities after donor strip harvesting and recipient site creation Physician control of graft position and spacing	Microscopic dissection contributes to slower procedure times Microscopic dissection requires training and time for technicians to become proficient An additional time disadvantage may be related to the separation of recipient site creation from graft insertion
The Choi implanter	Extremely fast implantation phase Very fast total case time Physician control of graft position and spacing	Extensive highly trained technical support is required for the implantation phase Choi implanters are disposable with short life spans, contributing to a higher cost to the physician Choi implanters may work better with coarse hair than with fine hair Grafts are made without the use of loop magnification, microscopic magnification, or backlighting, increasing the risk of follicular transsection The insertion phase utilizes physician participation

Reproduced with permission from: Stough D, Whitworth J. Hair restoration and laser hair removal – dermatologic clinics. In: Methodology of follicular unit hair transplantation, Volume 17, Number 2. Philadelphia: WB Saunders Co; 1999:297–306.

or no backlighting and simply a magnifying glass to cut donor tissue, or any number of possible combinations.

Currently, the present authors are proponents of the use of microscopes with backlighting for donor tissue dissection, in an effort to keep hair transection to a minimum (Figures 21.7–21.9).

Graft insertion

The recipient scalp is anesthetized in preparation of creating the incisions for graft placement. The present authors routinely perform a bilateral supraorbital nerve block, achieving anesthesia of the mid-frontal portion of the scalp. Subsequent local infiltration is

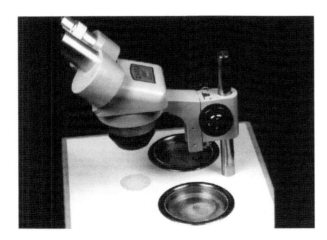

Figure 21.7 *A dissecting stereomicroscope utilizing 4× magnification and backlight illumination. The Petri dishes are positioned in an ice-bath which allows the grafts to be maintained at 1–3°C.*

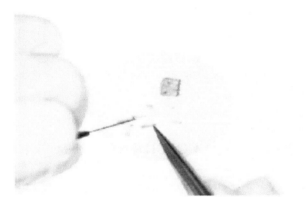

Figure 21.8 *Graft dissection is achieved with the aid of a dissecting microscope and backlight illumination. Jeweler's forceps and a number 10 blade are the present authors' choice for instrumentation.*

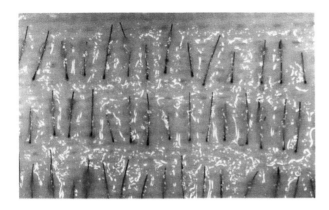

Figure 21.9 *Single hair grafts produced by follicular unit dissection.*

accomplished by employing 10 cm³ of 0.5% lidocaine with 1:200,000 epinephrine. Fifteen to 30 minutes before making the incisions, the area is injected with a mixture of 8 cm³ saline and 0.1 cm³ of 1:1000 epinephrine to inhibit bleeding. The final concentration of epinephrine is, therefore, 1:80,000.

The insertion phase of hair transplantation typically proceeds in one of two ways. In one method, all recipient sites for the grafts are created ahead of time, after which individuals performing the implantation of the grafts insert them, usually with a jeweler's forceps. In this method, graft position and spacing is dictated by the physician. The equipment typically used for the creation of the recipient sites may be either needles or blades.

Follicular unit hair transplantation surgery, when performed with appropriate regard to future hair loss and the patient's own hair characteristics, offers patients the most natural appearing hair restoration available (Figures 21.10–21.12). It is important to reiterate here in the strongest of terms that no hair transplant can duplicate the natural state. However, the present authors have noted many patients transplanted in the 1990s, with results which mimic nature so closely that their spouses and even hair stylists are unaware of their undergoing a hair transplant procedure.

Scalp reduction

A scalp reduction is simply an excision of bald scalp. With this technique, hair-bearing skin is brought closer together. There are many different designs employed in excising the balding area in a scalp reduction surgery. Reductions may be performed in conjunction with hair transplantation to the remaining bald scalp, so that in combination these two techniques allow for completion of the hair restoration process.

One problem that often arises after a scalp reduction is, with the passage of time and natural progression of hair loss, scars becoming noticeable. Another problem that can occur is the widening of scars after a scalp reduction, even when performed by experienced surgeons. Usually, more than one scalp reduction is necessary to effectively address a person's baldness. Although scalp reductions are a short-term solution to baldness, this efficacy diminishes due to

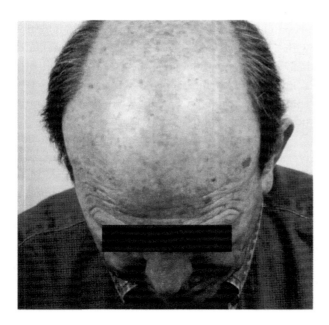

Figure 21.10 A 61-year-old male, prior to transplantation.

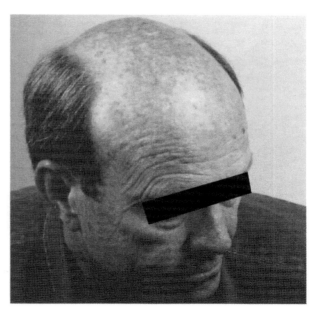

Figure 21.11 The patient shown in Fig 21.10 before transplantation.

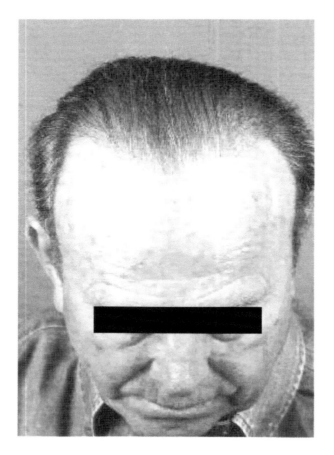

Figure 21.12 The patient shown in Figures 21.10 and 21.11 after transplantation of 4385 follicular units.

the unpredictable progression of hair loss in any given individual.

SHORT-TERM CONSIDERATIONS

Immediately after hair restoration surgery the surgeon should supply the patient with instructions on wound care and permissible activities.

LONG-TERM CONSIDERATIONS

One must remember that alopecia progression may impart a desire for further hair restoration procedures. Common observations that warrant these subsequent treatments are recessions along the temporal scalp, which results in the isolation of transplanted hair on the occiput and anterior scalp, or which may make reduction, lift, or flap scars more noticeable. Careful planning and appropriate candidate selection produce results that withstand the test of time – a realistic goal for the vast majority of patients. However, future hair restoration procedures may be required to maintain cosmesis.

CONCLUSIONS

The options available for the restoration of male or female pattern baldness are now plentiful. Countless patients the world over are tremendously satisfied with results attained from the described surgical techniques, as well as the medical treatments.

References

1   Stough DB, Jimenez F. Adverse consequences in hair restoration surgery. In: Stough DB, Haber RS, editors. Hair replacement surgical and medical. St. Louis: Mosby; 1996:299–305.

2   Bernstein RM, Rassman WR. Follicular transplantation: patient evaluation and surgical planning. Dermatol Surg 1997;23:771–84.

3   Reed W. Rethinking some cornerstones of hair transplantation. Hair Transplant Forum International 1999;9:133–9.

4   Stough DB. Consent for hair transplantation. In: Stough DB, Haber RS, editors. Hair replacement surgical and medical. St. Louis: Mosby; 1996:435–6.

5   Fiedler VC, Camara CR: Topical growth promoters of androgenic alopecia. Dermatol Therapy 1998;8:34–41.

6   Unger WP. The history of hair transplantation. Dermatol Surg 2000;26:181–9.

7   Limmer BL. Elliptical donor harvesting. In: Stough DB, Haber RS, editors. Hair replacement surgical and medical. St. Louis: Mosby; 1996:142–7.

8   Whitworth JM, Stough DB, et al. A comparison of graft implantation techniques for hair transplantation. Seminars Cutaneous Med Surg 1999;18:177–83.

22. Facial hair removal

Jean Luc Levy and Adeline de Ramecourt

INTRODUCTION

Techniques for the removal of excessive hair from the body vary according to its location and density; technological advances have also influenced the methods employed. Removal of facial hair is often requested because a person feels uncomfortable with an appearance that is viewed to be socially unacceptable; indeed, hair removal may be viewed as a beauty treatment. For women in particular, facial hair symbolizes masculinity and/or old age, even though there may be an underlying cause for its appearance, e.g. the menopause or anorexia.

The aim of this chapter is to review the various techniques of facial hair removal, which vary from patient to patient and according to the part of the face from which the hair is to be removed. Hair removal is complex, as hair regrowth must also be considered and is influenced by the method of removal. Some properties of the hair may change following hair removal, e.g. density (by unit area), the growth cycle, colour, and the length and diameter of the hair shaft. Patients may be affected by changes in the hair on its regrowth.

THE REQUEST FOR HAIR REMOVAL

Patients requesting facial hair removal may be suffering from psychosocial disorders produced by unease with their condition. In determining appropriate action the age and circumstances of the patient must be taken into account.

When dealing with adolescents it is important to establish if there is a diagnostic cause for excessive hairiness and, if so, to determine whether the condition can be treated; there may be lifestyle changes that the patient can adopt before resorting to hair removal.

Pregnant women may experience excessive hair growth; this may be agreeable when scalp hair becomes thick and lustrous but not so when previously dormant hairs appear on other parts of the face and body.

Women may also experience changes in hair growth patterns at the menopause; for example, large, pigmented terminal hairs may appear on the chin, natural down on the upper lip may become terminal hairs, white hairs may become more numerous, and the cheeks and neck may become covered with downy growth. These unwanted changes can cause much distress (Figure 22.1).

Following a rhytidectomy men may find that their beard in the preauricular area ceases to grow and this may lead to a request for removal of hair from the whole beard area.

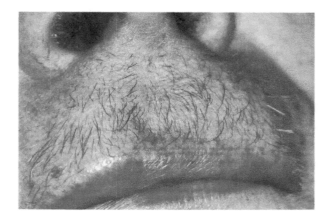

Figure 22.1 Hair developing after menopause.

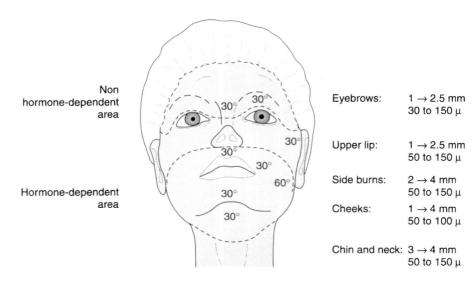

Non hormone-dependent area

Hormone-dependent area

Figure 22.2 *Common facial hair sites: depth and diameter.*

Eyebrows:	1 → 2.5 mm 30 to 150 μ
Upper lip:	1 → 2.5 mm 50 to 150 μ
Side burns:	2 → 4 mm 50 to 150 μ
Cheeks:	1 → 4 mm 50 to 100 μ
Chin and neck:	3 → 4 mm 50 to 150 μ

Transsexuals may request a reduction in facial hair either before or after sex-change surgery.

A clinical examination will allow an estimate of expected hair emergence and the evolution of the hair thereafter. Several facial zones can be distinguished, where a zone will contain hairs sharing similar characteristics such as diameter and depth, e.g. the upper lip (stopping at the nasogenien lines), the lower lip area, the chin, the submental area and the cheeks (Figure 22.2). Other secondary areas can also be identified, e.g. the inter-eyebrow area, areas above and below the eyebrows, and the ears (particularly in males). The clinician will note the hair type, its density, its rate of growth and the facial zone on which it is growing.[1] A possible cause for the excessive hair growth will be sought and either temporary or more lasting methods of hair removal to treat the condition will be suggested. Due to the unaesthetic qualities of facial hairiness, especially for women, a good outcome is desirable and psychological help may be required if techniques for its treatment are unsuccessful or unavailable.

A distinction is made between facial hirsutism and hypertrichosis (Table 22.1). Hirsutism is often associated with hyperandrogeny; if biological investigations and ovarian ultrasound scans are normal then the hairiness is considered to be idiopathic. Hypertrichosis has more varied causes.

In the next section the embryology, anatomy and physiology of hair will be reviewed; techniques of facial hair removal will then be considered (note that

Table 22.1 *Causes of facial hirsutism and hypertrichosis*

Hirsutism (post-puberty)
  Ovarian hyperandrogenic
  Adrenal hyperandrogenic
  Idiopathic

Hypertrichosis
  Idiopathic
  Diseases: porphyria, anorexia, hypothyroidism
  Medications: corticosteroids, androgen, cyclosporin, minoxidil, phenothiazine, PUVA therapy
  Congenital: congenita lanuginosa, hairy elbow, hairy ear, hairy becker hamartoma

Asian and African hair will be excluded from the following discussions).

EMBRYOLOGY, ANATOMY AND PHYSIOLOGY OF HAIR

Embryology

The germinal cells of hair come from two different cellular tissues: the mesoderm forms the dermal papilla and the connective sheath, and the ectoderm forms the epithelial sheath. Interaction between these two cellular tissues – by molecular adhesion, growth factors or cytokines – initiates a change in the hair.[2] The hair growth cycle appears to be regulated by stem cells in the hair bulge that have a slow cycle of growth.[3] As new cells are formed older cells are pushed upwards into the lower part of the matrix, and then form the root and shaft of the hair. Melanocytes (derived from embryonic pluripotential neural crest cells) in the epidermal layer of the skin give the hair its pigmentation. It is presumed that a relationship exists between factors controlling matrix activity and melanocytes but its exact nature is presently unknown. The dermal papilla has a rich network of blood vessels responsible for providing nutrition for the hair. The volume of the papilla is proportional to the height of the follicle and the diameter of the hair shaft.

In order to permanently eliminate a hair all of the growth structures must be destroyed.

Anatomy

A hair is composed of a bulbar region containing a matrix of dividing cells and the dermal papilla, and a hair follicle consisting of an outer cuticle, a cortex (forming the bulk of the hair and containing the hair pigment) and a central core (Figure 22.3). The hair follicle is at an oblique angle of 10–90° depending on the facial area in which it occurs. The dermal papilla is 1–5 mm deep depending on the type of hair.[4]

When using electrolysis, the excision line between the shaft and the epithelial sheath is easily determined in the dermal layer and a fine straight electrode can be used. However, when laser irradiation or pulsed light is used the lower parts of the papilla are sometimes missed, explaining incomplete destruction of the hairs.

The richness of sensory receptors around hair follicles in the dermal layer and the presence of nervous nets around erector muscles means that hair elimination cannot be painless. During electrolysis, needle insertion imposes greater damage to the hair follicle than that caused by laser epilation, which is centred on the pigmented cortex of the hair shaft. However, with increasing pulse duration of the laser beam, diffusion of heat is likely to raise the temperature around the hair follicle, thus increasing the level of pain experienced by the patient.

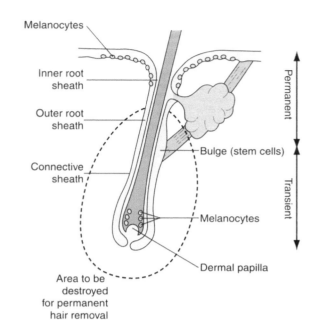

Figure 22.3 *Anatomy of hair.*

Different hair types have different physical properties. Vellus hair is unpigmented; the hair follicle is short in length and is 15–40 μm in diameter; the hair cycle lasts about 6 months. Middle-sized hairs are lightly pigmented; the hair follicle is slightly longer than that of the down and is 40–60 μm in diameter; the hair cycle lasts about 12 months. Terminal hairs are darkly pigmented; the hair follicle is 60–150 μm in diameter; the hair cycle lasts about 18 months. The density of terminal hairs is often lower than that of other hair types. Following repeated epilations, the hair cycle may lengthen and density may decrease. The depth and diameter of terminal hairs is similar for hairs occurring in the same area. The hair cycle varies between individuals and can vary depending on the season; there are also differences related to age, race and skin type.

Facial down cannot be reached by laser beams and electrolysis is only suitable if the hair is clearly visible and well defined. Middle-sized hairs can be treated with coloured lasers that strongly absorb melanin. Providing that the gradient of pigmentation is suitable for the skin type, terminal hairs are good candidates for treatment by laser.

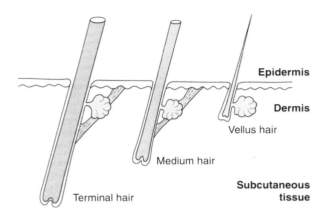

Figure 22.4 Pigmentation of different types of hair in the anagen phase.

Hair cycle

Each hair follicle has its own cycle, i.e. it is a non-synchronized process. The hair cycle has three phases: anagen, or growth, phase (Figure 22.4); catagen, or regression, phase; and telogen, or latent, phase. Following the end of telogen and the start of the next anagen phase there may be no hair for days to weeks, especially on the body.

On the face, the percentage of hairs in anagen at the time of the hair removal treatment is of great significance; ideally, 60–80% of hairs should be in this phase for long-lasting results. During anagen the increase in cellular activity in the cellular matrix leads to an increase in pigmentation and, in addition, the pigmented cortex of the hair follicle is in contact with the dermal papilla; these properties make this an ideal time for hair destruction with either laser treatment or electrolysis. Destruction of the middle part of the hair papilla, without causing damage to the dermal papilla, means that telogen will be quicker but that the hair follicle will not have been permanently destroyed.[6]

In determining the outcome of an epilation treatment the number of hair cycles without hair growth is of importance (this should be one or two 'missed' cycles), as is the hair count on regrowth. Any hair-free interval is viewed positively by the patient and this social benefit for the individual should not be forgotten.

Pigmentation

The cortex of the hair shaft contains pigment giving hair its colour. During anagen, functional melanocytes situated in the bulbar region of the follicle are active. Preventing melanocyte activity leads to cessation of hair growth, which explains why hairs in catagen and telogen are only lightly pigmented on the lower part of the follicle. Melanocyte activity starts early in anagen and stops just before it ends (Figure 22.5).

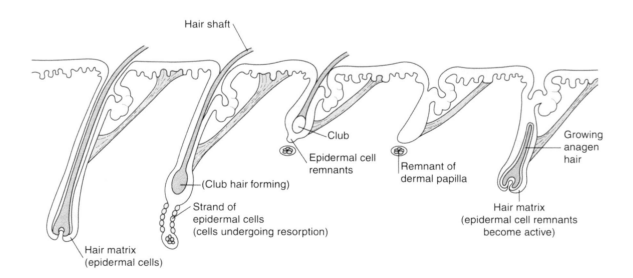

Figure 22.5 Hair in the anagen phase.

In Caucasians melanin is composed of two pigments: the brown and black eumelanin, and the yellow and red phaeomelanin. Most hair contains both pigments and its colour and composition is determined by the quantities of each type.[7] Black and brown hair contain large, ellipsoidal, heavily melanized eumelanosomes; red hair contains spherical phaeomelanosomes; blond and grey hair contain few melanosomes, or those present are incompletely melanized; and white hair contains no melanocytes and the epithelial sheath of the follicle thickens, although sometimes the hair shaft is white and the follicle is still grey. Phaeomelanin absorbs little radiation at wavelengths > 700 nm, so white hair cannot be treated by laser but electrolysis is suitable in this instance.

Physiology

The activity of hair follicles and not their number determines hairiness. Facial hair has a density of about 500 hairs/cm^2 but most hairs remain dormant. Hormonal or external stimulation, and sometimes a genetic predisposition, may cause this dormancy to cease, or cause middle-sized hairs to become terminal ones. The rate of change of hair growth depends on the sensitivity of the individual but it may develop very gradually.

At the menopause, female hormones decrease and that may lead to the emergence of hyperandrogenic-related hair growth, e.g. on hormone-dependent areas such as the chin, neck, cheeks and upper lip. Preventative medical treatments can be given but terminal hairs that have already formed will not respond to anti-androgen medication. The eyebrows may also change in character but this is not a hormone-dependent change; plucking with tweezers is the best solution, which may lead to a decrease in the number of hairs on regrowth although they may show an increased length.

The majority of patients seek permanent hair removal, having already tried various cosmetic therapies that give temporary results (Table 22.2). The remainder of this chapter will deal with the two main techniques currently available to the physician: electrolysis and laser.

ELECTROLYSIS

This method was first described in 1875 by CE Michel,[9] and since then it has been refined to be faster,[10] more effective[11] and safer.[12]

Method

Hair roots are destroyed by the application of a high-frequency electric current through a fine-wire electrode (needle). The technique is selective and minimum damage should occur to the surrounding tissues.

The channel into which the electrode must be inserted is noted from the emergence of the hair shaft through the skin. The diameter of the needle selected for use is chosen to be equal to that of the hair to be removed. The needle also has a protector to limit its depth of insertion.[12] Damage to

Table 22.2 *Cosmetic measures*

Methods	Effects and convenience	Side-effects/disadvantages
Shaving	Short-lived	Poor acceptance on face
	Synchronized hair growth cycles	Stimulates vellus to thick hair
Chemical depilatories	Cheap and easy	Skin irritation
Bleaching agents	Cheap and easy	Thick hair escape
		Stimulates increase in hair diameter
Plucking	Suitable only for some areas, e.g. eyebrows	Stimulates increase in the number of hairs, folliculitis, scars, crusting hyperchromia
Waxing	Longer lasting than plucking	Risks of hyperchromia

Recommendations for action before and after electrolysis.

> Preferably no plucking or waxing 1 month before treatment.
>
> Let hair grow to 1.5 mm.
>
> Use antiseptic solution and corticosteroid for 3 days after treatment.
>
> Use total sunscreen.

surrounding tissue depends on the current used and the duration of its application, and on the control the operator has over it. The energy delivered to the hair root is equal to the current intensity $\times$ duration. The end-point is reached when the hair can be extracted without resistance with the root attached; if force is required to remove the hair then it is being plucked, which means that it has not been properly destroyed. The treatment is most effective when used during anagen as needles can be inserted more precisely at this time and the cells are more active. The period between treatments must be less than or equal to the length of anagen.

Electrolysis is carried out under local anaesthetic, which enables the patient to undergo longer sessions of treatment and allows the operator to achieve greater accuracy and to use more powerful currents. However, the procedure may affect the diameter of surrounding blood vessels and care must be taken to adjust the duration and intensity of the voltage applied as necessary.[13]

Protocols for facial hair removal from various zones will now be considered (see box above).

Upper lip

For women, the hairs in this area tend to be high-density, and middle-sized. It is a particularly sensitive area and a large amount of local anaesthetic is required. It is also helpful if the hair is bleached a few days before treatment to make it more visible and the area is best lit obliquely. Due to the density of the hair growth, voltage of high intensity but short duration is required.

Chin

Hair growth on the chin is a distressing condition for women and so at the beginning of the treatment regime it may be necessary to perform electrolysis more frequently than would usually be the case. Between treatments, patients may be advised to cut the hairs to 1 mm and not to remove them by other methods, e.g. plucking.

The procedure is often performed under cryoanaesthesia. It is important that all the hairs are removed at each session of treatment. After 1 month of treatment hair regrowth is usually finer than before treatment; after 3 months of treatment up to 50% of the hairs may have been permanently eliminated. Treatment may be required for up to 18 months (Figure 22.6).

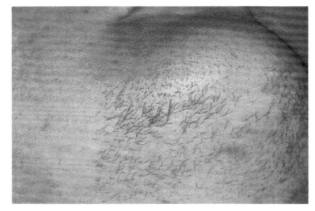

a

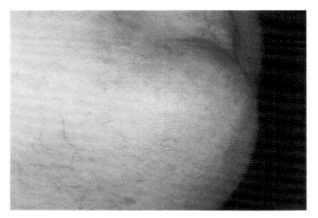

b

Figure 22.6 *Chin before and after seven sessions of electrolysis over a 14-month period: permanent result.*

Eyebrows

This is an area from which it is painful to remove hair and one that is not easily anaesthetized due to easy bruising. The best way to remove hair here is by plucking. The hair growth cycle of the eyebrow hair is about 8 months.

Down on the cheeks

This hair is unlikely to have been removed previously and so it can be treated over a short time period by electrolysis. Two or three treatments over a period of 2 months is usually sufficient.

Summary

Electrolysis is a useful technique for treating small areas quickly and efficiently, and it gives good long-lasting results. The results are best for fine hairs and hair that has not previously undergone temporary epilation techniques such as plucking and waxing. If the hair has not previously been removed by temporary methods then the elimination of hairiness over eight sessions of treatment follows an exponential decay curve producing permanent result (Figure 22.7). However, electrolysis is a laborious process and the outcome is operator dependent.

LASER HAIR REMOVAL

Background

Laser treatment for hair removal arose from the use of lasers in the field of dermatology. Early studies of epilation with Nd:YAG lasers in the naso-pharyngo-oesophageal area proved its efficacy as a treatment. The procedure itself was not painful and the hair removal was shown to be permanent. The technique has been refined to provide a method that is not painful for the patient, has minimal side-effects, has a good cost:efficacy ratio and is straightforward for the operator to perform.

In 1995 Grossman et al. reported the results of a study on 13 patients using long-pulse (0.3 ms) ruby laser treatment.[14] Three months after treatment a delay in regrowth of the hair was observed, and after 6 months regrowth was significantly less than before treatment. However, it was noted that injury to the follicles had occurred (Figure 22.8). A similar study by Dierickx et al. showed that a significant decrease in hair growth was achieved 2 years after treatment on sites that had been shaved as opposed to waxed prior to laser application.[15]

The Q-switched alexandrite laser is used to treat pigmented lesions and tattoos. This type of laser absorbs about 20% less melanin than ruby lasers; however, this is compensated for to some degree by

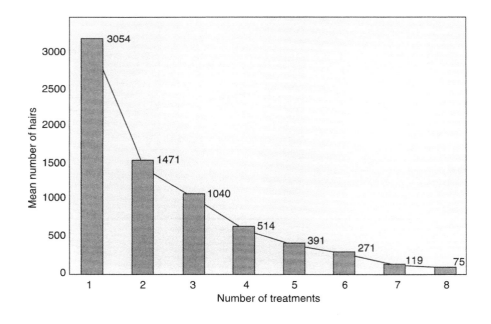

Figure 22.7 Electrolysis: efficacy on hirsutism and hypertrichosis of the face on 36 patients (personal data).

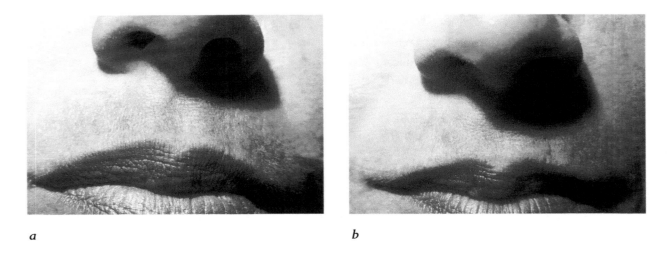

a   b

Figure 22.8 *Upper lip before (a) and after (b) three sessions with a long-pulse ruby laser (3 mm, 40 J/cm², no cooling).*

less scatter as the beam passes through the dermis. McDaniel reported on the use of long-pulse alexandrite laser treatment, which, 6 months after treatment, showed a reduction in number of hairs similar to that achieved with a ruby laser.[16]

Other studies also suggest that ruby and alexandrite lasers give similar results but differences arise with regard to skin type and epidermal protection. Further studies on different areas of the face and body need to be done.

High-powered diode lasers were the next type of laser treatments to find use in the clinical setting. Semiconductor diode lasers emit in the near-infrared range and are the smallest systems available. Williams et al. presented results showing the efficacy of this type of laser 9 months after treatment.[17]

Nd:YAG lasers have been shown to be superior in efficacy and safety in the removal of blonde hairs compared to ruby lasers.[18] The Q-switched Nd:YAG laser emits in the infrared at a wavelength of 1064 nm.

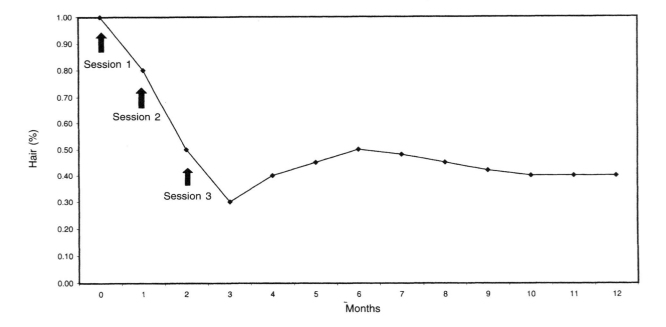

Figure 22.9 *Follow-up of hirsutism and hypertrichosis after long-pulse Nd:YAG laser treatment on 29 patients (personal data).*

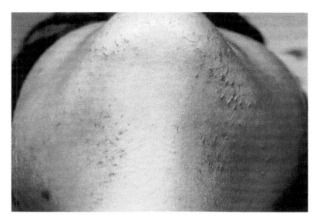

a

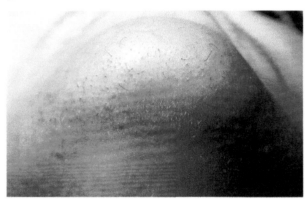

b

Figure 22.10 *Chin before (a) and after (b) three sessions of long-pulse Nd:YAG laser (3 mm, 70 J/cm², no cooling).*

Nanni and Alster used this laser in a study to determine the effectiveness of application of a carbon solution to an area before treatment;[19] the results suggested that an increase in efficacy was not produced using this protocol. It was suggested that a higher energy laser beam was required. Using a laser beam with an energy intensity of 1 J/cm² gave results similar to those achieved with other laser types 3 months post-treatment.[20] Another approach to improve efficacy is to increase the depth of penetration of the laser beam into the hair follicle by increasing the depth of penetration of dye applied pretreatment.[21]

The long-pulse Nd:YAG laser is a recent technique for hair removal. This laser is very reliable and cheap to manufacture. Nine months post-treatment the results are similar to those using a ruby laser. The wavelength of this laser (1064 nm) is not absorbed well by melanin but deeper penetration and higher energy beams mean that significant reduction in the number of hairs can be achieved (Figures 22.9 and 22.10).

Intense pulsed filtered light (i.e. a non-laser treatment) has also been shown to be efficacious in hair removal. An intense xenon flashlamp emits incoherent light in the 590–1200 nm range but filters enable wavelength selection; pulse durations of 2–5 ms are used.[22] To date, long-term studies have not been reported but it seems unreasonable to anticipate an efficacy similar to that of alexandrite lasers. However, flashlamps require an experienced operator and filters are difficult to manipulate (Table 22.3).

Methods used to cool the skin during and after treatment are not specific to particular laser treatments. A cooling device to protect the epidermis may be used, e.g. sapphire-tipped devices, or cryogen sprays may be applied to the skin.

Table 22.3 *Different systems of laser and light hair removal and their marketing perception*

	Ruby sapphire tip	Alexandrite gel scanner	Alexandrite cryogen	Diode sapphire tip	Long-pulse Nd:YAG sapphire tip	Long-pulse Nd:YAG, cooled air forced	Q-switched Nd:YAG without carbon	Flashlamp gel or water sapphire tip
Need experience	++++	++	++	+++	++	++	++	++++
Non-physician delegation	+	+++	+++	+	++	+++	+++	+
Quick	+	+++	+++	+	++	++	+++	+
Ergonomic	+	+++	+++	+	++	++	+++	+

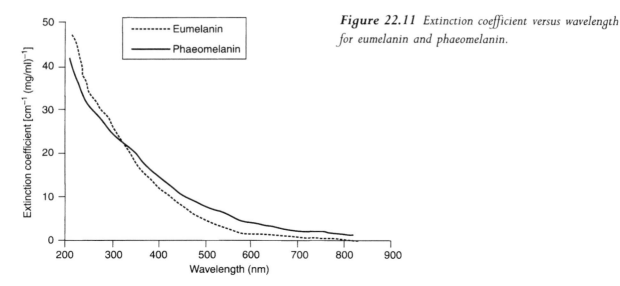

Figure 22.11 *Extinction coefficient versus wavelength for eumelanin and phaeomelanin.*

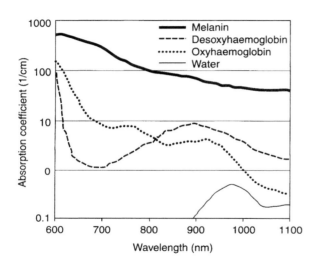

Figure 22.12 *Absorption coefficient versus wavelength for oxyhaemoglobin, desoxyhaemoglobin and water.*

Table 22.4 *Thermal relaxation time for different hair follicle diameters*

Hair diameter	Thermal relaxation time
50 μm	2 ms
100 μm	8 ms
200 μm	33 ms
400 μm	130 ms

Photothermal methods

Hair is a cylindrical structure and has a target diameter of 50–400 μm, a variable angle of hair emergence from the skin and an average depth (for males) of 1–50 mm.

The optical stage of the hair removal process is the absorption of the applied beam wavelength by the main chromophore of the hair, i.e. melanin.[23,24] It is unknown to what extent absorption is influenced by the amount of eumelanin and phaemelanin in the hair shaft (Figures 22.11 and 22.12). Chromophores absorb wavelengths in the 700–1100 mm range. Green wavelengths are absorbed well by chromophores but beam scatter in the dermis significantly reduces the depth of penetration.

During the thermal stage of hair removal, heat dissipates in the target area mainly by heat diffusion. The time taken to cool down to the ambient temperature is termed the thermal relaxation time. For hair follicles, the thermal relaxation time is 1–100 ms.

If long-term hair elimination is to be achieved, the growth centres of the hair must be destroyed. These areas are the dermal papilla, the matrix in the hair bulb and the 'bulge' that occurs on the outer layer of the hair follicle in the dermis, at the site of arrector pili muscle attachment. Due to the depth of the dermal papilla and the hair bulb, significant energy must be applied for hair destruction to occur. If cells in the 'bulge' are modified then hair growth slows down; if cells in the bulb are modified then hair regrowth is finer.[25]

By use of various combinations of laser energies, spot sizes, pulse widths and wavelengths it is possible

Table 22.5 *Passive and active cooling systems*

	Ice cube	Gel	Sapphire tip with water	Sapphire tip with cryogen	Cryogen spray	Cooled, air forced
Clinical efficacy	+	+/–	++	+++	+++	++

Table 22.6 *Lasers and light sources with Foods and Drugs Administration approval (source: Aesthetic Buyers Guide, April 2000)*

Manufacturer	Product name	Laser type	Wavelength	Energy output (J/cm²)	Pulse length	Price	Accessories
Aesculap-Meditec	RubyStar	Ruby	694 nm	up to 80 J	2 ms	$79,900	Q-switched for tattoos
	MeDioStar	Diode	800 nm	up to 60 J	5–30 ms	$89,900	Handpieces: 8, 10, 12 14 mm FDA approval pending Contact cooling: 16 mm handpiece
Altus Medical	CoolGlide	Long pulse Nd:Yag	1064 nm	10–100 J	10–100 ms	$69,500	ClearView handpiece: 10 mm Spot Contact cooling
Candela	GentleLASE Plus with Dynamic Cooling	Alexandrite	755 nm	10–100 J	3 ms	$72,500	Handpieces: 8-, 10-, 12-, -15, 18 mm
Coherent	LightSheer EP	Diode	800 nm	10–60 J	5–30 ms	$135,000	ChillTip handpiece
	LightSheer EC	Diode	800 nm	10–60 J	5–30 ms	$110,000	ChillTip handpiece
	LightSheer SP	Diode	800 nm	10–40 J	5–30 ms	$105,000	ChillTip handpiece
	LightSheer SC	Diode	800 nm	10–40 J	5–30 ms	$82,800	ChillTip handpiece
Cynosure	Apogee-40	Alexandrite	755 nm	107 J	5/20/40 ms	$114,500	Handpieces: 7-, 10 mm (12.5 mm option)
	Express	Alexandrite	755 nm	75 J	5/20/40 ms	$99,900	Scanner/cooling systems - option Handpieces: 7-, 10-, 12.5 mm
	Apogee-40 TKS	Alexandrite	755 nm	50 J	5/10/20 ms	$62,500	Handpieces: 7-, 10 mm (12.5 mm option) Scanner & cooling system - option
Diomed	LaserLite	Diode	810 nm	up to 350 J	50–250 ms	$77,500	Scanning handpiece
	A100	Diode	810 nm	up to 90 J	50–250 ms	$29,950	
ESC/Sharpian	EpiLight	Pulsed light	590–1200 nm	30–65 J	2.5–7 ms	$89,900	Handpieces:8×8 mm, 8×35 mm, 10×45 mm
	MultiLight	Pulsed light	515–1200 nm	10–90 J	2.5–25 ms	$129,900	
	VascuLight	Pulsed light	515–1200 nm	10–90 J	2.5–25 ms	$149,900	
	EpiTouch Plus Alex	Alexandrite	755 nm	up to 50 J	2–40 ms	$79,900	Scanner: 50 × 50 mm 1–10 mm handpieces
Continuum (ConBio)	Medilite IV	YAG	1064/532 nm	5–12 J	5–7 ns	$95,000	Q-switched
	Medilite	YAG	1064/532 nm	5–8 J	5–7 ns	$60,000	Q-switched
CoolTouch	Varia	Long pulse ND:Yag	1064 nm	up to 500 J	up to 200 ms	n/a	Pulsed cooling w/Thermal quenching *Intl sales only at present
Laserscope	Lyra	ND:Yag	1064 nm	100 J	10–50 msec	$69,995	Handpieces (3 mm, 5 mm) Scanner (up to 25 mm)
Nidek	EpiStar	Diode	800 nm	10–50 J	1–200 ms	$76,000	5 or 10 mm handpiece
Palomar	Palomar SLP1000	Diode	810 nm	100≠ J	50–1000 ms	$69,900	SheerCool contact cooling handpiece
	Palomar E2000	Ruby	694 nm	2–50 J	3 ms, 100 ms	$100–	
	EpiLaser	Ruby	694 nm	10–50 J	3 ms	150,000 $49,900	Subzero handpiece: 10 mm/20 × 20 mm adapter Contact cooling handpiece: 7, 10 mm

to provide sufficient thermal energy to damage the hair follicle whilst minimizing the damage to surrounding tissue, thus mimizing side-effects. This is the process of selective photothermolysis. The thermal relaxation time of the hair follicle is dependent upon its diameter (Table 22.4). For the epidermis this is 3–10 ms; for melanosomes it is 1 µs. Long wavelength lasers with long pulse widths are needed to cause damage deep in the skin. During such treatments cooling systems may be required to prevent epidermal damage. Cooling systems may be either active or passive, with the former appearing to be the most effective (Table 22.5).

For humans, 93% of incident light with a wavelength of 810 nm penetrates 1.5 mm deep.[26] However, with a spot size > 6 mm optical scattering means that there is a reduction in penetration and damage may be caused to the perifollicular skin. Lasers currently in use have the following wavelengths: ruby, 694 nm; alexandrite, 755 nm; diode, 780–810 nm; and Nd:YAG, 1064 nm. Sommer et al presented a study of the treatment of facial hirsutism using a ruby laser; after four treatments, 9 months later hair growth had been reduced by 45%.[27] These results were similar to those from two other long-term studies, one using a long-pulse Nd:YAG laser[28] and one using a diode laser.[17]

A wide variety of laser and light sources are produced, and many are approved by the Foods and Drugs Administration (Table 22.6). Manufacture of lasers is variable and the technical specifications of each instrument must be taken into account, e.g. the system of transmission of the sapphire beam on contact with or at a distance from the target, the height of the beam, the cooling system and the length of the unit. Clinical comparisons between lasers and their accessories (cooling system and scanner) show them to be of comparable efficacy in both long- and short-term studies. Clinical comparisons of cooling systems have not yet appeared in the literature.

Photoacoustic methods

Two studies with Q-switched ruby and Q-switched alexandrite photoacoustic lasers did not produce good results. A Q-switched Nd:YAG laser was studied with and without carbon solutions. Outcome was dependent on the composition and penetration of the carbon solution used, which highlighted the follicular target. It was of interest to compare absorption of melanin versus the chromophore. The delay of secondary hair growth was not as good as with photothermal methods. Powerful Q-switched lasers used without chromophores appear to have the same efficacy as photothermal methods but minus the side-effects.[29]

Patient safety

Due to the number of 'spots' of laser treatment, especially over a large area, the risk to patients' eyes is high. Nd:YAG lasers, whether Q-switched or not, emit radiation in the near-infrared part of the spectrum and so the beam is not visible to the eye. However, retinal damage to the unprotected eye is severe, causing blindness.

Ruby, alexandrite and diode lasers and non-laser flashlamps all emit radiation in the visible spectrum, and all are hazardous to the unprotected eye. During treatment it is essential that eye shields and goggles are worn by the patient. When being treated by flashlamp it is also advisable for the patient to close their eyes and turn their head away from the radiation source.

All treatment systems put the patient at risk of epidermal injury with permanent hyperpigmentation; textural changes and scarring are rare. However, it is prudent for the operator to avoid pulse durations of > 30ms, even when treating thick, high-density hair. With more vulnerable skin types it is best to decrease the energy intensity of the laser beam.

Summary (see box on the facing page)

- Facial areas respond better to treatment by lasers than other parts of the body. After 12 months the chin was shown to be the facial area that was least satisfactorily treated.
- Dark hairs respond better to laser treatment than light hairs; regrowth of dark hairs is significantly lighter.
- For all laser systems: the higher the energy intensity applied the greater the efficacy; small spot sizes are sufficient on facial areas; cooling the skin aids patient comfort.

Recommendations for action before and after laser hair removal.

> Preferably no plucking or waxing 1 month before treatment.
>
> No shaving or use of depilatory cream 2 days before treatment
>
> No suntanning before treatment.
>
> Offer to help use camouflage make-up to cover blemishes following treatment.
>
> Use antiseptic cream (Cu or Zn) after treatment.
>
> Use sunscreen with a very high SPF.

Strategy for facial hair removal.

> Low-density hair growth: first step, electrolysis (hairs should be 1.5 mm in length) on asking patient during the first 3 months.
>
> Hair density 30–50 hairs/cm^2: first step laser treatment. Three to six sessions at 3–6 week intervals.
>
> Maintenance, laser: note the hair-free interval and propose an acceptable decreased frequency of laser sessions. If hair density decreases significantly, then propose to finish treatment using electrolysis.

- Treatment on areas where hair has not previously been removed by temporary methods gives the best results.
- For a treatment regime, slow hair regrowth is viewed as being a favourable outcome.

RATIONAL APPROACH TO HAIR REMOVAL METHODS (see box above)

In diagnosing hairiness, the evolution of hair growth, density and contrast of hair, skin colour, and previous medical and technical treatments must all be taken into account by the clinician. Facial hairiness is usually viewed as a psychosocial complaint to be treated cosmetically.

When hair density is low (10–35 hairs/cm^2) electrolysis is usually the treatment of choice. For blond, white or grey hairs, or down, electric epilation is the preferred treatment method.

For higher density hair growth, and especially for thick, pigmented hairs, the treatment method of first choice is laser. Such treatment usually results in a significant decrease in hair density on regrowth and a slowing of the hair growth cycle; therefore the frequency of treatment is decreased and the patient achieves a greater sense of social comfort.

If hairiness is an evolutive process with a medically underlying cause, then a therapeutic treatment must precede hair removal. Once laser treatment has achieved a decrease in hair density and a slowing of the hair growth cycle, electric epilation may be considered the best method to keep the condition under control. The two methods can be considered to be complementary; laser treatment gives a higher efficacy but electric epilation is rapid and painless. The patient must be made aware of the fact that laser treatment will not offer a permanent solution and that perhaps a switch to electrolysis will be necessary.

SUMMARY

Hair removal by electrolysis and laser are complementary methods in the field of facial epilation. The upper lip, the submental area and the cheeks are areas that respond well to laser treatment; the chin, where hair growth is deeper, has less good outcomes.

In treating facial hairiness a balance must be struck between the following factors: the hair-free interval; pain control; and efficacy, which is related to the patient's expectation of outcome.

Technical developments and increasing knowledge of hair mean that there are still many challenges to be met by professionals in this field, which, it is hoped, will lead to improved epilation methods.

References

1. Lasker K. Determining efficacy of electroepilation treatments. Dermatol Nursing 1996;8:48–66.

2. Salomon D. Morphologie et physiologie du folliculle pileux en perpective de l'épilation laser. Nouv Dermatol 2000;19:12–18.

3. Richards RN, Meharg CE. Cosmetic and medical electrolysis and temporary hair removal. Toronto: Medric Ltd; 1997.

4. Cotsarelis G, Sun TT, Lavker RM. Label retaining cells reside in the bulge area of pilosebaceous unit; implications for follicular stem cells, hair cycle, and skin carcinogenis. Cell 1990;61: 1329–37.

5. Dawber R, Van Neste D. Hair and scalp disorders. London: Martin Dunitz; 1995.

6. McKinstry CT, Inaba M, Anthony JN. Epilation by electrocoagulation: factors that result in regrowth of hair. J Dermatol Surg Oncol 1979;5:407–11.

7. Ross VE, Ladin Z, Kreindel M, Dierickx C. Theoretical considerations in laser hair removal. Dermatol Clin 1999;17:333–55.

8. Richard RN, McKenzie MA, Meharg GE. Electroepilation (electrolysis) in hirsutism; 35,000 hours' experience on the face and neck. J Am Acad Dermatol 1986;15:693–7.

9. Michel CE. Trichiasis and districhiasis: with an improved method for their radical treatment. St Louis Clinical Record 1875;2:145–8.

10. Bordier H. Technique de l'épilation diathermique. Le Monde Médical 1932;Fév:78–81.

11. Hinkel A, Lind R. Electrolysis, thermolysis and the blend: the principles and practice of permanent hair removal. California: Arroway Publishers; 1968.

12. Kobayashi T, Yamada S. Electrosurgery using insulated needles: basic studies. J Dermatol Surg Oncol 1987;13:1081–4.

13. De Ramecourt A. L'épilation électrique: une méthode de référence. Nouv Dermatol 2000;19: 19–25.

14. Grossman M. Laser targeted at hair follicles. ASLMS 1995;221.

15. Dierickx CC, Grossman MC, Fannelli WA, Anderson RR. Permanent hair removal by normal-mode ruby laser. Arch Dermatol 1998;134: 837–42.

16. McDaniel D. The long pulse alexandrite: a preliminary report of hair removal of the upper lip, leg, back and bikini region. Laser Surg Med 1998;19:39.

17. Williams RM, Gladstone HB, Moy RL. Hair removal using an 810 nm gallium aluminium arsenide semiconductor diode laser: a preliminary study. Dermatol Surg 1999;25:935–7.

18. Dierickx CC, Grossman MC, Farinelli WA, Anderson RR. Comparison between a long pulsed ruby laser and a pulsed, infrared laser system for hair removal. Laser Surg Med 1998;10:42.

19. Nanni CA, Alster TS. Optimizing treatment parameters for hair removal using a topical carbon-based solution and 1064-nm Q-switched Nd:YAG laser energy. Arch Dermatol 1997;133:1

20. Kilmer SI, Chotzen VA. Q-switched Nd:YAG laser (1064 nm) hair removal without topical preparation. Lasers Surg Med 1997;9:31.

21. Sumian CC, Pitre FB, Gauthier BE, Bouclier M, Mordon SR. A new method to improve penetration depth of dyes into the follicular duct: potential application for laser hair removal. J Am Acad Dermatol 1999;41:172–5.

22. Gold MH, Bell MW, Foster TD, Street S. Long-term epilation using the EpiLight Broad Band Intense Pulsed Light Hair Removal System. Dermatol Surg 1997;23:909–13.

23. Lin TY. Hair growth cycle affects hair follicle destruction by ruby laser pulses. J Invest Dermatol 1998;111:107–13.

24. Kolinko VG, Littler CM, Cole A. Influence of the anagen:telogen ratio on Q-switched Nd:YAG laser hair removal. Laser Surg Med 2000;26:33–40.

25. Liew SH, Ladhani K, Grobbelaar AO et al. Ruby laser-assisted hair removal reduces the coarseness of regrowing hairs: fact or fallacy? Br J Plast Surg 1999;52:380–4.

26. Reinish L, Biesman B. Measured temperature profiles and thermal models of diode lasers for hair removal. ASLMS 2000;12:5.

27. Sommers S, Render C, Sheehan-Dare R. Facial hirsutism treated with the normal-mode ruby laser: results of a 12-month follow up study. J Am Acad Dermatol 1999;41:974–9.

28. Kilmer SL. Laser hair removal with the string pulse 1064 nm Coolglide laser system. ASLMS 2000;12:84.

29. Liew SH, Gault DT. Laser-assisted hair removal at 1064 nm without added chromophore. Br J Dermatol Surg 1999;52:322–30.

23. Minimally invasive procedures in periocular rejuvenation

Jean Carruthers and Alastair Carruthers

INTRODUCTION

Minimally invasive techniques of facial rejuvenation have gained increasing public acceptance. The baby-boomer population is expected to achieve life spans of 75–80 years or more, a marked contrast to the 47–48 year span averaged 100 years.[1]

In Chapter 15, the gold-standard treatment for mimally, invasive periocular rejuvenation – botulinum toxin (BTX) chemodenervation – has been discussed. In this chaper, perspectives on the rejuvenation of the brow and periocular region using surgical techniques are considered. These include upper eyelid blepharoplasty and several brow-lifting techniques, lower eyelid blepharoplasty and newer fat preservation, and lower eyelid redraping procedures, as well as periocular coherent and noncoherent light resurfacing modalities.

UPPER EYELID BLEPHAROPLASTY AND BROWLIFT

Thirty years ago, the upper face was generally ignored by surgeons performing facial rejuvenation surgery.[2] In today's upper face approach, both the upper eyelid and the brow/forehead complex must be considered simultaneously when the treatment plan is derived.

The normal resting position of the brow differs in adult men and women. In the female, the cilia are at or above the bony orbital margin, increasing in height as the brow is observed from medial to lateral aspect. This exposure of the bony superolateral margin of the orbit is a common determinant of a 'female' brow that is not seen in men (Figure 23.1). In addition, the female superior palpebral furrow itself is higher than in a man (7–12 mm compared to 4–8 mm), allowing

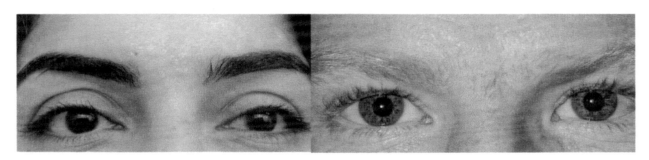

a　　　　　　　　　　　　　　　*b*

Figure 23.1 *(A) Female and (B) male brow anatomy.*

exposure of the tarsal platform which is then further accentuated by eyeliner, eye shadow, and mascara.[3]

The male brow in contrast, is normally 3–5 mm lower than a female's, being at or below the bony orbital margin. It is suspended from the much more prominent bony masculine supraorbital ridge, an effective superior umbrella camouflaging the male superior palpebral furrow and superolateral bony orbital margin. Generalized brow ptosis is a normal male characteristic, whereas medial, lateral or generalized brow ptosis in the female is perceived simultaneously as both a masculinizing and an aging feature.

Too high a brow is also an aesthetic and social concern in both men and women. A brow positioned higher than normal for each gender robs both of the facial expression of authoritative concern. In a woman, the impression is of a disinterested 'space cadet'; and in the man it is a potent facial feminizing feature. In addition, an overelevated brow removes the emotional visual center of attention from the visual and emotional axis of the eye to the huge upper sulcus,[4] thus further giving the observer the impression of social disinterest, coupled with total lack of responsible authority.

Brow surgery or upper blepharoplasty?

The sole indication for brow-elevation surgery is anatomical brow ptosis. The subgaleal coronal browlift was the original brow-elevating procedure, but it has relatively severe long-term sequellae due to the inherent surgical transection of the long branch of the supraorbital nerve with the planned bicoronal incision. This very important sensory nerve supplies sensation to the temporoparietal scalp.[5]

The endoscopic browlift as described by Fodor and Isse[6] neatly avoids this sequel by the placement of the scalp incisions to avoid the long branch of the supraorbital nerve. By careful release of the fascial attachments of the temporal fusion line, and the superolateral fascial attachments to the bony orbital margin, the forehead and anterior scalp are released. The scalp and forehead can then be redraped higher and more posteriorly, and permanently anchored by a variety of techniques including screws, sutures, and bone tunnels in the outer table of the skull.[6] Concomitant endoscopic removal of the corrugator

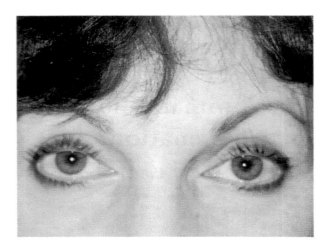

Figure 23.2 *Post endoscopic brow lift: attempting to frown.*

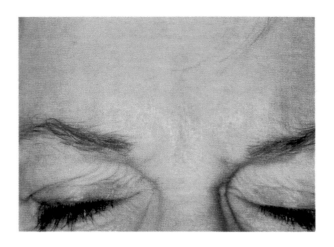

Figure 23.3 *Recurrent brow depressor activity after endo brow lift 3 years before.*

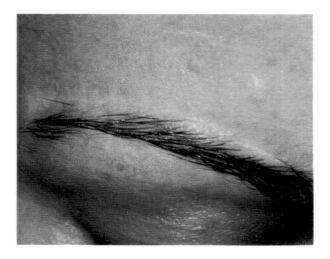

Figure 23.4 *Direct brow lift scar.*

and procerus muscles prevent dynamic recurrence of brow descent (Figure 23.2). BTX can also be used to restore brow elevation if, as in some individuals, the brow descends towards its presurgical position over time due to recurrence of brow depressor muscular activity (Figure 23.3).

Information is not included here on the direct browlift (incision immediately above the eyebrow cilia), trans forehead browlift (incision within a horizontal forehead line) or pretrichal browlift (incision immediately anterior to the frontal hairline) because the resulting incision scars are considered to be too intrusive for a truly aesthetic and perceived noninvasive result (Figure 23.4).

Other approaches to the ptotic brow and the 'baggy' upper eyelid coordinate the surgical incision with the anatomy. Stasior and Lemke[7] describe a lateral browlift of the descending temporal brow through the upper blepharoplasty incision. In approaching the superolateral orbital margin, a Desmarres retractor is used to expose the superolateral frontal periosteum. In a modification of their technique, the present authors use two 30-gauge needles inserted through the lateral brow cilia accurately site the deep suture placement in the lateral brow tissue. The 4:0 Mersilene suture is then gently passed through the periosteum of the frontal above bone for a measured disance (usually 3–5 mm) above the bony lateral orbital margin, lateral to the supraorbital notch. The sutures are inserted on both sides and gently tied with a double-throw and half-bow to facilitate adjustment of brow height between the two sides to achieve symmetry. Note that unlike the technique in an isolated upper blepharoplasty, the upper extent of the upper eyelid skin incision is not performed until the brow position is settled, because this will depend on the position achieved with the browlift. In this way, the lateral browlift and upper eyelid blepharoplasty can be safely performed at the same surgical intervention (Figure 23.5).

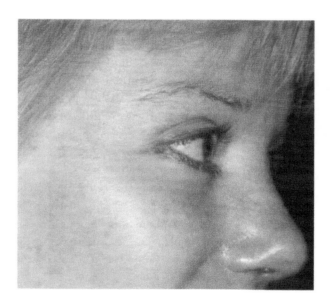

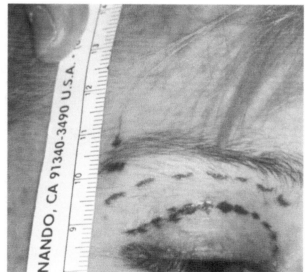

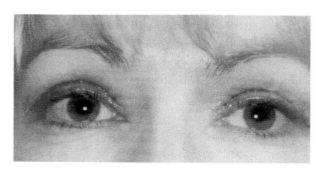

Figure 23.5 Transblepharoplasty browlift.

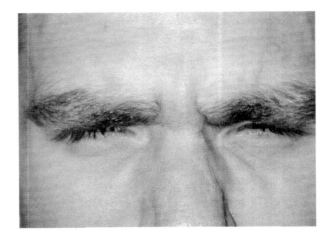

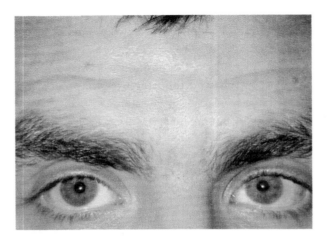

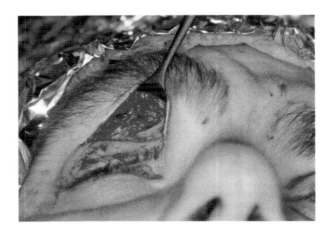

Figure 23.6 Transblepharoplasty corrugator extirpation.

In another trans upper blepharoplasty approach, the corrugator and procerus, muscles can be safely and gently debulked through a trans upper blepharoplasty incision. This procedure was described as a surgical alternative to glabellar BTX injection.[9] In the present authors' experience, subjects who have received repeated high dosage BTX to the glabellar musculature, with only short-term effects, benefit most from this procedure (Figure 23.6).

TEMPORAL BROWLIFT

The indication for a temporal browlift is lateral brow ptosis, often seen in combination with upper eyelid dermatochalasis in middle-aged patients. Simply taking more upper eyelid skin laterally in an upper eyelid blepharoplasty is not a good solution because the excessive skin removal simply serves to bring the lateral brow further forwards creating a permanent sad and disappointed expression. In the temporal browlift, a vertical scalp incision is made 1–2 cm behind the temporal hairline and down to the deep temporal fascia. A nick can be made in this fascia to observe the vertically oriented fibers of the temporalis muscle underneath. It is only when dissecting in this deep plane that the nonendoscopic surgeon is able to avoid the frontal branch of the facial nerve. The fascial attachments of the superolateral orbital margin are gently released, as are the attachments of the deep temporal fascial fusion line. Care should be taken not to damage the sentinel vein which is situated 2–3 cm lateral to the lateral canthus. The lateral brow is then elevated with multilevel closure of the anterior skin flap to the deep temporal fascia, and then skin to skin. There is no surgical dissection of the long branch of the ophthalmic nerve, so there is no resulting temporopanetal sensory dysfunction as with the traditional coronal lift. If the dissection is too superficial, the frontal branch of the facial nerve could be damaged, which can cause weakness of ipsilateral frontalis activation and corrugator function.

Results can be as succesful as with endoscopic and coronal lift, without the danger of medial overelevation. If it is co-performed with upper eyelid blepharoplasty, the browlift should be performed first so that the amount of skin to be excised can be judged accurately. This surgery is performed under local anesthesia 2% lidocaine with 1/100,000 epinephrine, as well as light intravenous sedation so the patient is able to sit up and cooperate with the surgeon to examine both brow and lid symmetry

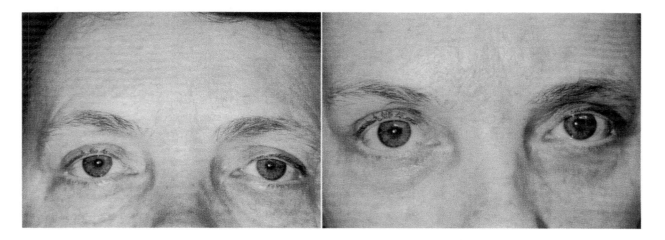

Figure 23.7 Non endoscopic temporal brow lift.

during the procedure to give the most balanced aesthetic result (Figure 23.7).

UPPER EYELID BLEPHAROPLASTY

If the eyebrow is not ptotic, the upper lid hooding is best addressed with a CO_2 laser-assisted or electro-surgical needle-assisted cosmetic upper eyelid blepharoplasty. The present authors prefer to mark the upper eyelid skin incision preoperatively with the subject in the sitting position and the eyes in primary gaze.

Greene forceps[10] are used to demonstrate the extent of full lid closure when the desired amount of skin is excised. In addition, it is believed that the subject should have a full preoperative ophthalmic evaluation, including the best corrected visual acuity, the Schirmer test and tear film break-up time to assess resting tear secretion, the measurements of the margin–reflex distance (2–4 mm), the height of the palpebral fissure (7–12 mm), the levator excursion with the brow fixed to prevent brow glide, which mimics the levator function, and the vertical distance between the lowest eyebrow cilia and the upper eyelashes with the upper lid in full downward excursion (20–25 mm is required to ensure upper lid closure).[11]

Preferably, the medial fat pad in the upper lid is addressed with gentle debulking or laser light vaporization only, using a 7 watts continuous wave beam in defocused mode. The same approach can be used to gently tighten the orbital septum rather than debulking the central fat pad. It is believed that preservation of orbital fat will become more and more important in cosmetic blepharoplasty surgery as our population continues to age and continues to wish to avoid the over-resected, gaunt, and skeletonized appearance of the excessively debulked orbit.[12] The skin is sutured with a running suture of 6:0 monofilament nylon to expedite removal in 6–7 days. A monofilament suture is a protective mechanism against wound infections as there are no 'suture craters' for bacteria to colonize (Figure 23.8)

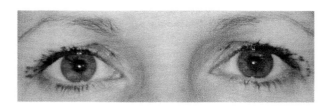 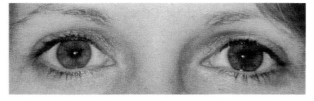

Figure 23.8 CO_2 laser upper blepharoplasty.

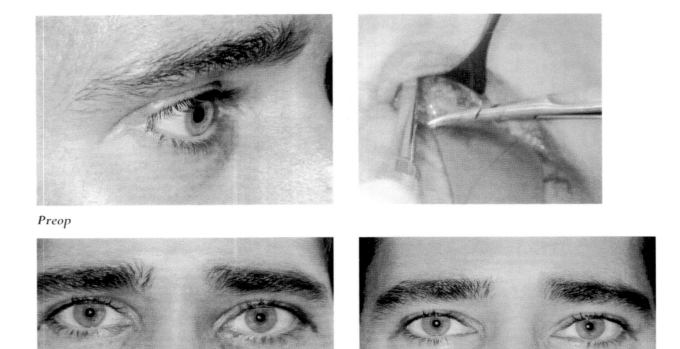

Preop

3 days post

6 months post

Figure 23.9 *Lower lid blepharoplasty with anterior fat transposition along arcus marginalis.*

In the past, infralash blepharoplasty was the gold-standard approach.[13] However because of the unacceptably high level of postoperative lower eyelid malposition,[14] the transconjunctival approach to the fat pads has become the more recent gold-standard,[15] as there is a 0% incidence of postoperative lower eyelid malposition. According to the patient's needs, the lateral, central and medial fat pads can be gently debulked with no visible scar.

In addition, the transconjunctival approach allows direct access to the periosteum of the arcus marginalis. The newer addition of the lower eyelid fat pad anterior transposition to transconjunctival lower eyelid blepharoplasty conveniently uses the subject's own vascularized orbital fat pedicle to support the valley of the nasojugal fold, which is, in turn, revealed by the descent of the malar fat pad (Figure 23.9).

The skin tightening that is needed can conveniently be given using a skin-pinch technique, or with an ablative or nonablative resurfacing technique. The additional skin tightening technique is found to add

refinement and 'polish' the final result, it is also well tolerated by patients. In subjects with type IV–VI skin, it is usually suggested that either the skin-pinch or the CoolTouch nonablative resurfacing technique is employed in order to avoid postoperative dyspigmentation that might possibly complicate ablative resurfacing.

LATERAL CANTHOPEXY

As time passes, the fascial framework supporting the lower eyelid in particular may become more lax. This may result in subjective symptoms of epiphora (tearing) when out of doors (e.g. skiing, running and walking in a cold wind, etc.). In addition, the physiologic snap test will be looser than normal and the lower lid will not reposition to its normal level upon release after distraction.

Many excellent surgical approaches have been used to effectively tighten the lateral retinaculum of the lateral canthal tendon to the lateral orbital tubercle. The

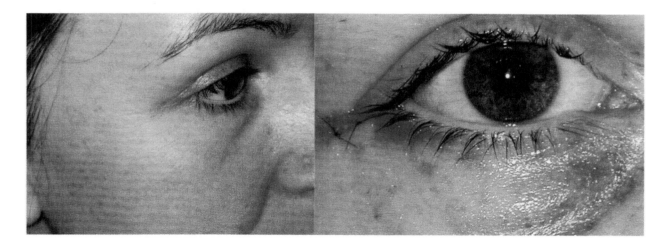

Figure 23.10 *Pre/day 1 post TCB/FT with lateral canthopexy.*

most direct approach is described by Baker and Pham.[17] A 4–5 mm skin incision is made over the lateral bony orbital margin at the level of the lateral canthus, not transecting the lateral commissure. Dissection is carried anteriomedially in the suborbicularis plane for c. 7–10 mm, in order that the lateral canthal tendon can be gently grasped with toothed forceps. The dissection is also carried posterior to the orbicularis at the level of the lateral orbital tubercle where the periosteum is easily visualized as a shiny white layer. A double-armed suture of 4:0 Mersilene is used to capture the lateral canthal tendon and to anchor it with appropriate tension to the lateral periosteum. The snap test is immediately tighter and the lower eyelid is gently resuspended. This technique is also very helpful in prophylactically preventing lower eyelid malposition after CO_2 laser resurfacing in which the anterior lamella of the eyelid is generally tightened (Figure 23.10).

COMPLICATIONS

What is left in is more important than what is taken out. This fact is generally so well appreciated that the most common complication of blepharoplasty – undercorrection – is actually a desirable result. In the first place, if the result is overdone then medical complications, such as the inability to close the eyes at night (nocturnal lagophthalmos) and keratoconjunctivitis sicca or dry eye, can result. The conversion of a cosmetically concerned to a medically compromised

patient is for a positive event. In addition, philosophically, if a patient is overdone the look is one of obvious treatment as opposed to one that is natural and fresh.

The most serious complication of blepharoplasty – blindness – occurs in 1/40,000 cases. This may be related to technique, such as clamping and cutting the fat upon removal, which can inadvertently tear the posterior fibrous matrix that supports the fat and the vascular matrix within the orbit, resulting in acute hematoma formation with increased intraorbital pressure that causes occlusion of the central retinal artery. In the present authors' opinion, all blepharoplasty surgeons must be able to recognize and treat acute orbital hemorrhage in a timely fashion in order to ensure the visual safety of the patient.[18]

Over-resection of orbital fat is a new cosmetic concern to both patients and surgeons. The hollowed and skeletonized orbit after a zealous fat removal blepharoplasty will become more of an aesthetic issue as the years go by and physiologic fat atrophy ensues. Autologous fat injection from hip or abdominal fat using tumescent local anesthesia can be effective over the long term in building up the concavities that develop in aging faces.[19]

ABLATIVE AND NONABLATIVE LASER RESURFACING AND REMODELING

The CO_2 laser ablates the photodamaged epidermis and dermis, allowing new dermal collagen and elastin

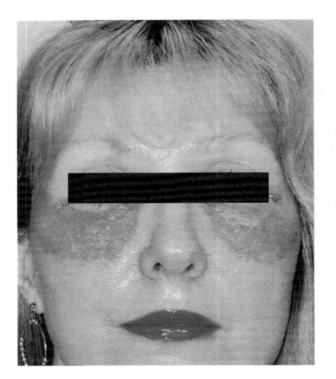
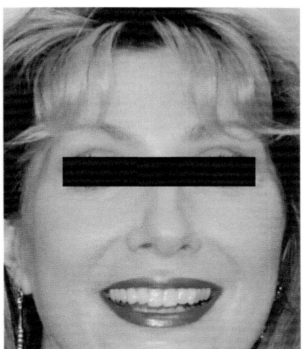

Figure 23.11 *Lateral canthopexy and CO$_2$ LR.*

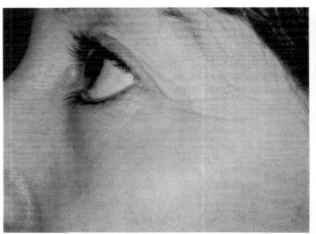
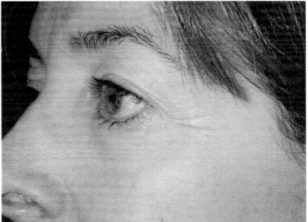

Figure 23.12 *Mild periocular improvement at rest, CoolTouch only between treatment 3 and 4.*

to form under the newly generated epidermis. The resulting erythema and weeping takes 10–14 days to re-epithelialize and a further 30–90 days to completely settle. This procedure, whilst effective, is not at all minimally invasive from the perspective of the recovery period alone (Figure 23.11).

The nonablative laser systems, such as the 1320 nm Nd:YAG CoolTouch system, may circumvent the issue of the recovery time by creating a dermal injury alone, as the epidermis is protected by refrigerant spray. Several treatments are needed to stimulate nonablative remodeling. It has been found that four to six treatments are required, but patients are very happy with the absence of any downtime (Figure 23.12).

In addition, the noninvasive rejuvenation of photodamaged skin using serial intense pulsed light treatments has recently found great acceptance because it treats the rhytides, the vascular telangiectasias the lentigenes, the pore size and the facial flushing.[20] This treatment can be combined with blepharoplasty and browlift and BTX to enhance the overall aesthetic result.

CONCLUSIONS

Minimally invasive aesthetic treatments are what is wanted by the current patient population. Blepharoplasty, canthopexy and browlift need more recovery time than BTX chemodenervation alone but, are well accepted as most subjects are back to their normal activities in c. 1 week, particularly if the dissections are made with the CO_2 laser beam or cutting bovie. Previous fat removal standards have changed dramatically so that fat transposition rather than removal has become the new area of surgical exploration. Combining treatments such as BTX, eyelid surgery and browlift with nonablative resurfacing procedures gives a pleasing fresh, youthful and harmonious aesthetic result. The timeliness of minimally invasive procedures is important to today's aesthetically concerned patient.

References

1 Kligman AM, Koblenzer C. Demographics and psychological implications for the aging population. Dermatol Clin 1997;15:549–53.

2 Knize DM. Reassessment of the coronal incision and subgaleal dissection for foreheadplasty. Plast Recon Surg 1999;103:1326–7.

3 McCord CD Jr, editor. Eyelid surgery. New York: Lippincott Raven;1995.

4 Berman M. 2001.

5 Knize DM. A study the supraorbital nerve. Plas Recon Surg 1995;96:564–9.

6 Fodor G, Isse N, editors. Endoscopically assisted aesthetic plastic surgery. Mosby Year Book;1996:57–61.

7 Stasior OG, Lemke BN. The posterior eyebrow fixation. Adv Ophthal Plast Reconst Surg 1983;2:193–7.

8 Beeson W. Video presentation of the Canadian Ophthalmological Society Annual Meeting, Halifax, Nova Scotia, 1999.

9 Knize DM. Muscles that act on glabellar skin: a closer look. Plast Recon Surg 2000;105:350–61.

10 Alt T. Lecture on cosmetic blepharoplasty at the Annual Meeting of the International Society of Dermatologic Surgery, Budapest, 1995.

11 Remington K, Carruthers JDA. Laser blepharoplasty. J Cutan Med Surg 1999;3:21–6.

12 Hamra ST. The role of orbital fat preservation in facial aesthetic surgery. A new concept. Clin Plast Surg 1996;23:17–28.

13 Shorr N, Goldberg RA. Lower eyelid retraction following blepharoplasty. Am J Cosmet Surg 1989;69:77–82.

14 Shorr N, Seiff S. Management of complications of lower eyelid blepharoplasty. In: Hornblass A, editor. Oculoplastic, orbital and reconstructive surgery, Volume 1. Baltimore: Williams and Wilkins; 1990:548–9.

15 Baylis HI, Long JA, Groth MJ. Transconjunctival lower eyelid blepharoplasty. Technique and complications. Ophthalmol 1989;96:1026–32.

16 Goldberg R. Fat repositioning. In: Putterman A, editor. Cosmetic oculoplastic surgery, 3rd edition. Philadelphia; WB Saunders: 1999.

17 Baker SS, Pham R. Lateral canthal tendon suspension using carbon dioxide laser. A modified technique. Dermatol Surg 1995;21:1071–3

18 Goldberg RA, Marmor MF, Shorr N. Blindness following blepharoplasty. Two case reports and a discussion of management. Ophthal Surg 1990;21:85–9.

19 Pinski K. Fat transplantation and autologous collagen: a decade of experience. Am J Cosmet Surge 1999;16:217–24.

20 Bitter PH. Noninvasive rejuvenation of photodamged skin using serial, full face intense pulsed light treatments. Dermatol Surg 2000;26:835–43.

COMBINATION TREATMENT (Nicholas J Lowe)

Indications	Potential combination treatments	Chapter reference
Periorbital skin laxity	Photoprotection	2
	Topical protection	3
Brow ptosis	Laser skin resurfacing	10,11
Upper eyelid ptosis	Non-ablative laser rejuvenation	13
Lower lid laxity	Botulinum toxin A	14,15
	Dermal fillers	17,18
	Endoscopic brow lift	25

24. Use of the endoscope in facial aesthetic surgery

Brian A Coghlan

Minimal-access surgery has swept through all fields of surgery. Unusually, plastic surgeons have been relatively slow to maximize the potential of the endoscope in cosmetic procedures. This chapter will review the current and possible future uses of the endoscope, concentrating on patient indications and its use in combination with other procedures.

The equipment required for a working system is a light source suitably cabled and channelled through one port of an endoscope, the image then illuminated being focused and transferred down another port of the rigid or flexible endoscope through an adapter to a camera (Figure 24.1). From here it passes to a camera control unit and is displayed on a monitor (Figure 24.2). Various recording devices such as video or digital disks can be used to allow later playback. It has only been with the miniaturization of electronic equipment and the improvements in image resolution that these systems have become affordable and less cumbersome. The surgical instrumentation includes a range of elevators with sharp tips, curved or angled

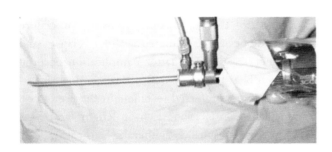

Figure 24.1 *The endoscope with adapter and camera mounted.*

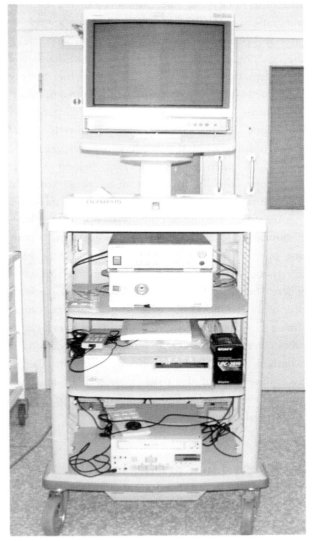

Figure 24.2 *A typical stack for processing, recording and displaying the endoscopic image.*

shafts, graspers, punches, and bipolar and monopolar coagulators which are specially designed to cope with the contours of the facial region.

Credit must be given to HH Hopkins, the British optical physicist who in 1950 described the Hopkins rod lens. The rigid glass rods with air lenses then and now form the basis of the optics for rigid endoscopes.[1] The flexible fibre endoscope, rather than the rigid scope, has not been widely used in aesthetic facial surgery.[2]

The advantages of endoscopically assisted procedures include: small, discreet incisions placed distant from the site of surgery, magnification of the operative site, bright illumination, the use of anatomical planes to minimize tissue trauma, visualization of vital structures (such as the supraorbital nerve) and integration with other surface treatments such as laser and peels. The disadvantages are the expense of the equipment, lack of stereo-optic field depth and the adaptation in surgical technique for remote instrument surgery with visualization from a monitor. Procedures can be split into those where the endoscope is the only surgical visualization, and endoscopically assisted procedures where part of the surgery is open and is in part helped by the endoscope, usually involving distal dissection that traditionally would involve longer or more incisions.

Anesthesia for endoscopic versus open procedures is similar except when tissue planes adjacent to bone are opened; the author's experience is that local anesthetic with sedation is insufficient for browlifts where the periosteum is extensively lifted, patients are more comfortable with a general anaesthetic under these circumstances. Where local anesthetic is administered, alone or supplemented by sedation, or whether a general anesthetic is used, the use of hydrodissection of the tissue planes aids hemostasis and provides a safer endoscopic passage parallel to anatomical layers.

TYPES OF PROCEDURE

For the purposes of the assessment and treatment of aging, the face can be divided into three sections: (1) the upper third, from the hairline to the opening of the eyes (endoscopic browlift); (2) the middle third is from the eye opening to the opening of the mouth

(endoscopic midface lift); (3) the lower third is from the mouth opening to the collarline (endoscopic necklift).

The exact surgical details and their variations are outside the scope of this chapter; instead the general indications and an outline of each procedure and how it can be used in combination with surface treatments will be covered.

UPPER THIRD OF THE FACE

The forehead lift

This is the most common endoscopic facial procedure. The primary indication for its use is brow ptosis with overhanging skin resting on the upper eyelids. Procerus, depressor supercilii and corrugator muscle overactivity in the region of the glabella can be reduced by direct resection during the endoscopic browlift, although botulinum toxin injections will also achieve a similar, but temporary, functional effect. Horizontal lines on the forehead respond well to treatment with CO_2 laser resurfacing, either alone or in combination with an endoscopic browlift. Forehead asymmetries in brow height and prominence should be noted preoperatively and can usually be improved with the browlift procedure. The browlift is usually performed in conjunction with an upper blepharoplasty procedure. Patients with a brow height (eyebrow to hairline) > 6.5 cm and a pupil to brow height > 2.5 cm may not be suitable for the standard endoscopic browlift because of the amount of lift involved and access from the scalp to the orbital rim.

In patients with male pattern baldness, previous hair transplants or high foreheads the use of the trans-blepharoplasty forehead lift has been described, assisted by the endoscope to allow fixation of the lateral brow to the temporal fascia.[3] Complications particular to the endoscopic browlift procedure include alopecia, asymmetrical lift, relapse and frontal nerve palsy. The latter complication occured as frequently as two cases out of three in one series.[4]

The author's preferred technique is the use of two paramedian scalp incisions 1 cm in length and orientated anterior–posteriorly within the hairbearing scalp away from the hair parting and about 4 cm apart. These allow central forehead undermining in a subperiosteal plane to within 2 cm of the supraorbital ridge. Two temporal incisions are made, 1.5 cm long to give access to the temporal area and to link with the forehead dissection. The periosteum is raised, under vision with the endoscope, extending around the supraorbital ridge to the temporo-zygomatic suture, and beyond if esthetically indicated. The periosteum is then divided and the glabella musculature exposed to allow resection. Care is exercised to identify and avoid the supraorbital and supratrochlear nerves and to prevent depression at the glabella from overresection of the procerus/corrugator muscles (this can be corrected with fat transfer at the time of the browlift). Fixation of the advanced brow is with 13 mm screws introduced percutaneously at the predetermined lift points to act as posts; the tension of the lift is adjusted to match the aesthetic ideal. Alternatives include resorbable screws[5] or fibrin sealant.[6] The temporal lift, important to address hooding of the lateral brow, is by advancement of the temporoparietal fascia over the deep temporal fascia and securing with strong but dissolvable sutures. Scalp

incisions are closed with staples; no drains are used. The percutaneous screws and staples are removed on day 12 postsurgery (Figures 24.3 to 24.7).

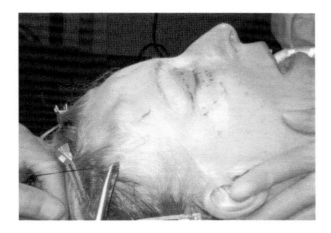

Figure 24.4 The temporal incision made during the endoscopic browlift with the flat-bladed dissector lifted to show its position.

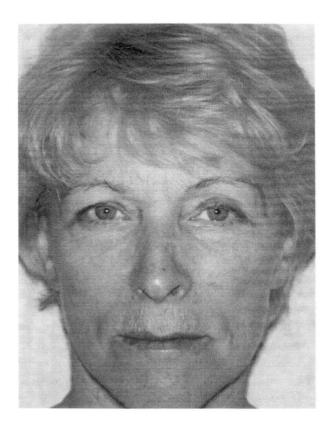

Figure 24.3 Patient pre-endoscopic browlift and upper blepharoplasty.

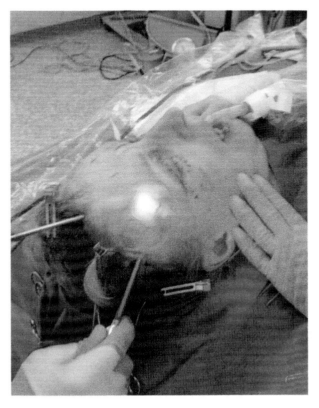

Figure 24.5 Introduction of the endoscope through a paramedian portal to allow dissection under vision.

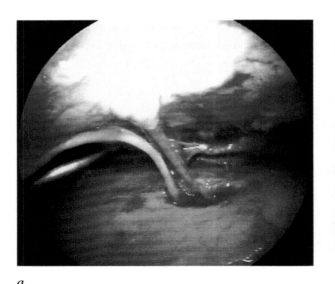

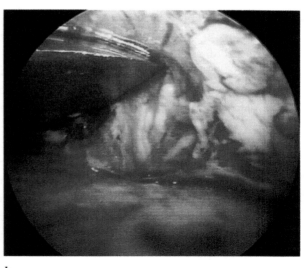

a   b

Figure 24.6 *(A) Endoscopic view of supraorbital nerves emerging from their bony foramen. (B) Endoscopic view of supratrochea nerve fibres adjacent to the glabella.*

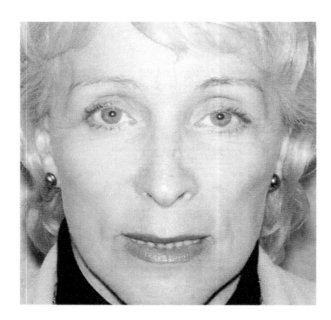

Figure 24.7 *The same patient as in Figure 24.6 3 months later.*

THE MIDDLE THIRD

The endoscopic assisted midface lift

This procedure replaces the standard subperiosteal or mask-type facelift and is particularly appropriate for those with brow ptosis, descent and wrinkling of the lateral canthal region and a heavy middle third of the face without excessive superficial rhytides. It is indicated in younger patients where there has been soft tissue ptosis but minimal sun damage. There is no skin removal during the procedure, and midface ptosis usually has elements of ageing of the upper third of the face and is commonly performed with a browlift, and often a lower blepharoplasty.

The temporal incision is shared with the browlift but the endoscopically assisted dissection allows visualization of the intermediate temporal fat pad which leads to the zygomatic arch and beyond to the origin of the masseter muscle. This allows a continuous cavity by joining with the midface dissection. Access to the maxilla can be from the exposure through the open lower blepharoplasty approach or from the upper buccal sulcus. The whole of the periosteum is lifted from the maxilla and body of the zygoma, extending to the piriform aperture but avoiding the infraorbital nerve.

Fixation of the lifted midface structures after adequate release can be at one or all three sites: suborbicularis oculi fat (SOOF), inferior malar periosteum (IMP) and Bichat's fat pad (BFP); the number and direction depends on the esthetic aims (Figure 24.8). Fixation of the superficial musculo

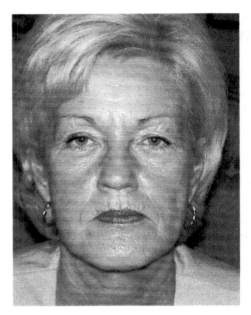
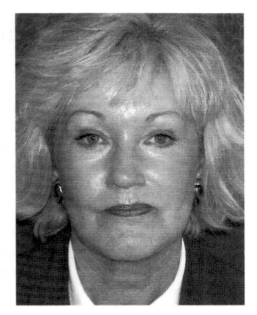

a   *b*

Figure 24.8
(A) Patient prior to endoscopic face- and browlift and laser resurfacing. (B) The same patient 6 months later.

aponeurotic system (SMAS) layer is usually performed in an open procedure but a subcutaneous temporofacial lift combined with SMAS suspension using the endoscope has recently been described.[7] Depending on the direction and amount of lift achieved, there can be bunching of the lower eyelid skin as a secondary occurrence and this may need treatment, although this lift can be therapeutic for periorbital rejuvenation.[8]

Complications and their incidence need large series to document numbers; in one series of 72 patients who had undergone endoscopic upper and midface rejuvenation there were 11 cases of temporary numbness, three cases of lower lid retraction, three relapses of brow elevation (requiring reoperations) and brow asymmetry in two patients.[9]

LOWER THIRD

Endoscopically assisted cervicoplasty

All neck procedures that do not excise skin rely on good quality skin that will redrape without wrinkling. Ramirez[10] begins the neck dissection in a standard fashion with a 3–4 cm incision posterior to the submental crease; subcutaneous fat is separated from the platysma muscle in the triangle bounded by the sternocleidomastoid muscles. The endoscope is used to allow adequate vision with a small access incision. The submental muscular sling is recreated by suturing the platysma and the digastric muscles in the midline. Occasionally an interlocking suspension suture between the mastoids is needed to aid cervicomental definition.[11] This can be modified for suspension of the submandibular salivary gland and to avoid large incisions in young patients.

OTHER USES OF THE ENDOSCOPE IN AESTHETIC FACIAL SURGERY

Endoscopic removal of benign lesions

Congenital dermoids adjacent to the temporozygomatic suture at the lateral end of the eyebrow have been removed endoscopically using a similar dissection to that for the temporal part of a browlift.[12] A subperiosteal approach for these lesions allows them to be removed from their bony attachment and removed intact. A previous history of infection or trauma to the area, suggesting extensive scarring, can make the dissection more difficult and all patients should be asked for their consent for an open procedure if endoscopic techniques fail. Midline nasal dermoids should be fully investigated and imaged to exclude the possibility of extension into the nasal septum and skull base but may be suitable for endoscopic removal.[13]

Lipomas of the forehead usually occur between the galea/frontalis and the loose areolar tissue that separates this layer from the periosteum. Central forehead exposure using the same technique as endoscopic browlift can allow either direct removal or liposuction under vision to completely remove these lesions without the skin incision directly over the fatty deposit.

Osteomas and bony irregularities of the cranium and supraorbital ridge can be smoothed with guarded burrs attached to flexible drives that can fit within an endoscopic port. This can be a procedure on its own or in combination with an endoscopic browlift, especially in men, to reduce the heaviness and overhang of the brow.

COMPLICATIONS OF ENDOSCOPIC FACIAL SURGERY

Patients should be warned of the general risks of surgery and those which are specific to the endoscopic procedure. All patients can expect some swelling and bruising, although this can be marked and prolonged in midface surgery. Besides the risks of anesthesia, other surgical complications include haematoma, infection, unpredictable scarring with possible temporary or permanent alopecia and nerve injury. In endoscopic browlift the frontal branch of the facial nerve and the supraorbital and supratrochlear nerves are at risk, for the endoscopic facelift the zygomatic and buccal branches of the facial nerve and the infraorbital nerves. Neck surgery entails risk to the marginal mandibular nerves and sensation over the lower cheek and neck. With careful technique these complications should be < 5% for temporary loss and < 1% for permanent loss. Where additional procedures are performed, such as blepharoplasty, the potential risks are well documented in relevant texts on the subject. Relapse of the lift achieved using the endoscope is difficult to quantify but is probably related to the method of fixation and adequacy of release of the supporting structures.

COMBINATION OF ENDOSCOPIC SURGERY WITH OTHER TECHNIQUES

Maintenance of blood supply is the major key to early healing. Ramirez has laser resurfaced 26 patients at the time of rhytidectomy or browlift.[14] He reported three herpes simplex infections and two cases of minor skin sloughings, but concludes that experienced laser practitioners can safely laser over undermined skin flaps. The subperiosteal minimally invasive laser endoscopic rhytidectomy (SMILE) facelift aims to reposition the deeper facial tissues to a more youthful location using endoscopically assisted techniques whilst using the laser for resurfacing.[15] Early facial edema seems to be more extensive than either procedure alone but eventually improves.

An understanding of the three-dimensional shape of the youthful face has encouraged the use of augmentation of the skeleton or soft tissues. Bone grafts and alloplastic skeletal recontouring of the malar region and chin are the most common sites and these can be placed with the help of the endoscope. For instance, fat transfer techniques along the supraorbital ridges can be used to assist the browlift and prevent a flattened appearance.[16]

Many of the endoscope-only procedures without skin excision need elastic skin to adapt to the repositioning and tension. Before and after surgery, patients benefit from entering a skin program with moisturizers, sunblocks and facial peels to maintain the benefits achieved. Patients who are fully healed and beyond 6–8 weeks post-procedure would be suitable for surface laser treatments over the undermined skin without undue concern about skin necrosis. This would address the fine wrinkles, solar elastosis, damaged collagen and pigmentary changes covered elsewhere in this book.

FUTURE DEVELOPMENTS

After a late start in endoscopic techniques, plastic surgeons have embraced the principles of minimally invasive surgery and reports of well-known procedures being achieved with smaller incisions and new operations being designed on previously untried surgical planes represents the future of surgical innovation. Manufacturers are developing narrower endoscopes with more light transmission and improved resolution. One-chip cameras now achieve similar image qualities of the expensive and bulky three-chip cameras of last year. The adoption of advances pioneered in general and urological surgery with disposable instrumentation and ultrasonic dissectors will allow less tissue trauma. The use of robotics and identification of the position of the endoscope tip superimposed on computer tomograms or magnetic resonance imaging will allow exact placement of sutures and implants in a previously remote and inaccessible site.

References

1. Krause DE, Grybauskos VT, Friedman M. Instruments and equipment for endoscopic sinus surgery. Otolaryngol Clin North Am 1989;22: 4703–11.

2. Honig JF. The fifer endoscope with guidable and flexible working instruments for endofacelift: a new instrument in facial surgery. Aesthetic Plast Surg 1994;18(4):373–5.

3. Ramirez OM. Transblepharoplasty forehead lift and upper face rejuvenation. Ann Plast Surg 1996;37(6):577–84.

4. Burnett CD, Rabinowitz S, Rauscher GE. Endoscopic-assisted midface lift utilizing retrograde dissection. Ann Plast Surg 1996;36(5): 449–52.

5. Eppley BL, Coleman JJ 3rd, Sood R, Ha RY, Sadove AM. Resorbable screw fixation technique for endoscopic brow and midfacial lifts. Plast Reconstr Surg 1998;102(1):241–3.

6. Marchac D, Ascherman J, Arnaud E. Fibrin glue fixation in forehead endoscopy: evaluation of our experience with 206 cases. Plast Reconstr Surg 1997;100(3):704–12.

7. de la Fuente A, Santamaria AB. Endoscopic subcutaneous and SMAS facelift without preauricular scars. Aesthetic Plast Surg 1999; 23(2):119–24.

8. Dardour JC, Ktorza T. Endoscopic deep periorbital lifting: study and results based on 50 consecutive cases. Aesthetic Plast Surg 2000; 24(4):292–8.

9. Celik M, Tuncer S, Buyukcayir I. Modifications in endoscopic facelifts. Ann Plast Surg 1999;42: 638–43.

10. Ramirez O. Cervicoplasty: nonexcisional anterior approach. Plast Reconstr Surg 1997;99:1576–85.

11. Giampapa VC, Di Bernardo BE. Neck recontouring with suture suspension and liposuction: an alternative for the early rhytidectomy candidate. Aesthetic Plast Surg 1995;19(3):217–23.

12. Huang MH, Cohen SR, Burstein FD, Simms CA. Endoscopic pediatric plastic surgery. Ann Plast Surg 1997;38(1):1–8.

13. Weiss DD, Robson CD, Mulliken JB. Transnasal endoscopic excision of midline nasal dermoid from the anterior cranial base. Plast Reconstr Surg 1998;102(6):2119–23.

14. Ramirez O. Laser resurfacing as an adjunct to endoforehead lift, endofacelift, and biplanar facelift. Ann Plast Surg 1997;38(4):315–21.

15. Ramirez OM. Subperiosteal minimally invasive laser endoscopic rhytidectomy: the SMILE facelift. Aesthetic Plast Surg 1996;20(6):463–70.

16. Guerrerosantos J. Long-term outcome of autologous fat transplantation in aesthetic facial recontouring: sixteen years of experience with 1936 cases. Clin Plast Surg 2000;27(4):515–43.

25. Rejuvenation of the neck

William R Cook, Jr and Kim K Cook

INTRODUCTION

The appearance of the neck is often a matter of prime cosmetic concern to patients. Undesirable changes with age may take two forms: changes in the shape and contour of the neck, and changes in the skin. These two types of changes are often found together in a single patient, but they are treated in different ways.

The shape and contour of the neck may alter with age, developing sagging, bagging, 'double chins', 'turkey neck', and so on. Until recently, the only treatment method available for such changes was rhytidectomy, or facelift – an extensive surgical procedure which requires a prolonged recovery period and may leave significant scars. But exciting developments over the past 10 years, particularly the advent of tumescent liposculpture and the introduction of reliable surgical lasers, now offer the possibility of an alternative approach. Described in this chapter is a combined liposculpture and laser surgical procedure for rejuvenating the appearance of the face and especially the neck, which is termed the Cook Weekend Alternative to the Facelift™.[1,2]

In addition, the skin of the neck often shows age and sun damage, reflected in wrinkling and roughening of the skin, keratoses, discolorations and 'age spots'. When these changes occur on the face, they often respond well to treatment with a chemical or laser peel. In properly selected patients, a chemical or laser peel to the face can help to decrease wrinkling, smooth the skin texture, and lighten pigmented lesions. The skin of the neck is sometimes treated with the same agents, but non-facial skin in general has proven more likely to peel than facial skin.

The present authors have developed a combined chemical peel, using glycolic acid gel in combination with 40% trichloroacetic acid (TCA), which has proven to be safe and effective on the neck and other non-facial areas. This method is called the Cook Total Body Peel™.[1,3] The term 'Total Body Peel' does not mean that the entire body is treated, but rather that the technique can be used on most parts of the body. This technique has been used successfully on the neck as well as the chest, arms, hands, legs, back, abdomen, and balding scalp. The technique may also be used on the face when a somewhat lighter peel is desired than that achieved by 40% TCA alone.

The two modalities of treatment may be combined for optimal cosmetic improvement (Figure 25.1).

THE COOK WEEKEND ALTERNATIVE TO THE FACELIFT™

The face and neck are a prime focus of cosmetic concern to most patients. For many years the authors' practice has been devoted to improving the cosmetic treatment of the face and neck, resulting in the Cook Weekend Alternative to the Facelift™. This technique will usually produce a much better cosmetic result than liposculpture alone. In many cases it may give a result which is comparable to that from traditional rhytidectomy – without the

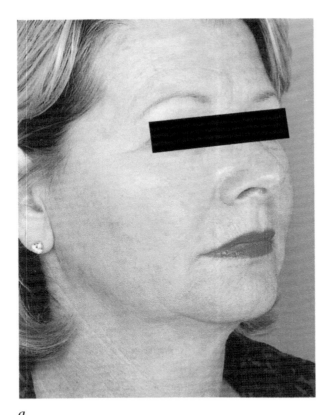
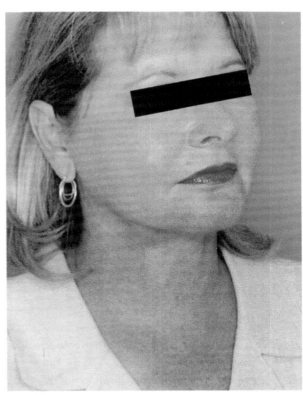

a   *b*

Figure 25.1 (A) Patient before and (B) patient after the Cook Weekend Alternative to the Facelift™ with chin implant, laser peel to the face, and Cook Total Body Peel™ of the neck. No makeup on neck.

prolonged healing period which rhytidectomy requires. The average patient can undergo this procedure literally 'over the weekend', with surgery on Thursday or Friday and a return to work the following week (Figure 25.2).

This procedure uses tumescent liposculpture to remove excess fat from the face, jowls, and neck.[4] With the tumescent technique, the operative area is infiltrated with a large volume of very dilute lidocaine solution which also contains epinephrine. The large volume of solution causes the operative area to swell, or tumesce, which greatly improves the surgeon's ability to precisely shape the area. For this reason, the tumescent procedure may be referred to as liposculpture rather than liposuction. The epinephrine helps to minimize blood loss and also slows the spread of lidocaine to the rest of the body, resulting in a much greater margin of safety. Of course, it is important to precisely control the quantities of fluid, lidocaine, and epinephrine which are infused.

In addition to liposculpture of the face, neck, and jowls, the Cook Weekend Alternative to the Facelift™ also includes: resurfacing of the dermis from the underside to promote tightening of the skin; plication of the platysma muscle to reduce neck banding; and transection of the septae of the anterior and lateral neck so that complete redraping of the skin will occur. Where indicated, a chin implant is also inserted. Using laser technology, these surgical procedures can be performed under tumescent local anesthesia at the same time as the liposculpture.

Indications

The Cook Weekend Alternative to the Facelift™ may be indicated to correct lipodystrophic changes of the lower face and neck, including 'turkey neck' and 'double chin'. This procedure is especially useful for patients who display poor cervico-mental angles, lax platysma, and mildly to moderately lax skin.

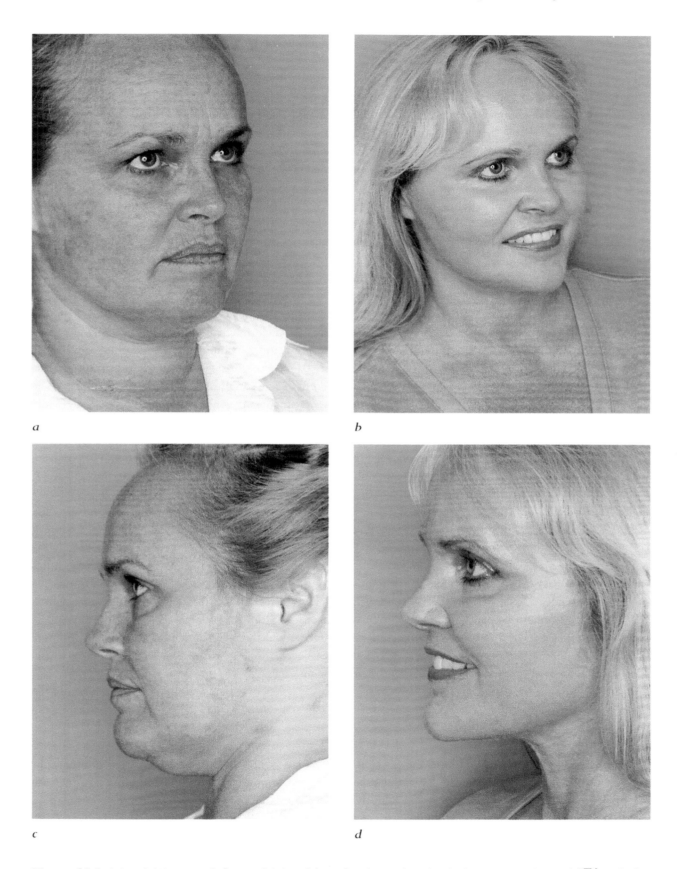

a

b

c

d

Figure 25.2 *(A) and (C) Patient before, and (B) and (D) after the Cook Weekend Alternative to the Facelift™ with chin implant and laser peel.*

However, the technique will not help a person whose skin is inelastic beyond repair. In some cases, individuals with poor elasticity in the skin of the face and neck may be helped by first performing a skin peel (see below), after which they can be evaluated for the Cook Weekend Alternative to the Facelift™.

Changes in the face, neck, and jowls can occur at any age but generally become more pronounced with aging. The present authors have performed face and neck liposculpture on patients ranging in age from 15 to 75 years. Patients at the younger end of the spectrum generally desire correction of an inherited pattern of fullness of the neck and face, and perhaps a recessive chin, which in many cases was also present in their grandparents and parents. Older patients seek treatment for changes in the appearance of their face and neck that develop with maturity. Beginning in middle age, the submental fat pad may become more prominent, the platysma muscle is weaker, and the skin begins to lose its elasticity. A 'double chin' may develop, with horizontal platysmal bands forming a ringlike configuration around the neck in several folds. Or the jowls become thickened and begin to sag. In many cases, these effects of time, gravity, and heredity can be helped by the Cook Weekend Alternative to the Facelift™.

As with any liposculpture procedure, careful consultation and evaluation of the patient is necessary with regard to clinical findings, goals, and realistic expectations on both the surgeon's and the patient's parts. Patients need to understand that, although significant improvement is seen within days, the final results will not be achieved until 2–3 months postoperatively. In some cases the patient's appearance will continue to improve gradually for 6–12 months or more.

Preoperative evaluation

In planning a liposculpture procedure, the distribution of the patient's facial adipose layer must be carefully evaluated. It is important to consider the general facial characteristics of that individual and also to evaluate the family history. In some cases the principal problem is bulging of excessive fat; in other cases the problems are mostly caused by lax skin and muscles. In particular, the 'turkey neck' deformity needs to be evaluated as to its fat content versus the effect of the platysma muscle. Sagging jowls may be caused by excess fat or a hypertrophic masseter muscle. The position of the larynx and hyoid bone should also be considered, and the bony structure of the face needs to be considered. Enlarged submandibular glands should be noted and pointed out to the patient, because these glands will remain after surgery.

The role of the platysma muscle is of particular clinical importance in addressing any age-induced changes that have occurred in the appearance of the neck. The platysma tends to become more redundant and lax with the aging process, and this contributes to the appearance of bands in the submental area.

One should also consider whether the cervicomental angle might be improved by inserting a chin implant and suctioning the ptotic chin pad (Figure 25.3). When assessing the patient for a chin implant, no firm rules apply as to the size of the implant. The most important consideration is not to overcorrect the patient so as to produce too drastic a clinical change in appearance. Generally, the authors use either Silastic® implants (Dow-Corning Corporation, Midland, MI) or Gore-Tex® implants (W.L. Gore & Associates, Flagstaff, AZ). These implants are commercially available in various shapes and sizes and are well tolerated by the patient. The implantation is performed through the same submental incision as is utilized for the remainder of the procedure. With this approach the physician can accurately carry out the subperiosteal pocket dissection to whatever height is required for the prosthesis. This preserves the integrity of the buccal sulcus and allows the implants to be positioned with minimal risk of injury to the mental nerve.

In selected patients, additional rejuvenation of the appearance may be achieved by performing a blepharoplasty (Figure 25.4).[1]

In addition to the direct examination, clinical evaluation may be aided by the use of photographs and/or computer imaging. It is important that the angle of the head and the position of the camera be in a consistent, specified position, both to facilitate planning, and to achieve comparable before and after photographs. Mathematical models may be used in assessing the patient's facial features and profile.[5]

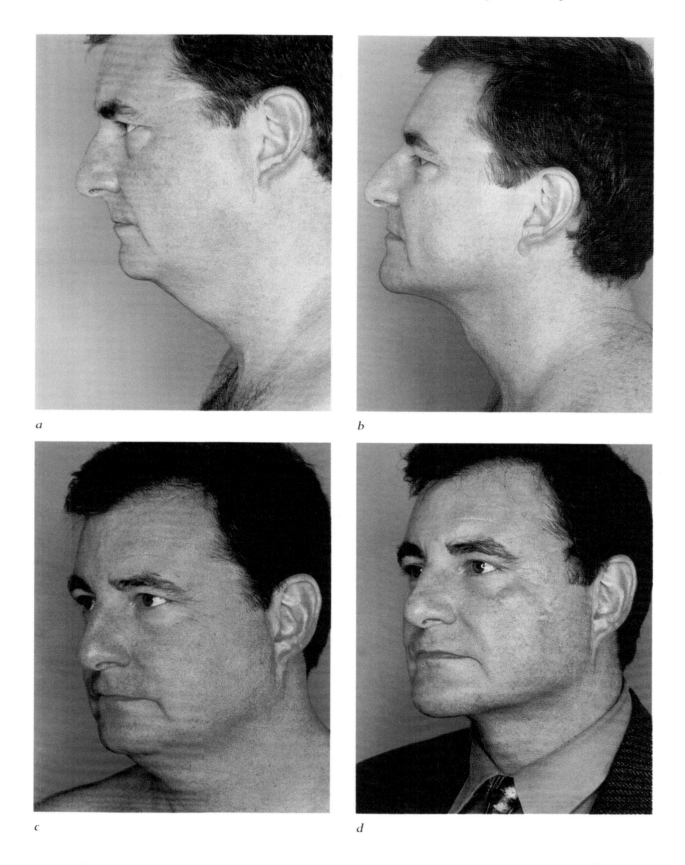

a

b

c

d

Figure 25.3 *(A) and (C) Patient before, and (B) and (D) after the Cook Weekend Alternative to the Facelift™ with chin implant and TCA peel.*

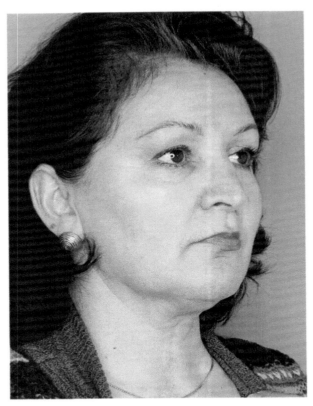

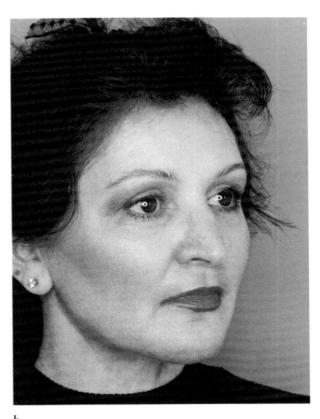

a   b

Figure 25.4 (A) Patient before and (B) after the Cook Weekend Alternative to the Facelift™ with upper blepharoplasty, periocular laser peel, and upper lip laser peel.

Surgical procedure

Precautions

It is important that the surgeon be adequately trained before undertaking this procedure. It is of particular importance that the surgeon and all other operative room personnel be thoroughly trained in the use of the surgical laser, since lasers involve important safety issues. These include electrical safety, fire prevention, respiratory precautions, and eye protection for both staff and patient.[6]

Summary

The Cook Weekend Alternative to the Facelift™ is a 10-step technique for tumescent cosmetic surgery to the face, neck, and jowls. The steps may be summarized as follows:

1. Tumescent liposculpture to the lower third of the face, the jowls, excess fat in the ptotic chin, and the entire anterior and lateral neck, covering an area from the mandible to the base of the neck and laterally to the anterior border of the sternocleidomastoid muscle. This removes fat and allows redraping of the submental skin.

2. Laser resection of a small ellipse of excess submental skin.

3. Complete transection of septae on the anterior and lateral neck, so that complete redraping occurs.

4. Separation of the insertions of the platysma muscle to the horizontal bands of the neck, which reduces, and in some cases eliminates, horizontal bands of the neck.

5. Tumescent liposculpture of the subplatysmal fat pad.

6. Laser vaporization of remaining fat globules on the platysma and undersurface of the skin of the neck.

7. Laser resurfacing of the fascia of the platysma muscle to help lift the ptotic submandibular glands.
8. Laser resurfacing of the underside of the dermis to produce tightening of the skin of the neck and jowls.
9. Insertion of a chin implant, when indicated.
10. Plication of the anterior border of the platysma muscle to produce maximal tightening and reduced platysmal bands, followed by closure of the submental incision.

Equipment

The authors use a Coherent UltraPulse® 5000 pulsed CO_2 surgical laser (Coherent Medical Group, Palo Alto, CA) for the surgical portions of this procedure. Such an ultrapulsed laser is recommended for superior surgical results. Ultrapulsed lasers produce less heat, less coagulation necrosis, less injury to tissues, less bruising, and a greatly shortened recovery time compared to non-pulsed surgical lasers or traditional metal scalpels.

A Klein infiltration pump (Wells Johnson, Tucson, AZ) is used for infiltrating the tumescent solution. For performing tumescent liposculpture, a mechanical vacuum pump (Wells Johnson, Tucson, AZ) and a variety of Klein and Capistrano cannulas (CKS, San Juan Capistrano, CA) are used.

Marking

The lower face, jowls, chin, and neck are marked with a gentian violet pen with the patient in a sitting position (Figure 25.5). Markings should clearly show the extent of the planned suctioning, any elevations or depressions, the midline of the chin, and the location of underlying bony structures such as the mandible.

Incision points should be clearly marked at this time. The incisions include: two 1mm incisions in the submental crease; two infra-auricular incisions; and two incisions in the lateral aspect of the mucosal surface of the upper lip. The incisions for infiltration and liposculpture should be kept as small as possible, ideally 1 mm up to a maximum of 2 mm in size.

Anesthesia

Before beginning the procedure, the patient is given intramuscular and sublingual sedation. The intramuscular sedation generally consists of midazolam

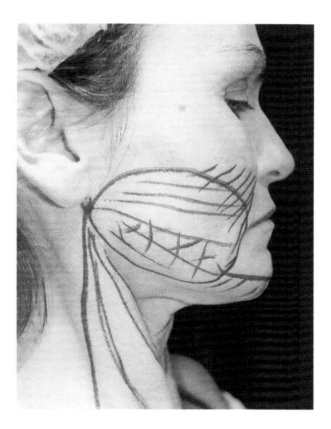

Figure 25.5 *Patient marked for the Cook Weekend Alternative to the Facelift™.*

(Versed), 2.5 mg if the patient is over 60 years of age, or 5 mg if younger than 60; meperidine (Demerol), 50–100 mg; and hydroxyzine (Vistaril), 25–50 mg. In addition, meperidine (Valium), 5mg, is administered sublingually. In most cases this initial dose of sedation is all that is required, but additional Versed, Demerol, or Valium can be given during surgery if necessary. No intravenous or inhalational general anesthesia is used.

The authors use a standard tumescent solution, which contains 0.1% lidocaine, 1:1,000,000 epinephrine, 10 mEq/l $NaHCO_3$, and 10 mg/l triamcinolone acetonide (Kenalog). The tumescent solution is made up fresh on the day of use. Before infiltration, it is warmed to approximately 39–40°C.

The solution is infiltrated through small incisions in the submental and infra-auricular areas. The entire anterior and lateral neck, jowls, and lower third of the face should be infiltrated. The average face and neck will require 500–800 ml of fluid to achieve good tumescence for this procedure.

Ultrasound

If indicated, external ultrasound may be applied to the tumescent areas after infiltration is complete.[7] Preoperative treatment with external ultrasound may help to promote patient comfort and speed healing. It may also make the liposculpture procedure somewhat easier for the surgeon to perform.

Step 1

After waiting at least 20 minutes to allow good vasoconstriction, tumescent liposculpture is begun through the submental incision sites, using two small incisions approximately 1 cm lateral to the midline on each side in the submental fold or the area which will be utilized for the submental incision. (In some patients who require a chin implant, the submental incision will be placed inferior to the submental fold. When the chin implant insertion elevates the submental fold, the incision will still be hidden in the submental area.) Having two incisions approximately 2 cm apart permits good crisscrossing during liposculpture of the neck. It also guarantees that the exact line for incision will be maintained, since in many cases the markings may be erased during the suction process, and the skin fold that one would normally choose for the incision may disappear due to tumescent expansion of tissues. Using first a 16-gauge and then a 14-gauge Klein spatula cannula, liposculpture is performed in the submental region, crisscrossing the area and forming a honeycomb pattern in the sites of involvement.

After this initial submental suctioning is completed, the infra-auricular incision is used to suction the lower third of the face, the jowl area, and the adjacent area of the lateral neck. Usually, 16-gauge Klein and Capistrano cannulas are used, making carefully spaced precise passes. This is done in the mid- or deeper plane to avoid ridging of the cheeks.

The next area of suctioning is through an incision, approximately 1 mm in size, in the mucosal surface of the lateral aspect of the upper lip, approximately 1.5 cm medial to the lateral commissure. A 16-gauge Klein spatula cannula and a 16-gauge Capistrano cannula, either 4 or 6 inches in length, are used to suction the mound portion lateral to the nasolabial fold, if indicated. The authors never use larger than a 16-gauge cannula in this area, so that the incision site

will close nicely without suturing and leave no apparent cosmetic defect.

After the initial liposculpture is completed, an additional 50–100 ml of tumescent solution is infiltrated into the neck region. This reinfiltration helps to expand the working space and provides additional vasoconstriction. The neck region is now sculpted using 14-gauge Klein spatula cannulas, first 4 inches and then 6 inches in length, and finally 12-gauge Klein spatula cannulas, first 4 inches and then 6 inches in length. During this final sculpting, one should thoroughly cover the areas from the mandibular ridge down to the base of the neck, so that all apparent excess fatty tissue is removed.

Step 2

The submental incisions are now connected with a gentian violet marking pen to outline a 2.5-cm submental ellipse approximately 2–3 mm in width. The primary goal of this excision is to provide a working window to allow the surgeon to perform the remaining steps in the procedure, rather than to remove a significant amount of excessive skin. Removal of excess amounts of skin may lead to poor wound healing at the incision site, due to increased stress on the wound edges. What may appear to be redundant skin in the area will be reduced by skin contraction from the dermal laser resurfacing described below.

The Coherent UltraPulse 5000 laser, with initial settings of 15 mJ and 4 W, is used to make the initial skin incision of the ellipse. This 'pulsed' mode produces a smaller, usually bloodless, incision with minimal tissue damage. The 7-W setting is then used to excise the elliptical piece of skin.

Step 3

A Toledo tissue dissector (Byron Medical, Tucson, AZ) is inserted into the submental incision and is utilized to break all visible septae in the entire anterior and lateral neck. The plane of dissection is important, staying relatively superficial. Hemostasis is achieved with both standard cautery and suction cautery, using a Valley electrosurgical unit (ValleyLab, Boulder, CO).

Step 4

The Toledo tissue dissector is then utilized to separate the insertion of the platysma muscle into the horizontal bands of the neck. Hemostasis is achieved with a Valley electrosurgical unit equipped with a special suction cautery tip.

Step 5

The mid portion of the platysma muscle is now infiltrated with a solution of 2% lidocaine and 1:100,000 epinephrine, approximately 1.5–2.0 ml injected directly into the muscle. This will provide anesthesia and vasoconstriction for the subplatysmal suctioning described below.

A small incision is made in the midline of the superior aspect of the platysma muscle. The subplatysmal fat pad is carefully visualized through this small opening and is gently aspirated using a 12-gauge Klein spatula cannula. The fat in this area is very soft, and extreme caution and very slow movements of the cannula are needed so as not to traumatize any of the adjacent structures. Following suctioning, the area must be carefully monitored for good hemostasis.

After the subplatysmal pad is removed, direct visualization is made of the jowl areas. Any residual globules of fat in this area are carefully removed, using the same 12-gauge Klein spatula cannula with the openings toward the skin surface.

Step 6

Any persistent fat lobules on the platysma and undersurface of the skin are spot vaporized with the laser. It is important to use the most defocused handle position and the minimum time necessary to vaporize the globules.

Step 7

The UltraPulse 5000 laser, in a defocused mode on a 7W setting, is used to gently and minimally resurface approximately 10–20% of the anterior surface of the area of the platysma muscle which covers the submandibular lymph nodes, using a crisscrossing randomized pattern. This tightens the fascial surface of the platysma.

Step 8

To tighten the skin, the undersurface of the dermis is carefully resurfaced in a crisscrossing randomized fashion, using the UltraPulse 5000 laser on a 7W defocused setting. Care must be taken to keep the laser beam moving continuously. The amount of resurfacing done on the undersurface of the skin will depend upon the skin laxity, the skin thickness, and the amount of tightening desired. Resurfacing should only be done on 20–30% of the skin undersurface. It helps to evert the skin and hold the non-dominant hand behind the area being resurfaced, to stabilize the skin and to guard against any areas of heat, which would indicate the need to adjust the laser concentration for the thickness of the skin in that particular area.

Step 9 (optional)

In patients with slight to moderate microgenia, the mandible may be augmented to maximize the cervico-mental angle. The implant procedure is initiated at this time by using the UltraPulse 5000 laser on the 7-W continuous setting to carefully separate the platysma muscle in a horizontal line proceeding down to the periosteum on the mandible, corresponding to the desired position for the implant. The periosteum is then incised with the UltraPulse 5000 laser. A Rich periosteal elevator (Byron Medical, Tucson, AZ) is utilized to create a pocket subperiosteally along the border of the mandible. The pocket for the implant should be located so that the implant will sit comfortably and squarely over the chin prominence, and will not extend higher than the natural labio-mental groove. The pocket must accommodate the prosthesis comfortably; otherwise the implant will slide inferiorly over the symphysis and rock back and forth.

Once the pocket is freed and hemostasis is achieved, the implant is positioned and secured to the periosteum with 4-0 clear nylon sutures. The fibers of the platysma muscle are then reapproximated with 4-0 Vicryl sutures (Ethicon, Inc, Somerville, NJ).

Step 10

Platysmal tightening is then performed to further improve the cervico-mental angle and to reduce neck banding. After liposculpture, severing of the septae, and removal of the platysmal insertions into the skin of the neck, the pattern of the particular individual's platysma muscle can clearly be noted. Because of the support given by the platysma and its role in the creation of the cervico-mental angle, there is no substitute for a very thorough plication of the medial platysma to create the best results in the neck.

The medial borders of the platysma muscle are carefully sutured together using a plication stitch of 3-0 Vicryl and a vertical mattress type of suture. By the time this suture is absorbed, there will be good firm support of the muscular filaments and the overlying fascia. The number of sutures and their placement will vary considerably, depending on the anatomy of the underlying platysma muscle.

Below the point of plication, a small horizontal wedge of muscle is resected from each of the anterior platysmal borders to break the continuity of the band and allow the creation of a sharp cervico-mental angle. Alternatively, a small cross-cut can be made into the platysma muscle to help demarcate the crease at the cervico-mental angle. This allows the muscle to conform to the cervico-mental angle rather than forming a 'bowstring' across it.

With good hemostasis achieved in all areas, the submental incision is closed with 4-0 Vicryl sutures in the subcutaneous layer, and 5-0 clear Monocryl absorbable sutures (Ethicon, Inc, Somerville, NJ) in the skin surface. Steri-Strips (3M Company, St Paul, MN) are also applied. The small incisions in the infra-auricular and lip areas are left open to promote drainage.

Postoperative considerations

Postoperative care

Stretch foam tape is applied to the neck and lower facial areas. The stretch foam tape must be positioned very carefully so as not to induce any folds in the skin. The tape is then covered by an elastic neck support to hold the tissues in the appropriate position.

Patients must leave the office after surgery with a responsible adult, who will drive them home and remain with them for the remainder of the day and night. Upon returning home, the patient is advised to rest for the remainder of the day, with the head elevated and ice-packs in position over the lower face and neck, 15 minutes 'on' and 15 minutes 'off'. This will help to reduce tissue swelling and prevent ecchymosis of the areas. Good hydration should be maintained through adequate water intake.

The first full postoperative day should be spent in quiet activities, with periodic rest and head elevation. Patients are instructed to leave the stretch foam tape in place and keep it dry until it is removed by the physician, and to wear an elastic chin strap 8–12 hours a day for 1–3 days. Excessive activity immediately after surgery is not recommended.

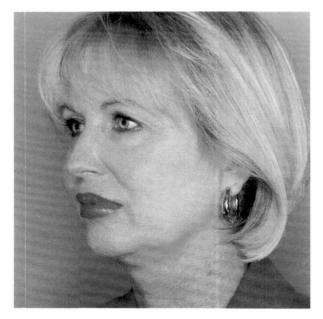

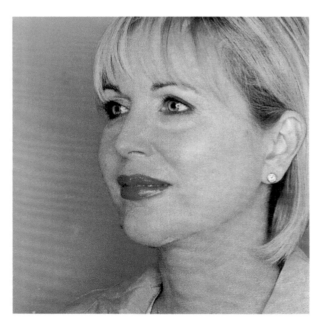

a

b

Figure 25.6 (A) Patient before and (B) after three days after the Cook Weekend Alternative to the Facelift™ with chin implant. Note submental sutures with Steri-Strips still in place.

The day after surgery, patients return to the physician's office for changing of the tape. Most patients return again on the second postoperative day and the tape is removed at that time (Figure 25.6). After this, they can return to work and normal activities. However, they should avoid vigorous exercise or immersion in water such as a swimming pool, hot tub, or bath tub until all the incisions have closed and the sutures have dissolved (approximately 3 weeks).

Complications and sequelae

Patients undergoing this procedure generally experience minimal postoperative ecchymosis or discomfort. Occasionally, the chin implant site may be tender for 1–2 days postoperatively. Patients are usually able to return to work and social activities on about the third postoperative day. Strenuous exercise of any type should be avoided for the 2–3 weeks postoperatively, particularly in patients who have received a chin implant.

Although patients will show significant cosmetic improvement as soon as the tape is removed, the final result of the surgical procedure may not be apparent for 2–3 months postoperatively. This must be emphasized before the operation, so that the patient's expectations will be in line with the natural healing processes which will take place.

The authors have had no serious complications to date. Some individuals will recover more rapidly than others, depending on the amount of skin retraction which must occur. Rarely, a small seroma may develop during the postoperative period. It may be easily drained, and recovery will then proceed uneventfully with generally excellent clinical results.

Individuals with a history of hypertrophic scarring or keloid formation need to be monitored and treated with intralesional Kenalog as indicated.

Results

The Cook Weekend Alternative to the Facelift™ creates a natural-looking cosmetic improvement that is far superior to that which can be achieved with liposculpture alone (Figures 25.7 and 25.8). In many cases the results are comparable to those achieved using rhytidectomy procedures. After this procedure, sagging or fatty neck areas are transformed by good tightening of the neck, marked reduction in skin laxity, and reduction of the platysmal bands. In general, patients have a more youthful appearance. Patients with round and heavy appearing faces gain a slimmer, more attractive look. The cheekbones appear more prominent, the mandible is more sharply defined, and facial features are in better balance. The cosmetic improvement, which can be dramatic, coupled with the rapid recovery period will generally result in great patient satisfaction.

THE COOK TOTAL BODY PEEL™

The procedure described above is primarily effective in reshaping the contour of the chin and neck, and tightening the skin. Many patients also desire cosmetic improvements in the texture and appearance of the skin of the neck. They usually hope for a firmer, smoother skin texture, decreased roughness and wrinkling, and elimination or lessening of pigmentary abnormalities. In many cases these desirable changes can be achieved by use of the Cook Total Body Peel™ on the skin of the neck, sometimes in conjunction with a chemical or laser peel of the face. This peel may be performed either as a stand-alone procedure or in combination with the Cook Weekend Alternative to the Facelift™.

The Cook Total Body Peel™ is primarily designed to be a safe and effective peel for non-facial skin. It utilizes a combination of 40% trichloroacetic acid (TCA) and 70% glycolic acid gel as peeling agents. It is important to use glycolic acid gel because it acts as a partial barrier to TCA penetration; liquid glycolic acid does not perform this role, so that combining it with TCA can result in too deep a peel on the body. The authors have found the 40% TCA formulation to be preferable to a lower strength, because it enables TCA to penetrate deep enough into skin lesions such as keratoses and lentigines.

A copious amount of sodium bicarbonate solution is used to neutralize the acids and stop the peeling at a time determined by the physician. The method permits precise timing, so that the extent and depth of the peel are almost entirely technique dependent. The result is a peel which can range in depth from superficial to deep, and can be used on most areas of the body and most skin types. Careful physician attention to the timing of the peel and prompt neutralization at

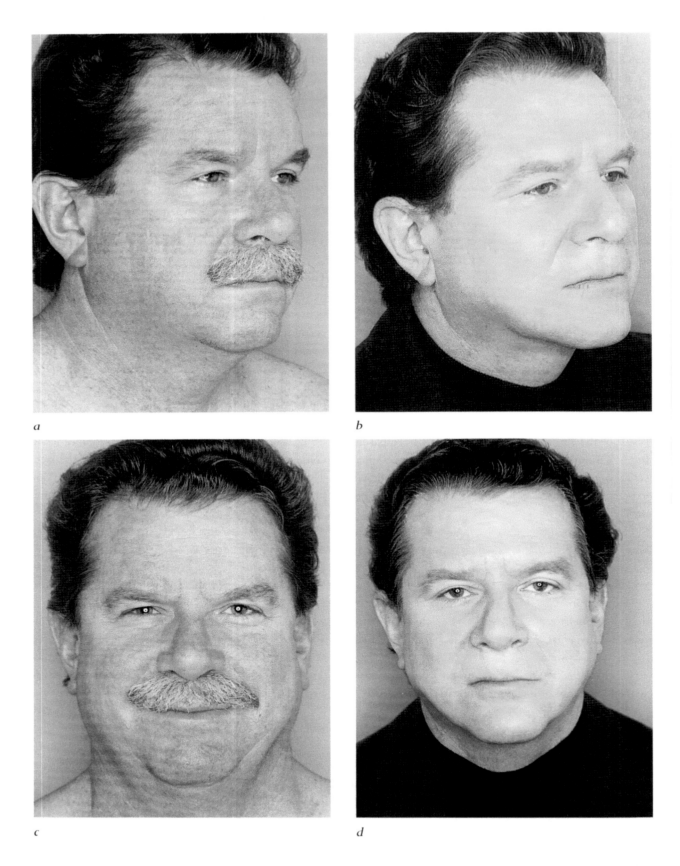

Figure 25.7 *(A) and (C) Patient before, and (B) and (D) patient after the Cook Weekend Alternative to the Facelift™ with chin implant.*

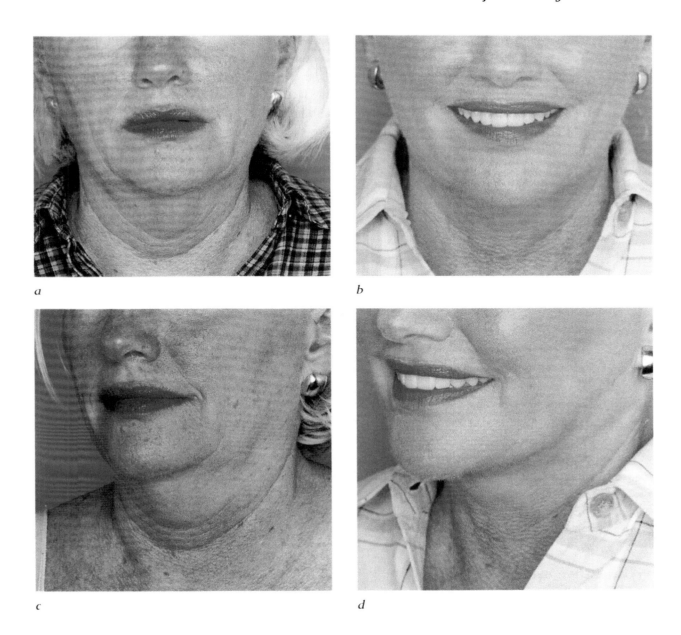

a *b* *c* *d*

Figure 25.8 *(A) and (C) Patient before, and (B) and (D) 1 month after the Cook Weekend Alternative to the Facelift*™*, with laser peel of the face and Cook Total Body Peel*™ *of the neck.*

the proper end-point are critical to the consistent success of this technique.

Indications

Cosmetic surgery patients often show epidermal and dermal lesions on the neck. These may include irregular pigmentation, lentigines, keratoses, wrinkling, roughness, and other problems caused by sun damage and aging skin. When cosmetic problems like these

occur on the face, they are generally treated with a variety of laser or chemical peels.[8,9] Facial peels can help to minimize wrinkles, smooth the skin texture, and lighten pigmented lesions. Skin resurfacing can also help give the skin a more vigorous, glowing, and youthful quality, due to the formation of new collagen and reorganization of the elastic fibers in the skin.

The benefits of peeling have proven somewhat more difficult to apply to the skin of the neck. Some agents, such as glycolic acid alone, may not penetrate deep enough to achieve the full effect. Other agents, like high concentrations of TCA alone, may penetrate too deeply when applied to the skin of the neck and body, so that they may cause undesirable reddening after treatment and may result in postinflammatory pigmentation. When properly performed, the 'controlled' peel, which the present authors have developed, seems to combine the deeper peeling of TCA and the lessened after-effects found with glycolic acid.

The great majority of patients in this office who receive a facial peel of any type are also given a TCA/glycolic acid gel peel (the Cook Total Body Peel™) to the neck, chest, and hands. Other body areas such as the arms, legs, abdomen, and back are also treated when appropriate.

The authors use this technique at the same time as a traditional peel of the face. For the facial peel a laser or a TCA chemical peel may be used, depending on the patient; in some cases, the TCA/glycolic acid gel technique is used to peel the patient's face as well as selected areas of the body. The combination of neck peeling with a facial peel allows good blending from one area to another. It can reduce or eliminate the sharp, rather unnatural-looking, contrast which may occur between treated facial skin and untreated neck and chest skin.

Preoperative evaluation

Patients should be evaluated carefully before treatment. Factors to be considered include the patient's general health; Fitzpatrick skin type;[10] the degree of actinic or age damage;[11] current medications, including isotretinoin (Accutane, Roche Pharmaceuticals, Nutley, NJ) and tretinoin (Retin-A, Ortho Dermatological, Raritan, NJ); the degree of sun exposure that the patient currently experiences and will experience in the future; and the degree and extent of poikiloderma on the neck. A relevant medical history must be obtained, including any history of prior cosmetic surgery, hypertrophic scarring, keloids, allergies (including 'sensitive skin'), or acne. As with any cosmetic surgery, it is important that the patient has realistic expectations.

Before this, or any, skin resurfacing procedure, patients are placed on prophylactic antibiotics and

antiviral medication, starting the day of the peel and continuing for 2 weeks. If patients can tolerate Retin-A, they will benefit from preoperative application to the face. Alpha-hydroxy acids and hydroquinone may also be used. However, care must be taken if patients use high concentrations of alpha-hydroxy acids or tretinoin on the neck skin during the week prior to the procedure, since these substances can increase the speed of penetration of the peeling chemicals.

Procedure

Peeling

The authors prefer to peel one individual area of skin all the way to neutralization, then the next area, and so on, treating each area separately to maximize control of the end-point.

No pretreatment with local anesthetic is needed before this peel. No sedation is required for procedures which include just the face, neck, chest, hands, and arms.

Glycolic acid gel 70%, non-neutralized, is purchased in ready-to-use form (Sun Laboratories, Roslyn, PA); TCA, 40% weight/volume, unbuffered, and sodium bicarbonate, 10% weight/volume, are made up by a local pharmacy (Figure 25.9).

The skin area to be treated is cleansed with acetone. Then 70% glycolic acid gel is applied to one selected area with a folded 3 × 3 gauze (Nu-Gauze, Johnson & Johnson, Fort Washington, PA).

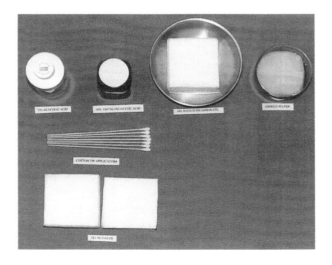

Figure 25.9 *Peeling supplies and equipment ready for use.*

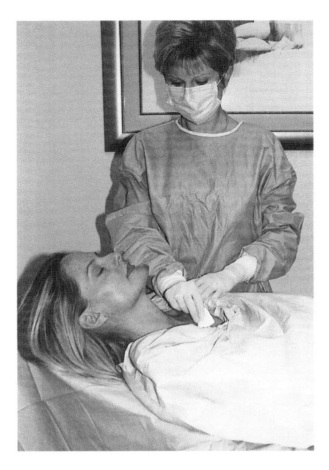

Figure 25.10 *Chemical peeling solution being applied to the chest.*

Immediately, 40% TCA is applied to the same area with a folded 3 × 3 gauze (Figure 25.10).

The skin is observed carefully throughout the process, so as to achieve the desired depth of peel. When the particular area being peeled has reached the desired end-point (see Visual end-point, below), the peeling process is immediately stopped by neutralizing the entire area. If only a small part of the area has reached the desired end-point, that part may be neutralized and the remaining areas observed carefully until they also reach the desired end-point.

If the desired end-point is not reached after approximately 3 minutes, a small test area of the skin is neutralized by wiping it clean with the corner of a 3 × 3 gauze soaked in 10% sodium bicarbonate solution, and the area is observed visually. In approximately one-quarter of patients, the test area will show signs of a deeper end-point only after it has

been neutralized. In these cases, the rest of the area is immediately neutralized as well. The entire area will usually show a similar reaction to the test spot, i.e. it will show visual evidence of the end-point only after being neutralized.

Approximately one-third of patients will reach the end-point within 3 minutes. If after 3 minutes the skin has not yet reached the desired end-point, a small neutralized test spot does not show end-point, and the patient is not complaining of a burning sensation, then an additional coat of TCA may be applied and the process allowed to continue. Several additional coats of TCA may be applied at 3-minute intervals, after again evaluating a different test spot and if the patient is still not experiencing a burning sensation, to attain the desired end-point.

When the end-point is reached, the peeling process is halted by neutralizing with a copious amount of 10% sodium bicarbonate solution. The sodium bicarbonate solution is applied at least five times with 3 × 3 gauze and gentle wiping. Sodium bicarbonate solution is used rather than water, because of its neutralizing effect. Care should be taken to remove all glycolic acid gel from the skin and to neutralize at least 3 inches beyond the treated area on all sides.

Visual end-point

Determination of the proper end-point is crucial for this technique to be successful. The physician must determine the appropriate end-point for each area according to the patient's skin type, actinic damage, and 'age damage'. The primary method for determining the end-point is by direct observation of the skin.

When undergoing a chemical peel, the skin goes through a series of color changes, primarily caused by the TCA in the formulation. Careful attention to the color change is key to obtaining the best cosmetic result. These color changes have been described by Rubin as 'levels of frost'.[8] First, the skin may become pink or erythematous (Stage I; Rubin's level 0). Then small white speckles develop (Stage II; Rubin's level 1; Figure 25.11a). The speckles increase in number and size until the skin reaches a 'frosted' appearance, with the underlying pink still showing through (Stage III; Rubin's level 2; Figure 25.11b). If a peel is taken even further, the skin will 'blanch', becoming first opaque

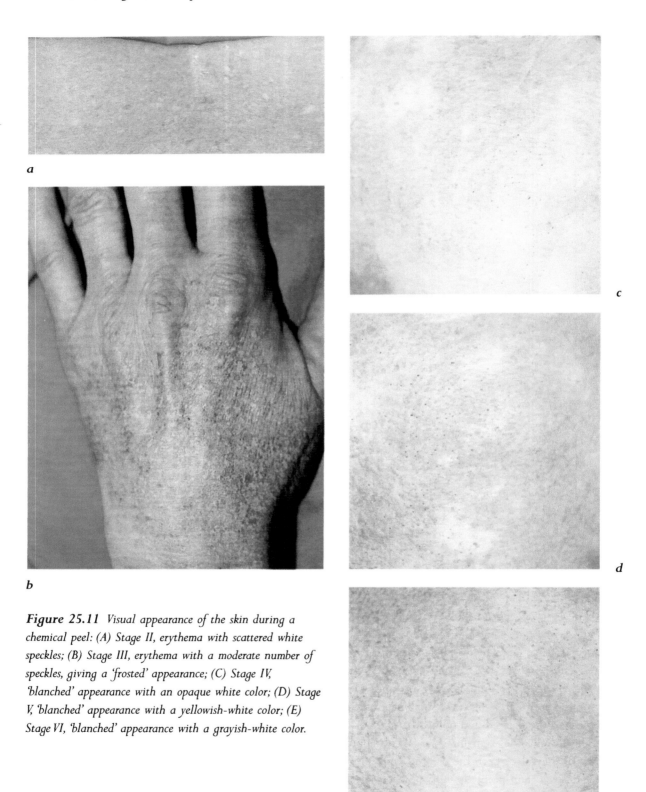

Figure 25.11 *Visual appearance of the skin during a chemical peel: (A) Stage II, erythema with scattered white speckles; (B) Stage III, erythema with a moderate number of speckles, giving a 'frosted' appearance; (C) Stage IV, 'blanched' appearance with an opaque white color; (D) Stage V, 'blanched' appearance with a yellowish-white color; (E) Stage VI, 'blanched' appearance with a grayish-white color.*

white (Stage IV; Rubin's level 3; Figure 25.11c), then yellowish-white (Stage V; Figure 25.11d), and finally grayish-white (Stage VI; Figure 25.11e).

A typical end-point for this technique is in the range of Stage II–III, depending on the degree of skin sensitivity and the amount of skin damage that has occurred.

In patients with darker skin types, the physician may wish to limit the depth of the peel to Stage I. Sensitive skin with mild to moderate sun damage should be peeled only to Stage II, which is characterized by erythema with small scattered white speckles, or an expression by the patient of a slight burning sensation. 'Tough', weathered, or sun-damaged skin can be taken to a more speckled or lightly frosted end-point (Stage III), which indicates a deeper peel. In general, the non-facial skin is rarely peeled past Stage III, to the point where it would begin to blanch to an opaque white.

In most patients, the authors peel the upper neck more deeply than the more distal areas of the neck, so as to blend better with the treated areas of the face. The upper neck may sometimes be taken slightly beyond Stage III to an early Stage IV.

Some skin areas may require more time or more TCA than neighboring areas to peel to the same stage. Similarly, different areas of the body may require different degrees of treatment to reach the same end-point. The peel is allowed to proceed more deeply in areas that have suffered more damage.

The artistry of this technique lies in the blending between one cosmetic unit and another, so as to achieve consistency in the final appearance of the skin. It is particularly important to create a smooth transition between the skin of the face, the upper neck, the lower neck, and the chest. Training and experience will help the physician learn to blend these areas into each other, so as to achieve a natural-looking result.

Postoperative considerations

Immediately after the procedure, an emollient such as Theraplex® (Medicis Dermatologics Inc, Phoenix, AZ) is applied to the treated areas. Patients will continue to apply this emollient twice a day until peeling is completed. They are told to wash the areas gently, without trying to remove all the emollient, and not to pick at the area as it peels.

Depending on the area treated, the skin will flake and scale for 2–4 weeks postoperatively (Figure 25.12). Patients can return to work and normal activities promptly after this procedure, but should strictly avoid sun exposure for at least 1 month. They are advised to use retinoic acid and hydroquinone after the skin has peeled.

This peel can be repeated as often as every month, as soon as the flaking process is complete. In the authors' experience, most patients are satisfied with the improvement seen after a single peel to the face, neck, chest, and hands. A few patients desire further treatment, and additional peels will usually bring additional benefit. A repeat peel tends to be more

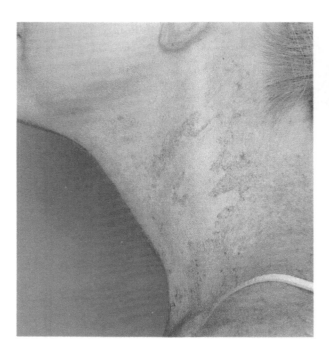

a

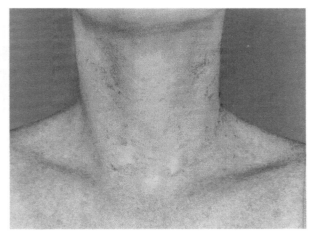

b

Figure 25.12 *(A) and (B) Patient 10 days after a Cook Total Body Peel™ of the neck. Note decreased pigmentation on areas already peeled.*

effective if it is performed as soon as the previous peel has healed (generally around 1 month after the initial peel), as compared to a repeat peel done after 6 months or more.

Results

The authors have performed the Cook Total Body Peel™ on thousands of patients. Virtually all of the facial peel patients receive this treatment on their neck, chest, and hands. When appropriate, the authors may also treat the arms, scalp, legs, abdomen, and back.

This method has produced consistently good results on the neck and chest (Figure 25.13). The skin has a smoother texture and there is a significant decrease in irregular pigmentation, lentigines,

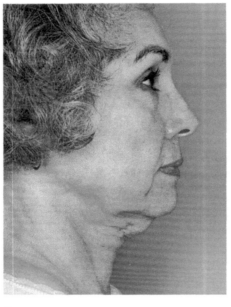

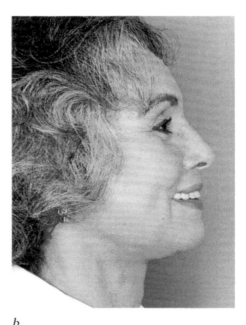

a   *b*

Figure 25.13 Cook Weekend Alternative to the Facelift™, laser peel, upper blepharoplasty and Cook Total Body Peel™ of the neck: (A) patient before and (B) patient after one peel.

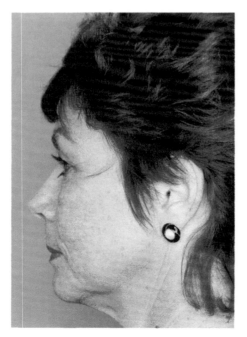

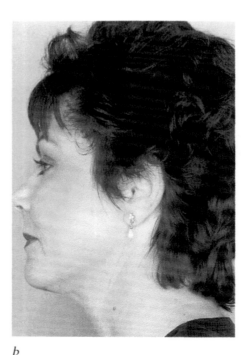

a   *b*

Figure 25.14 CO_2 laser peel of the face with upper eyelid blepharoplasty and Cook Total Body Peel™ of the neck: (A) patient before and (B) patient after one peel.

wrinkling, and actinic keratoses. However, 'flat' seborrheic keratoses usually show less improvement.

The results of this peel are particularly impressive in patients with freckled or actinicly damaged necks, chests, and hands. The technique promotes good blending between the facial skin and the skin of the neck. Patients can achieve a more youthful appearance while avoiding an abrupt 'demarcation line' between treated facial skin and adjacent untreated skin (Figures 25.14 and 25.15).

This technique shows a minimal incidence of postinflammatory pigmentation. The authors have not seen any depigmentation, scarring, or other major complications in their patients.

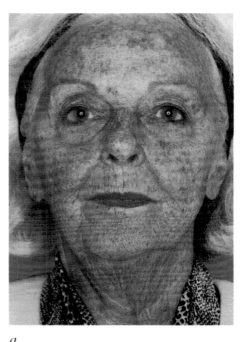

a

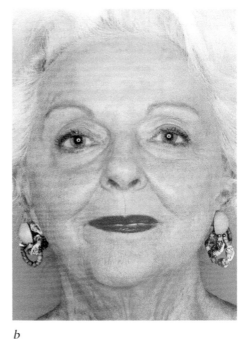

b

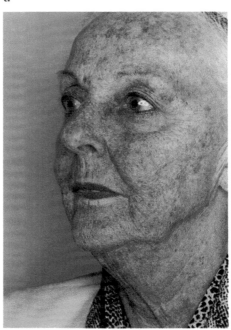

c

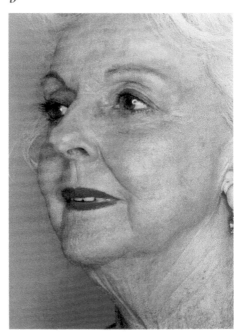

d

Figure 25.15 CO_2 laser peel of the face with Cook Total Body Peel™ of the neck: (A) and (C) patient before, and (B) and (D) patient after one peel. Note that some areas on the neck are still peeling.

References

1. Cook WR Jr, Cook KK. Manual of tumescent liposculpture and laser cosmetic surgery. Philadelphia: Lippincott Williams & Wilkins Publishers; 1999.

2. Cook WR Jr. Laser neck and jowl liposculpture including platysma laser resurfacing, dermal laser resurfacing, and vaporization of subcutaneous fat. Dermatol Surg 1997;23:1143–8.

3. Cook KK, Cook WR Jr. Chemical peel of nonfacial skin using glycolic acid gel augmented with TCA and neutralized based on visual staging. Dermatol Surg 2000;26:994–9.

4. Klein JA. The tumescent technique for liposuction surgery. Am J Cosmet Surg 1987;4:263–7.

5. Farkas LG, Sohm P, Kolar JC, Katic MJ, Munro IR. Inclinations of the facial profile: art versus reality. Plast Reconstr Surg 1985;75:509–19.

6. Alster TS. Manual of cutaneous laser techniques. Philadelphia: Lippincott-Raven Publishers; 1997.

7. Cook WR Jr. Utilizing external ultrasonic energy to improve the results of tumescent liposculpture. Dermatol Surg 1997;23:1207–11.

8. Rubin MG. Manual of chemical peels: superficial and medium depth. Philadelphia: Lippincott-Raven Publishers; 1995.

9. Brody H. Chemical peeling. St Louis: Mosby-Year Book; 1997.

10. Fitzpatrick TB. The validity and practicality of sun-reactive skin types I through VI. Arch Dermatol 1988;124:869–71.

11. Glogau RG. Chemical peeling and aging skin. J Geriatr Dermatol 1994;2:30–5.

26. Reproducible photography for the aging face

Douglas Canfield

DOCUMENTING CHANGE

Serial photography provides physicians with a means to record the change in a patient's appearance over time. The effects of facial rejuvenation are best appreciated by comparing post-treatment photographs of a patient to those taken prior to treatment. In order for such a comparison to be meaningful, the only observable difference from one image to the next should represent a direct result of the treatment in question. Good serial photography removes all other variables from consideration.

A number of factors may affect the usefulness of a photographic series as an objective medical record. These range from technical issues like lighting and exposure to extraneous elements such as makeup and hair color. Reproducible photography is achieved only when all possible variables in the photographic process are controlled. Such control may be accomplished by following a standardized methodology for patient photography. The number of technical decisions made during each photographic session should be minimized. For those elements of the photographic process that must be altered from one patient to the next, all pertinent settings should be recorded for reference at later sessions (Figure 26.1).

PATIENT PREPARATION

The first step in obtaining consistent photographic documentation is ensuring consistency in the subject being documented. There are many aspects of a patient's appearance that have no medical significance. Makeup, hair, clothing and jewelry provide no information about the condition of a patient's skin. At best, they create an unnecessary distraction. At worst, they may mask information that is of value. Whenever possible, these elements should be removed from the area to be photographed.

Of these factors, makeup is the most likely to obscure clinically relevant data. Foundations, concealers, powders and colors will obviously have a noticeable impact on the appearance of the skin. This is, after all, their purpose. All patients – male and female alike – should wash their faces prior to photography. Not only will this remove makeup, but it will also help reduce the reflective glare caused by oily skin. It is

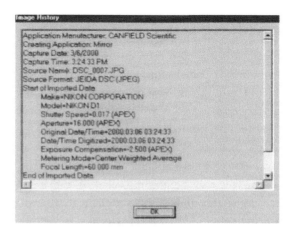

Figure 26.1 All camera settings should be recorded and stored with an image. This may be done automatically with some digital systems.

important, however, not to wash the face *immediately* before the photographic session. The cleansing process itself may introduce erroneous information such as mild erythema. A delay of 10–15 minutes is generally recommended between washing and photography.

Hair color and hairstyle can have a significant effect on a patient's overall appearance. A naturally gray-haired patient, for instance, will tend to look younger with dyed hair. Since the goal of facial rejuvenation is to improve a patient's appearance, any change in hairstyle or color may make it difficult to objectively assess a patient's progress. Also, some hairstyles cover parts of the face. The use of a black headband will keep hair out of the way and will promote a consistent look in photographs. It is important that the headband hold the hair off of the face without pulling, as tension on the scalp may alter the appearance of the patient's face.

While less of an issue than makeup and hair, clothing and jewelry do present an unnecessary distraction in medical photographs. This is particularly true in serial photography, as patients are unlikely to wear the same clothes and jewelry at every visit. Any jewelry on or around the face (earrings, hair accessories, etc.) should be removed prior to photography. Shirts should be covered with a black collar drape.

Eyes can sometimes present the greatest distraction of all. As any portrait photographer or artist knows, a subject's eyes command more attention than anything else. Eyes do not, however, provide much information regarding the condition of a patient's skin. Furthermore, an open eye has tremendous potential for variability. Eyes may be wide open, droopy or captured in the act of blinking, and the pupils may wander to different locations. The most objective patient record will be created if the eyes are closed gently during photography. (It is important that the patient's eyes be closed in as relaxed a manner as possible, with no straining or distortion of the facial musculature.) In cases where a more natural, open-eyed appearance is desired, every attempt must be made to capture the eyes in a neutral and repeatable expression. It may be helpful to instruct the patient to blink a couple of times just prior to taking the photo and to direct their gaze at a stationary target (a tape mark on the wall, for example). It is also advisable to capture multiple exposures in case of blinking.

FRAMING AND COMPOSITION

Distracting elements do not always need to be removed from the patient. Instead, it is often possible to remove distractions from the final photograph through proper image composition. For example, when photographing the entire head, the use of a solid-colored backdrop will keep all details of the examination room out of the image. Also, capturing such an image in a vertical format, rather than horizontal, will minimize the amount of background that appears in the photograph. In many cases, tighter cropping may be used to eliminate the background altogether. If treatment is localized to a specific portion of the face, then the image should be framed to include only the area of interest. However, a certain degree of vigilance is required, as an element that is cropped out of the final photograph may still impact the captured data.

As mentioned earlier, a black collar drape should be used for all facial photography. This is true even if the patient's shoulders do not appear in the photo. Due to the proximity of a shirt to the face, it is possible for light reflected from brightly colored fabrics to impart a color cast to the skin. A black drape prevents such potential color aberrations by absorbing all light that strikes it.

Facial expression is another consideration in determining proper image composition. For example, when documenting periorbital wrinkles, it might seem best to capture a horizontal image that includes only the areas immediately inferior and lateral to the eye. Indeed, such framing does an excellent job of eliminating extraneous details. Unfortunately, it may also crop out one very important piece of data: facial expression. The expression of a patient's mouth can have a profound impact on the appearance of wrinkles around the eyes. When a patient smiles, periorbital wrinkles are much more pronounced than when the mouth is relaxed. It is important, therefore, to include the mouth in the photograph. This may be accomplished by capturing a slightly larger area and/or by switching to a vertical image format.

For serial photography, image composition must be consistent. All photographs in a series should be framed in exactly the same manner. The best way to accomplish this is to have the baseline photograph on

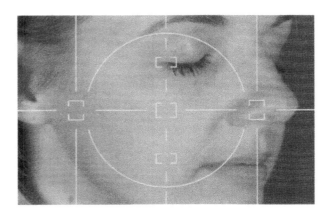

Figure 26.2 *The gridlines overlaid on this digital image correspond to gridlines on a custom focusing screen in the camera. This makes it easy to consistently line up facial landmarks.*

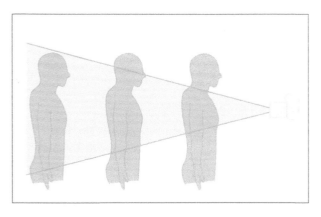

Figure 26.3 *The size of the captured area increases with camera-to-subject distance.*

hand for reference at each follow-up session. Gridlines and the standardized use of facial landmarks can further ensure uniformity in image composition. Returning to the example of periorbital wrinkles, one might choose to always position the lateral canthus at a point halfway across and one-quarter of the way down from the upper corner of the image. Most professional single-lens reflex cameras can be equipped with custom focusing screens that provide gridlines in the viewfinder. The integration of digital imaging can make gridlines even more useful. The baseline image may be viewed on the computer monitor with a grid overlay matching that in the viewfinder. This makes it very easy to line up facial landmarks in a consistent manner (Figure 26.2). As discussed later in this chapter, the use of a stereotactic face device can greatly simplify the process of framing facial photographs in a repeatable manner.

MAGNIFICATION

The use of gridlines addresses proper image framing in two dimensions; it is also necessary to maintain consistency in a third dimension. In order to assure uniformity in image magnification, the camera-to-subject distance must be kept constant from timepoint to timepoint. A direct relationship exists between distance and magnification. The viewable area of a camera may be thought of as a cone that

starts at the lens and expands outwards as the distance in front of the lens increases. The size of this cone is determined by the focal length of the lens and the size of the camera's image sensor. If the focal length remains constant, the captured area becomes larger as the camera-to-subject distance increases (Figure 26.3). The dimensions of the image sensor, on the other hand, are fixed for a particular camera.

In a 35-mm camera, the image sensor is a 36×24 mm area of film. If the subject is far enough away from the camera that the area captured measures 72×48 mm, then the image is one-half life size. In other words, the *reproduction ratio* of an image captured at this distance is 1:2. As the subject is moved further away from the camera, a point will be reached at which an area of 144×96 mm is captured. At this point, the reproduction ratio is 1:4, and the image is one-quarter life size. By definition, the reproduction ratio expresses magnification by relating final image size to original subject size. In practice, reproduction ratio is more commonly used to describe the captured area. For instance, a 1:6 vertical image captures a patient's full face with fairly tight cropping. A 1:8 vertical image captures the entire head with some background visible all around. For a given camera and focal length, each reproduction ratio corresponds to a specific distance between the camera and the subject.

The first step towards achieving consistency in image magnification is to limit the number of different reproduction ratios used to a finite set of specific values. For

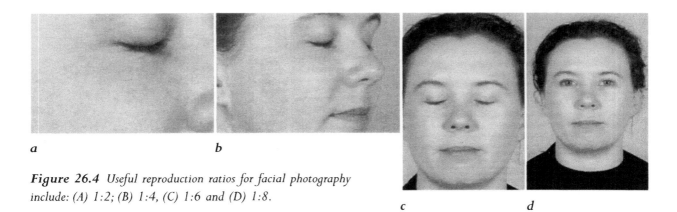

a   *b*   *c*   *d*

Figure 26.4 *Useful reproduction ratios for facial photography include: (A) 1:2; (B) 1:4, (C) 1:6 and (D) 1:8.*

facial photography, appropriate reproduction ratios include 1:2, 1:4, 1:6 and 1:8 (Figure 26.4). The camera lens should be indexed so that it may be set to these four reproduction ratios in an easy and repeatable manner. This may be accomplished through the use of color-coded marks on the focus ring. On many lenses, the manual focus ring is disengaged when autofocus is used. Once such a lens has been indexed, it is important to leave the lens permanently set to manual focus mode, as switching back and forth between auto- and manual focus will render the index marks invalid.

During a photographic session, the focus ring on the lens is set to the appropriate index mark and then left alone. (The 'appropriate' mark is determined by the area to be captured or, in the case of follow-up photographs, by the reproduction ratio used in the baseline image.) As stated earlier, the lens setting will establish a camera-to-subject distance. With the camera held at approximately this distance from the patient, the photographer looks through the viewfinder and moves the entire camera forward and back until the image appears sharp. This technique – termed 'body focusing' – is contrary to the method typically employed by photographers outside the fields of science and medicine. In most situations, the camera-to-subject distance is held constant and the focus ring is rotated to create a sharp image. Body focusing is preferable for serial photography as it ensures a fixed magnification from one session to the next.

CAMERA-TO-PATIENT REGISTRATION

Repeatable image composition is complicated by the fact that the human face is a three-dimensional object. From timepoint to timepoint, the spatial relationship of the camera to the patient's face must remain the same. Whether this is thought of as camera angle or as patient positioning, it is a variable that must be controlled for proper patient documentation. Ideally, the camera should always be held such that the imaging plane is parallel to the plane of the subject. Since the face presents a curved surface, however, it can be difficult to identify the appropriate target plane.

Consistency is best achieved through the use of a stereotactic face device (Figure 26.5). Such a device registers the patient's anatomy using several fixed contact points. While the exact orientation of the face may vary slightly from patient to patient, the device ensures that, for a particular patient, the head will always be positioned in the same manner. The angle

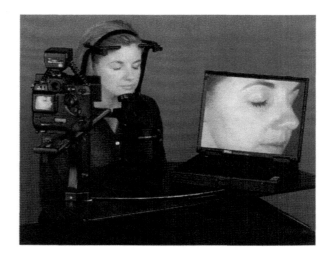

Figure 26.5 *A stereotactic face device ensures consistent camera-to-patient registration.*

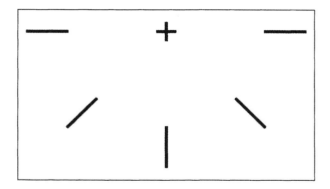

Figure 26.6 *Tape marks on the floor are useful for patient positioning.*

of the camera relative to the patient positioning apparatus does not change. The camera is restricted to lateral movements only along three axes for the purposes of properly framing and focusing an image.

In situations where a face device is not available, good results may still be obtained by following a strict photographic methodology. Tape marks should be placed on the floor of any room that will be used for photography. (A standard pattern for tape marks is shown in Figure 26.6.) It is also helpful to place vertical tape marks on the walls in line with the floor markings for lateral and oblique angles. For facial photographs, the patient should be seated on an adjustable-height stool placed on the center cross in the tape pattern. With the stool at a comfortable height, the patient sits with feet together and on either side of the appropriate tape mark for a frontal, oblique or lateral view. While sitting up straight, the patient looks directly ahead at the corresponding tape mark on the wall. The patient's midsagittal plane should be aligned with the floor marking and the head should be in a comfortable, neutral position.

The photographer, too, must be properly positioned. Like the patient, the photographer should be seated on an adjustable-height stool. In addition, the photographer's stool should be equipped with wheels. This provides a good balance of mobility and camera stability. Tape marks on the floor may be used to establish approximate camera-to-subject distances and to keep the camera on the proper axis. The height of the stool should be adjusted for each patient such that when the photographer is seated with the target area properly framed, the lens barrel is parallel to the floor.

LIGHTING

No single element in the photographic process warrants more careful consideration than lighting. 'Photography', after all, is the recording of light. An image is captured when the light reflected from a subject strikes a photosensitive imaging surface. How a patient appears in a photograph is determined as much by the nature of the light falling on his or her face during photography as by the actual condition of the skin. The color, intensity and direction of this light are important variables to be considered.

The use of either a camera-mounted flash unit or studio strobes is the only way to ensure complete control over how a patient is lit. A strobe or flash unit emits a brief burst of very bright light that is synchronized to the opening of the camera shutter. The short duration of the burst minimizes the impact of camera shake. The high intensity of light delivered allows for the use of a small aperture, thus maximizing the depth of field. Most importantly, the use of a flash minimizes the effect of ambient light on the final image. Ambient light is a combination of the light emitted by fixtures in the room and light entering the room through windows or open doors. Such light is prone to a high degree of variability in color and intensity. The light streaming through the window on a sunny day, for example, is very different to that on a cloudy day, and daylight has different characteristics than the light from either an incandescent or a fluorescent fixture. This can lead to variability not only from timepoint to timepoint, but even within a single photograph. For a given type of light, e.g. daylight, incandescent, fluorescent, etc., accurate color rendering may be achieved through the use of an appropriate film or by selecting the proper white balance setting on a digital camera. It is not possible, however, to adjust for the color profiles of several different types of light in a single image.

The angle at which light strikes a three-dimensional object determines how the form and surface texture of that object are rendered in a two-dimensional image. The appearance of highlights and shadows provides the viewer with important visual data. Careful attention to this fact is crucial for the accurate documentation of facial rejuvenation. By merely changing the position of a light, it is possible to show a reduction in the severity of a patient's

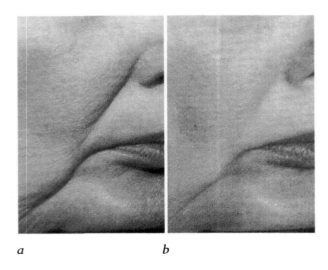

a   *b*

Figure 26.7 *(A,B) The apparent improvement in this patient's condition is due to a change in lighting angle.*

wrinkles, even if no actual change in the skin has occurred (Figure 26.7). It is also possible for a genuine improvement in a patient's condition to be completely lost in pre- and posttreatment photographs due to a poor choice in lighting.

While shadows provide valuable information in a clinical photograph, shadows that are very large or especially dark may actually obscure important data. Good lighting strikes a delicate balance, providing sufficient shadow detail without causing unnecessary distraction. This may be achieved by the use of twin light sources positioned symmetrically on either side of the lens. The distance between each flash head and the center of the lens determines the incident angle of light on the patient's skin. Flash heads positioned too close to the lens will produce a flat lighting that creates no shadows to mark fine lines and wrinkles. On the other hand, shadows cast by the gross features of the face may become overly large if lights are moved too far apart. The ideal flash position can be determined through trial and error, and may vary slightly with different patient views. It is important that any adjustments to the flash heads be accomplished in a measurable and repeatable manner. This

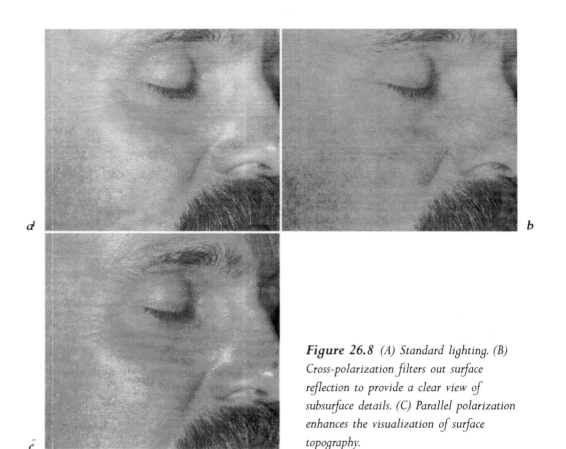

d   *b*

c

Figure 26.8 *(A) Standard lighting. (B) Cross-polarization filters out surface reflection to provide a clear view of subsurface details. (C) Parallel polarization enhances the visualization of surface topography.*

is easier with an indexed, camera-based flash system than with completely independent light sources.

Sometimes, the clinical information of greatest interest lies not in the ridges and furrows of the skin, but in the pigmentation and vascularity beneath the surface. Special lighting techniques are available to improve the visualization of these characteristics. Vascular details such as erythema and telangiectasia are best photographed using cross-polarization to filter out surface reflection. Linear polarizing filters placed over the flash heads ensure that the patient is illuminated by light waves oriented in parallel planes. Light waves reflected directly from the surface of the skin retain their original orientation and are blocked by a linear polarizing filter over the lens that is set perpendicular to those on the flash heads. Light waves that penetrate the skin are scattered by collagen fibers and other structures of the dermis. Some of the scattered light waves are reflected back towards the camera in random orientations (i.e. scattering depolarizes the light). The majority of these waves are able to pass through the polarizing filter on the lens. The resulting image captures subsurface details of the skin with none of the surface highlights and shadows that would normally obscure this information (Figure 26.8).

Ultraviolet (UV) reflectance photography is useful for documenting changes in the pigmentation of the epidermis. UV-pass filters placed over the flash heads block most of the visible spectrum, so that the patient's face is illuminated primarily by UV light. This light passes through the epidermis and is reflected off of the dermis back to the camera. Any melanin in the epidermis absorbs UV light, thus creating dark patches where pigment is present in high concentrations (Figure 26.9). This technique is employed mainly for the documentation of photodamage.

EXPOSURE AND METERING

To capture an image of acceptable quality, the photoreceptor [film or charged coupled device (CCD)] in a camera must be exposed to the proper amount of light. Insufficient light levels result in underexposure, with photographs appearing dark and

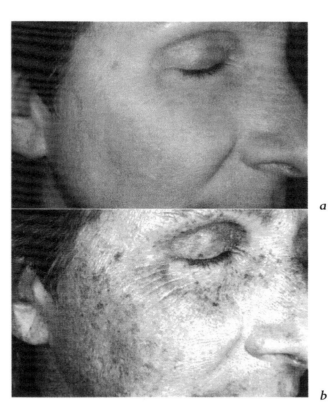

Figure 26.9 *(A,B) UV reflectance enhances the appearance of epidermal pigmentation.*

muddy overall and lacking detail in the darker areas of the subject. Excessive amounts of light lead to overexposed images that appear washed out and lacking detail in the highlight areas. The quantity of light required for proper exposure is dependent upon the sensitivity of the image sensor.

In the case of film photography, sensitivity is a property of the film used and is expressed as an International Organization for Standardization (ISO)/American Standards Association (ASA) rating. Higher ISO numbers indicate faster films that require less light. The sensitivity of a digital camera is determined by the capabilities of the CCD and the camera's on-board image processing. Digital camera sensitivity is typically expressed as an ISO equivalency and, in most digital cameras, may be adjusted to one of several values. Clinical photography is best performed using the lowest available sensitivity setting on a digital camera or using film with an ISO rating of 64 or 100. Lower sensitivity helps to minimize the impact of ambient light on the final photograph. Furthermore, an inverse relationship exists between sensitivity and image quality. Low sensitivity equates to finer film grain or, for digital images, a better signal-to-noise ratio.

The amount of light that reaches an imaging surface is a product of three factors: the intensity of light reflected from the subject, the duration of exposure and the size of the opening in the lens through which the light must pass. When a flash is used, these three elements are controlled by adjusting flash power, flash duration and aperture. The shutter speed used for flash photography is significantly longer than the duration of a flash burst, and is not adjusted to control exposure.

The simplest approach would be to use a fully automatic camera system that controls both the flash and the aperture without direct user intervention. With most modern cameras, this approach will often yield acceptable exposures. However, shooting in full program mode generally produces photographs with a shallow depth of field. This is especially evident at the working distances used for facial photography and may lead to images in which the eye is in sharp focus but the nose is not. To maximize depth of field, the photographer must take control of the aperture adjustment by setting the camera to either aperture-priority or manual mode.

In aperture-priority mode, aperture (measured in f-numbers) is set by the photographer and flash output is adjusted automatically by the camera. By using small aperture settings (large f-numbers) it is possible to increase depth of field. For each reproduction ratio used, an optimal f-number setting may be derived through trial and error. Once these values have been established, they become the starting point for all patients. (In some cases, the use of exposure compensation may be necessary.) The complexity added to the photographic process by using aperture-priority instead of full-program mode is minimal, and is easily justified by the improvement in image quality.

A photographer who wishes to have complete control over exposure may choose to shoot in manual mode. With a camera set to manual, the photographer is responsible for adjusting both aperture and flash output. Provided all settings are properly recorded and reproduced at each timepoint, this method can produce very consistent exposures. However, using a camera in manual mode may introduce a high degree of operator error and may not be appropriate for all practices. This becomes less of an issue when using a digital camera, as the immediacy of the results allows for a trial-and-error approach to proper exposure.

COLOR FIDELITY

In addition to being properly exposed, clinical photographs must accurately and consistently render the color of a patient's skin. This is arguably the most challenging aspect of photographic documentation. A number of variables exist in the production and processing of color film that are entirely beyond the control of the photographer. The differences from one roll of film to the next, or from batch to batch of processing chemicals, make it impossible to achieve perfect color. Steps may be taken, however, to minimize the degree of variability.

First, it is important to always use the exact same type of film. Switching from one brand or type of film to another will significantly impact color. The photo laboratory used to process film should also remain the same, and should be a facility geared towards professional photographers rather than general consumers. It is helpful, too, to reduce the number of steps involved in processing by using slide film rather than print film. Finally, photographing a color standard on each roll of film can provide a useful reference. While this will not ensure correct or consistent colors, it does provide an indication of what kind of color cast is present on each roll of film.

Compared to film, digital imaging offers several distinct advantages with regard to the accuracy and consistency of recorded color. Most notably, both the image sensor and processing are built into a digital camera – they do not change unless the camera is replaced. This eliminates the major causes of color variability that are inherent to film. In addition, a color standard may be used in conjunction with appropriate software to perform precise and objective color correction to digital images after they have been captured. While this does not provide a 'cure-all' for poor lighting or improper white balance settings, standardized digital color correction can eliminate minor imperfections in color rendering.

Unfortunately, the consistency and objectivity of digital images exist only on a mathematical level. A digital image is, after all, just an array of numbers that represent color values. Viewing a digital image requires the use of an output device such as a monitor or printer. Much of the allure of digital imaging involves the wide variety available of such output devices. Each type of device has certain characteristics related to the specific technology it uses to display an image. It would be unrealistic to expect the glowing phosphors of a cathode-ray tube monitor to stimulate the retina in exactly the same manner as light reflected from the colored pigments on a printed page. If properly calibrated on a regular basis, however, one particular output device can render images that are accurate and consistent within the limitations of that device.

SUMMARY

The visible characteristics of a patient's skin are best documented through photography. Images, therefore, constitute a valuable part of a patient's medical record. As such, the accuracy of photographic records warrants as much consideration as the accuracy of any other piece of documentation in a patient's chart. This does not require artistic talent or creativity – clinical photography is more of a science than an art. Armed with the proper equipment and a basic understanding of the concepts presented in this chapter, any medical professional should be able to capture good patient photographs.

27. Digital photography

Joseph Niamtu, III

Strange times these are! Anyone reading this chapter is living through a paradigm shift. A paradigm shift occurs when an excepted method or model, such as film photography, is replaced by a new method or model, in this case digital photography. When a paradigm shift occurs, all the previous rules change and the new technology is often met with skepticism, as it requires people to change their thinking and the way in which they do things. Sometimes people are so ingrained in the previous technology that they are blinded by the benefits of the new technology and miss progress.

The Swiss watch-making industry invented the quartz liquid-crystal timepiece but did not even patent the idea. Their leaders were blinded by this new technology and did not take it seriously; after all, it was a departure from their paradigm. It could not be a timepiece; there were no moving parts, no jewels, and no movement. This watch needed no winding, was 1000 times more accurate and was cheap to manufacture. The Japanese saw this potential and snatched the patent and the rest is history; the Swiss lost dominance in the timepiece industry. The moral here is never underestimate a paradigm shift. Go with the new technology!

The new technology of digital photography is in its Stone Age infancy but it is advanced enough for every contemporary cosmetic surgeon to convert yesterday. Many people are hesitant to make the conversion from film photography to digital photography and they offer many excuses: 'The technology is changing too fast', 'The resolution is not high enough', 'I am computer illiterate', etc. Remember it is natural to fear a paradigm shift.

With all this in mind, it must be remembered that technology cannot be outraced, so a point at which to jump in must be chosen. This point occurred in about 1997. It is now easy, accurate and affordable to use digital photography in medical practice.

DIGITAL CAMERAS

Film photography was popularized in the early 1800s and, with notable refinements, has essentially remained the same. The process involves a lens that focuses on a subject and a shutter that controls the amount of light that is shed on a photosensitive medium. This entire process is a mixture of light and lens. The photosensitive medium is then wet processed into negatives, slides or photographs. Not much has really changed since the Civil War.

Digital photography, although new, also relies on light and lenses. The front half of the digital camera is not much different to a conventional film camera; the main difference lies in the photosensors within the camera. These sensors are called charged coupled devices (CCD) and function by processing focused light into a digital mode – ones and zeros to be specific. The higher the bit of the CCD, the more shades of color will be seen, i.e. a 12-bit CCD chip is superior to an 8-bit CCD. An 8-bit CCD chip will record 16.7 million colors while a 12-bit chip will record 68.7 billion colors, which is true photographic photography. The colors increase exponentially with the increase in bits. Each pixel has a code for various colors and this combination allows the picture to be assembled. Since the number of pixels is proportional to the amount of digital information, the higher the number of pixels, the more information within the photograph. For all practical purposes, this information is called resolution and one can basically say that the higher the number of pixels, the greater the resolution and the better the picture.

There are a myriad of digital cameras available and they change weekly. Like most high tech hardware, the same product will probably not be in use 48 months later. Digital cameras can be classified into three main types: toys, consumer grade and professional. The inexpensive digital cameras with 640×480 resolution were the first-generation cameras. They are still sold for several hundred dollars and are fine for e-mailing pictures to family and friends, but will not suffice for clinical digital photography. Consumer-grade digital cameras run the full gamut of price and accessories. Most cameras that will suffice for clinical digital photography are in the $800–1500 price range. Professional-grade digital cameras are in the $5000–15,000 price range and are usually out of the reach of most cosmetic surgeons. Just because a camera is expensive does not mean that it is ideal for clinical photography. However, it is important that a good consumer-grade digital camera should perform as well as the professional counterparts, and it can if the basic important functions are present. There are several critical requirements for clinical digital photography, which will now be discussed.

Resolution

Resolution is one of the major misunderstandings in digital photography. Many people feel that resolution is the only important factor in digital photography, and mistakenly assume that the higher the resolution, the clearer the picture. While this statement holds some truth, resolution actually relates to the size of an image. An image captured at 640×480 pixels will print out at about the size of 7×9 inches (16×22 cm). This is the same resolution as an National Television Standard Committee (NTSC) video signal or the same size as that played on a VCR. An image about twice the size (1024×1280 pixels) will print out at about 14×18 inches (36×45 cm). The gold standard for resolution is still 35-mm slide film, the resolution of which is approximately 3000×4000, which would theoretically equal 12 million pixels. The maximum resolution of consumer-grade digital cameras at the time of publication is 3.3 million pixels. With this in mind, half of the resolution barrier has been conquered in about a decade. Certainly, the next decade will breach the gold standard and develop extreme resolutions. Figure 27.1 illustrates the relative size in digital resolution as compared to 35-mm slide film.

As resolution has increased, so has the demand for memory. Higher resolution images may be 10–80 megabytes (MB) and storage solutions are much needed. In the early 1990s a laptop computer with a 170MB hard drive was a cutting-edge machine. At the time of publication laptops are available with 30 gigabyte (GB) hard drives. There is no doubt that image resolution and storage capacity will increase concomitantly. This raises the question of how much resolution is required for medical photography. A resolution of 1280×1024 pixels is adequate for accurate detail. This minimum standard will constantly increase in concert with digital camera resolution and soon minimal resolution will be an obsolete phrase.

The author currently uses a resolution of 1280×1024 pixels, which is a mid-range resolution provided by most high-end consumer digital cameras. This resolution works well in terms of detail, does not overpower the Windows operating system and is suitable for most academic applications, including clinical archiving, multimedia lecturing, and scientific publications.

Through the lens focusing

Through the lens focusing (TTL) is another important requirement. Most practitioners are used to taking clinical images with 35-mm single-lens reflex (SLR) cameras. These cameras have focusing systems that allow the user to view the same image that will be registered on the film, i.e. it is essentially a WYSIWYG (what you see is what you get) system. Rangefinder types of cameras are not TTL and there is a phenomenon known as parallax in which the same image

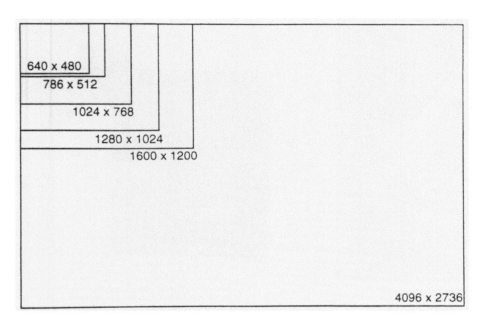

640 x 480
786 x 512
1024 x 768
1280 x 1024
1600 x 1200
4096 x 2736

viewed through the rangefinder lens is not the exact image registered on the film. This can be very frustrating, especially with macrophotography, as the image seen may not be the same as the picture produced, e.g. the edge may be cut off or it may be off center.

Flash location

Flash position is another important feature. As with any camera, the flash will frequently make or break an image. Since most cosmetic surgeons require close-up images, a digital camera should be versatile in that respect. Cameras with flashes that are mounted far from the focusing lens can be problematic because the closer the camera is held to the subject, the further away the flash will be. In a real situation, a flash mounted 5 inches from the lens is fine for a full-face or full-body image, as the flash will be far enough away from the subject to disperse and shower the entire area with light. If the same camera is used to focus on the ear at a distance of 2 inches, the flash will be positioned 5 inches away and light up the nose but not the ear (Figure 27.2). With this in mind, the closer the flash is to the lens, the better the arrangement for macrophotography. Obviously, macroflashes can solve this problem but, in the author's experience, the proper digital camera can take 99% of clinical images without specialized flashes or lenses.

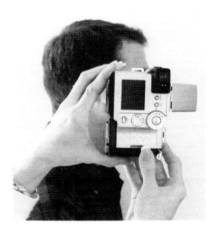

Figure 27.2 *The problem of a flash attachment being mounted too far away from the lens is illustrated; the closer the flash is to the lens, the better suited the camera is to macrophotography.*

Macrolenses

Macrolens capability is paramount for a suitable clinical camera. Inexpensive cameras may advertise 'macro' capability but produce distorted images. With lenses, you get what you pay for and the higher end cameras usually have superior lenses, e.g. the Olympus C2500L can focus to 0.8 inches. A good

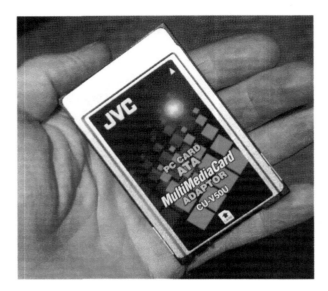

Figure 27.3 PCMCIA cards are excellent storage devices for digital images and can easily be attached to all current notebook computers and to desktop computers with an appropriate slot.

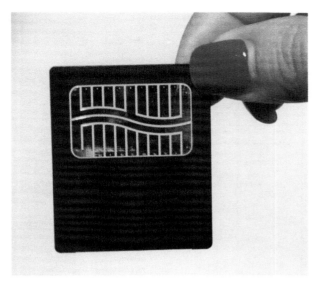

Figure 27.4 The SmartMedia storage card is a wafer-thin storage medium that has become increasingly popular in various digital cameras.

means of evaluating the quality of a macrolens system is to take a picture of text from a book; if the periphery of the image is significantly distorted then the macroimages will be too. Many digital cameras offer diopter lens kits that allow the user to screw on macrolenses of various magnifications. The biggest problem with taking good macroimages is the camera flash, as mentioned previously.

Liquid-crystal display

A liquid-crystal display (LCD) monitor is an absolute necessity for a clinical digital camera. The main advantage of digital photography is the ability to immediately preview an image. One of the greatest disappointments with 35-mm photography was photographing that rare clinical lesion to find out a week later that the image was out of focus or that the processor destroyed the film. Without an LCD monitor on the digital camera, it is not possible to know whether the image just taken is adequate or not. With digital photography there is no reason to ever take a bad picture, because it can be previewed and a better image retaken if necessary. That ability is lost without a monitor and this will result in disap-

pointment when images are downloaded to find out that the out-of-town patient blinked and had their eyes closed in the picture that is needed today. *Do not* purchase a digital camera without an LCD display.

Removable memory

Image storage is also another important thing to consider. *Do not* purchase a digital camera that does not have some type of removable storage medium. There are various storage media available. Personal Computer Memory Card International Association (PCMCIA) cards are credit-card sized memory cards that will work on all laptops or desktops with a special card reader (Figure 27.3). They function well and, depending upon the configuration, can be purchased with 8MB to hundreds of megabytes of memory. These were popular on the earlier digital cameras but are quickly being replaced by more compact media. SmartMedia cards are wafer-thin memory cards about the size of a matchbook cover and are currently very popular. In addition, some cameras have CF (CompactFlash) memory slots for future technologies, or to use as a secondary CF memory slot – CF memory cards are about half the size of PCMCIA cards. The author has

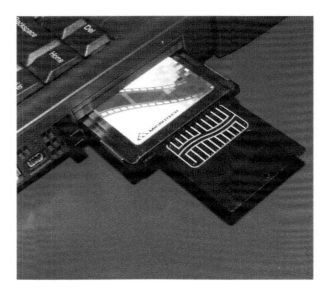

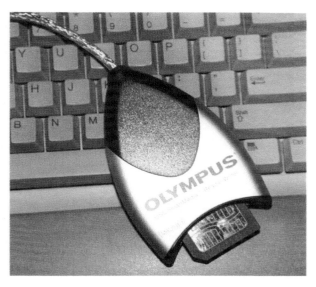

Figure 27.5 *PCMCIA card-readers are available for the SmartMedia storage cards. The SmartMedia card simply inserts into the PCMCIA card which, in turn, inserts into the computer.*

Figure 27.6 *USB card-readers are a great and portable alternative for reading SmartMedia cards and other types of digital camera storage cards. Most new computers have USB ports which enable the use of this type of card-reader.*

experimented with all major digital camera systems and prefers a SmartMedia type of storage system, which is used by Olympus and other manufacturers (Figure 27.4). This wafer-thin storage medium is placed into the camera and used to store the images. The amount of memory currently ranges from 8 to 128MB. Depending upon the selected resolution of the camera, anything from several to several hundred images may be stored in a single media card. The media card is then removed from the camera and placed in some type of reading apparatus. Various types of card-readers are available. A specialized 3.5-inch floppy disk card-reader is very popular, as most end-users are comfortable with this interface; they are easy to use and are relatively expedient at image transfer. Since floppy drives are not terribly fast, it may take up to 1 minute to transfer images; however, it is a tremendous advantage over cable transfer. Most digital cameras have cables that connect most frequently to a serial port for image transfer. Although this is inexpensive, it is very slow and takes several minutes per image, making it a waste of time, and time is money. Newer cameras may incorporate a universal serial bus (USB) adapter, which enables extremely rapid image transfer. Still, one must deal with cables and adapters.

The PCMCIA interface is familiar to all laptop users, as modern laptops usually have two PCMCIA slots. PCMCIA card-readers are credit-card sized devices that accept the SmartMedia card and plug into the PCMCIA slot on laptops, or into PCMCIA card-readers for desktop units (Figure 27.5). The PCMCIA interface is rapid and the images are read as an additional drive on the computer; image transfer is virtually instantaneous with this interface. One problem that the author has encountered is that each card has a separate driver. Most cards will be recognized by Windows Plug-and-Play applications and will function with a default Windows PCMCIA driver. However, in the author's experience, if one uses multiple cards from multiple companies, serious driver conflicts may result that can be very difficult to resolve. The author has been forced to initialize his hard drive several times due to PCMCIA driver conflicts. Whilst still using them, the author tries to use only a single card and if an additional card is used for another camera then it is one from the same manufacturer; this has worked well so far.

The newest type of card-reading device is the external USB card reader (Figure 27.6). These powerful devices are inexpensive and can fit in the palm of the hand. They plug into the USB port on laptop or desktop computers. USB readers are available that read PCMCIA, smart card and SmartMedia formats.

Function control

Automatic and manual camera modes are also important with clinical photography. While most clinicians are interested in fully automatic functions, there may be times where lighting requirements warrant manual modes. The author has found this to be true especially when photographing in the operating or emergency room. Even using the camera in different office treatment rooms with varied lighting can make a difference. In order to standardize the images, sometimes it may be necessary to adjust the flash, shutter speed and the analog of International Organization for Standardization (ISO) settings, exposure and white balance. The more automatic features that are available, the better, because there is nothing easier to use than a 'point-and-shoot' camera.

Accessories

Accessory adaptation may be an important feature for many clinicians. If one desires to use macro flashes, slave or background flashes or conventional 'hot-shoe' flashes then having a flash port or a hot-shoe adapter is important. These allow synchronization with the shutter, as do professional cameras. Other adaptations include a direct current (DC) input, which will allow the use of house current instead of batteries. Most digital cameras have data-transfer ports. One useful connection is a video-out port that allows the user to project the images directly onto a television screen. This can be useful in consultations or in an environment when a computer is unavailable. The author highly recommends purchasing two sets of nickel–cadmium (Ni–Cd) rechargeable batteries so that fresh power is always available. Digital cameras are very draining on conventional batteries; a camera can be used for an entire week on a Ni–Cd charge.

COMPUTERS FOR IMAGING

Laptop computers have already been mentioned several times thus far and the point should now be made that the author recommends laptops for medical imaging for many reasons. The author takes about 4000 images each year and in earlier times had these images only on the office desktop computer. It seemed that so many times images were needed at home or on the road. The author then began copying images and transferring them to the home computer, and it did not take long to confuse which images were duplicates and which images were on which computer. Worse than that, there was no convenient access to images whilst traveling.

As laptop memory and processor speed increased, one was used solely for imaging. This was an emancipating event for progress. All images could be stored on one machine, which could be taken home, to various satellite offices, to the hospital and, most importantly, on trips. Digital imaging is more than a function, it is a hobby! For those who rely upon images for clinical and academic reasons, one must continually download, process and archive these images. Although it takes some time every night, or several times per week, it pays off exponentially when the images are required to work for you. State-of-the-art imaging software will automate much of this work but none the less one must stay abreast of archiving. As the old adage goes, 'garbage in, garbage out'.

When discussing the ability of a digital media camera card to store images, more is good but not always better. Some of the media cards can hold hundreds of pictures and it is definitely human nature for us to not download our images until we have to. In view of this, if the media card malfunctions (and you know it will at some point), you will lose all of the images that have not been downloaded. Also, a big problem with allowing images to pile up is that by the time you finally download them, archiving becomes a big problem. You are now staring at perhaps 100 images and it is usually impossible to remember whose eyelid it is or how many days after surgery another image was taken. As already stated, most esthetic surgeons are very serious about their images and good doctors will spend regular time attending to them.

It is human nature to try and use what we have, but skimping on an imaging computer is bad business. Computers are like cars, motorcycles, boats and airplanes in that you will be sorry later for not purchasing enough power. As image resolution

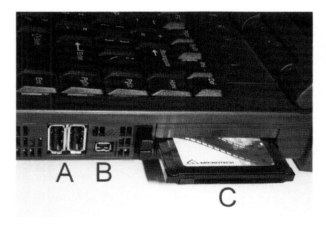

Figure 27.7 *The versatility of today's portable computers is illustrated: (A) USB ports; (B) a 'firewire' port; (C) a dual PCMCIA slot.*

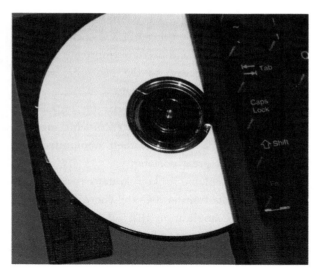

Figure 27.8 *A removable CD recorder with a notebook computer is the author's choice for mobile data backup.*

continues to increase, computer processor speed, RAM memory and hard drive size have increased as well. At the time of this publication, the author recommends a notebook computer with a 700-MHz processor, 256MB of RAM, a 30GB hard drive and a 15-inch LCD screen. A computer of this stature will retail for between $3000 and $4000. Other important options to look for when buying a computer for imaging (whether notebook or desktop) are the presence of USB ports, composite and Super Video (S-video) inputs and outputs, and an Institute of Electrical and Electronic Engineers (IEEE) 1394 (firewire) port (Figure 27.7). These interface ports will allow for uploading and downloading not only digital camera images but digital video, which is the next vista in clinical photography. Many brand name computers have these interface options built into the computer, while others accomplish this hook-up through docking stations or port replicators.

BACKUP STRATEGIES

For any clinician who has amassed a large collection of Kodak slides, it would be devastating to lose this entire collection, as it takes many years to accumulate and organize. Short of a house fire, it would be difficult to lose one's collection, but none the less devastating. It must constantly be kept in mind that

an entire digital slide collection could be lost in a matter of seconds from a computer virus or malfunction. The 'Love Bug' virus that swept the world in May 2000 is a good example. This virus was attached to an e-mail and, when activated, searched one's entire hard drive for JPEG images and corrupted them. The author personally lost several thousand images, but had luckily backed them up the previous week. However, the images that were not backed up were lost and some of these images were from the operating room and of unique pathology, and can probably never be replaced. Unfortunately, there were thousands of computer users without any backup strategy who lost everything. If this has never happened to you, I can guarantee that it is a feeling of extreme violation. Don't be stupid; backup your images! The best strategy is to backup on a regular basis. The author tries to do this before going to bed at night so that next morning the job is complete.

There are multiple means to back up image data, varying from floppy disk to much larger storage media. The author prefers a laptop computer with a CD-recordable removable drive, as 700MB of data can be backed up on a single disk and it is an extremely stable medium. The portability is also paramount as one can backup on the road (Figure 27.8). The author has about 5000 images on his computer and it currently requires two CD-recordable drives to back up these files. Digital versatile disk

(DVD) recordable units are commercially available but are, at the time of publication, very pricey. As this technology improves and becomes more affordable it will become mainstream in the end-user arena. A single DVD can store 7GB of data.

Zip drives are also very popular for backing up data; they are cheaper than CD recordable medium but slower. One advantage is their diminutive size, which allows for great portability.

Another acceptable backup strategy is computer-to-computer data transfer. PC Anywhere™ is a brand name software application that allows the user to access remote computers from any location with a telephone modem service. One can activate PC Anywhere™ from the office computer to the home computer and so can begin downloading images when leaving work; the images will be backed up automatically on the home computer. The problem with this type of transfer is usually speed, as modem transfer is slow. As cable modems and ISDN services become more popular this option will be more appealing. Another advantage of PC Anywhere™ or similar software is that it allows data to be accessed from a remote location. The author was once giving a lecture in Phoenix, AZ, and the night before the lecture realized that one of the presentations about face peels had been forgotten. This was a big lecture and the author was very upset. Luckily, PC Anywhere™ was installed on the notebook computer and allowed connection from the hotel to the office (in Richmond VA), and the forgotten lecture material could be uploaded. It was that day that the author realized the true power of digital imaging. The newer Windows operating system will have remote access capability as a function.

Again, whatever the interface, plan to backup often, as it is guaranteed that at some time one will be faced with data loss or corruption.

IMAGING SOFTWARE

The entire advantage of digital photography is having the ability to instantly process an image and have total control over the editing of that image. Imaging software has become very sophisticated during the past decade. Imaging software has gone from $20,000–30,000 systems to systems that are < $1000

today. In examining imaging systems it is important to compare like with like. Some very high-priced systems cannot outperform lower priced systems and some low-priced systems have very limited imaging functions. It is important to know what to look for when purchasing imaging software. Some of the most important features are considered below.

Archiving software

The primary function of any imaging software is to make it quick and easy to download images from a digital camera. This should be through a fast interface such as a USB port or a PCMCIA card; slower interfaces such as serial cables should be avoided. The archiving software should allow the images to be read instantaneously as a separate computer drive. Archiving software should also allow real-time image transfer between folders on the hard drive – an image is of no use if it cannot be found. Good archiving software should allow all image files to be viewed as thumbnail images, so that it is known what the image is and where it is. More sophisticated archiving software systems will also allow basic image editing directly through the archiving software. Simple image manipulation such as rotation, brightness and contrast, and cropping, may be performed directly through the archiving application. The archiving software should allow image properties such as extension format, size, and date taken, to be viewed. Advanced archiving software also allows for 'drag-and-drop' transfer of images between applications. This allows the user to simply move an image from any folder and drop it into a word-processing document or a PowerPoint presentation.

Image editing software

The true workhorse of any imaging system is the image editing capability. Powerful image editors allow professional image manipulation in a user-friendly interface. The image editor is used to perform a multitude of important imaging functions such as image resizing, duplication, cropping, cutting, copying, pasting, enhancing brightness and contrast, hue and saturation, color balance, adding text and arrows, making before and after pictures, adding special effects, retouching and image print management.

Morphing

Morphing is the ability to change a digital image to simulate a given surgical result. Morphing is commonly used to illustrate augmentation, reduction, rhytid and scar effacement, suspension and lifting techniques, anatomical rotation, and other predictive illustrations (Figure 27.9). Image morphing is very interesting as many patients may wish to have some idea of what to expect from a surgical procedure, although it can be a double-edged sword, as a patient may be very disturbed if their surgical result is not as was graphically predicted. A good general rule is to 'not let your mouse write a check that your scalpel can't cash'! All patients should be advised in writing that these 'computer cartoons' are merely estimations and that no result is implied. The author is familiar with at least one case of litigation involving an implied result of predictive morphing. Morphing software varies and some companies offer very complex morphing. It is the author's experience, after being heavily involved in the imaging industry for a decade, that many doctors buy imaging systems for the 'bells and whistles', including morphing. They initially morph everything on everybody but this novelty soon wears off. If the remainder of the system is weak then they are left dissatisfied. The moral is not to purchase an imaging system for the 'bells and whistles' but to look at the total package. In addition, some morphing applications are, in the author's opinion, unnecessary. Some companies offer morphing software to illustrate post-laser erythema by overlying the face with red tones, but it would be more realistic simply to show the prospective patient actual post-laser pictures of laser patients. The author has a computer slide show that shows the post-laser erythema from 24 hours to 30 days postoperatively. The author also shies away from complex and frequent morphing for most surgical procedures and instead shows the patient digital slide shows of actual before and after surgery that he has performed. This not only gives a realistic idea of what can be accomplished but also shows the author's proficiency as a surgeon. The author feels that there is a place for clinical morphing, but it is not as popular as it was a decade ago and it is no longer a novelty or a sign of advanced technology, as it is available for free as shareware and on children's software.

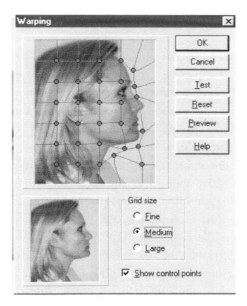

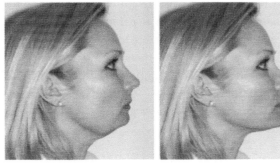

Figure 27.9 *An example of image morphing, which has become very popular for demonstrating presurgical computerized predictions of outcome.*

Presentation software

Merely having images does little; making images work does more. With the sophistication of quality imaging software, it is easy to make digital presentations, slide shows, patient education programs, and before and after pictures, add images to referral letters and pamphlets, and perform a multitude of desktop publishing applications. Computer digital presentations using Microsoft PowerPoint™ and other programs are becoming the standard for most professions. The advantages over carrousel slide presentations are obvious. Some imaging systems offer standalone presentation programs that allow the user to make sophisticated multimedia presentations simply by clicking on the images they wish to include. In the author's practice, digital-image presentation shows for the major procedures performed have been made. If a patient presents for a laser resurfacing consultation, they are taken to the consultation room, handed a mouse and can then proceed through a multimedia presentation at their own pace. This presentation shows the causes of the pathology, the actual procedure (with a full-motion video), the postoperative appearance and care, the various phases of healing, multiple pre- and postoperative cases, and a discussion of complications. When the consultant re-enters the room, say 10 minutes later, the patient has a good idea of what resurfacing consists of and the personal consultation time is decreased. More importantly, the patient has a much clearer idea of what to expect and what not to expect. This is some of the most important time spent with the patient. If the patient desires, they are presented with a CD of the presentation to show their friends or spouse. In the reception room a continuously looping digital presentation of the causes of facial aging and the various cosmetic procedures available is played.

Databasing software

The more advanced imaging systems offer front- and back-end databases that enable the user to add fields to each image, and then have the ability to search for these fields. For instance, a doctor may have an image and attach fields for the patient name, referring doctor, insurance company, procedure, date, complication, place of service, etc. If the surgeon wants to perform a search for all patients treated over a given period who were, for example, Asian females with breast augmentation who experienced capsular contraction with a specific implant, this can be done with several mouse clicks. The problem with databases is that one must enter all the data for each image, which is very time consuming. This is beyond the desires of most clinicians, but those involved in research or specific projects will appreciate this ability.

There are a multitude of other functions that are offered by imaging companies but the aforementioned applications are the most important ones.

MAKING DIGITAL IMAGES

Many problems that existed with conventional film and slide photography have been eliminated with digital photography. The frustration of taking pictures and getting them back from the processor a week later and having important images out of focus, patients with their eyes closed or improperly exposed images was known to all clinicians. There is no need to take a poor image with today's digital camera. The ability to preview all images will allow the doctor to simply retake an improper image.

Standardization is by far the most important single factor in making clinical images. Standardization has been greatly improved by digital technology, in that one can post-process images to adjust for some parameters that were not standardized at the time the image was taken.

Image standardization should be the main goal of every clinician, as it is much simpler to take controlled images rather than to spend time editing each image. The following represents some of the more important factors in image standardization.

Background

Background is perhaps the most important variable when taking consistent images. It is unfortunate that some doctors do not pay attention to backgrounds, producing images showing office equipment or doors as the unfocused background. The author uses a white flat-finish, non-reflective wall as a photographic background. White is preferred because if printing out images a color or black background wastes ink or toner. Shadow control is the biggest problem with light colored backgrounds, which can be corrected by various means. Slave or background bounce flashes are techniques utilized by professional photographers. Simply rotating the digital camera to the vertical position can control the angle at which the flash approaches the image. The author rotates the camera vertically when taking profile images so that the flash presents in a direction so as not to cast a shadow from the nose and chin (Figure 27.10). If the author is photographing a right profile, the camera is held vertically to the right so the flash is directed towards the patient's anterior profile. Another trick that may prove handy is not to use any flash. The more expen-

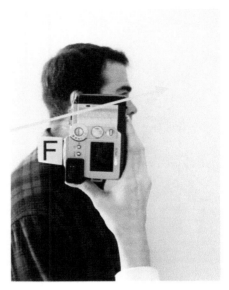 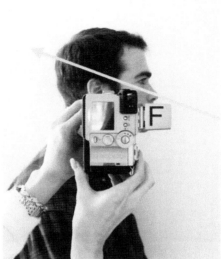

Figure 27.10 Although ring-, point-, slave- and background-synchronized flashes are available, simply positioning the camera to control the flash angle can eliminate shadows. When taking a profile image, having the flash horizontal, or coming in from the back of the head (left frame), will cause a shadow; simply rotating the camera, so that the flash comes in towards the patient's profile, will prevent shadowing.

sive digital cameras have excellent exposure capabilities and, providing the room lighting is sufficient, may not need any flash to expose the image. In the case of no flash, there is no shadow.

Focal distance

The distance from the camera to the subject should be the same for all images. This can be controlled by marking a place on the floor for the photographer to stand. Another means is to attach a piece of string to the end of the camera and always hold that string the same distance from the subject.

Ambient lighting

Ambient room lighting can severely influence the quality of any photograph. There are significant color differences between incandescent and fluorescent lighting and compensations must be made. The reflections from surrounding walls, furnishings and clothing may also influence the color and quality of the image. Although an advantage of digital photography is portability, it is convenient to do most photography in one room that has been set up for color and light standardization. Most high-quality digital cameras offer a vast array of exposure and ISO settings that can compensate for photographic

variables. The trick is to experiment until an acceptable control is achieved, and then maintain that variable control for all images. When attending meetings, many participants judge the competency of a presenter by the quality of his or her images.

WHAT DOES THE FUTURE HOLD?

Digital photography, although still in its infancy, has progressed exponentially in less than a decade from a novelty to the touchstone of clinical record keeping. This technology will continue to improve and one of the drawbacks about keeping up is the rapid obsolescence of current technology. The good news is that the computer will enhance our professional lives, including photographic records.

A big question in everyone's mind is how will digital images be standardized? In order for them to stand as medical records, an unalterable and secure format is required. Attempts to find an image-protection standard have begun, as many see the necessity for unalterable images. Also important is a universal standard for all machines and devices to be able to recognize shared data. Digital imaging and communications in medicine (DICOM) is a format being phased in at medical centers and hospitals, and its eventual penetration into all health-care services is

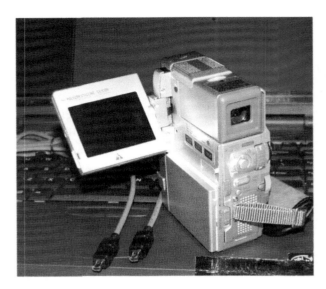

Figure 27.11 Affordable digital camcorders and new technologies enable the use of full-motion video in clinical and academic applications.

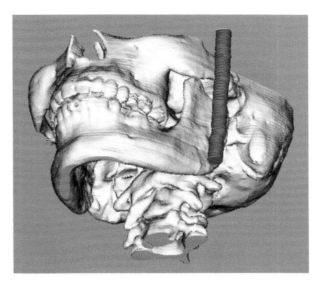

Figure 27.12 A spiral or 3D computerized tomography scan of the skull. This technology has existed for over a decade and is valuable for diagnostic purposes as well as CAD–CAM implant construction.

likely. The DICOM standard is being developed so that one vendor's product can communicate with another vendor's devices. The DICOM system also uses a modular tagged-file format, which allows the storage of vital medico-legal and diagnostic information relating to that specific image. This information is referred to as unique identifier (UID). The information can include a record of the patient visit, the patient's vital statistics, detailed information on how the image was made, what device was used to make the image, the patient's personal information and reams of other information.

Full-motion video is more powerful than still images because it allows procedures to be illustrated in real time, with narration. Digital camcorders are now available with the qualities and capabilities to transfer full-motion video to computer presentations. The main limitation is the intensive memory required. As more powerful compression schemes continue to develop, academic medicine will be enhanced by the ability to add full-motion video to presentations (Figure 27.11).

Three-dimensional applications are being developed, which allow the clinician to view the patient in this mode, with the ability to rotate the virtual patient in space. Although this technology has existed

in radiology in terms of scan reconstruction (Figure 27.12), the ability to perform this with photographic methods is in its infancy. At present this requires expensive and cumbersome hardware, but will soon become the standard and two-dimensional images will probably fade away with BetaMax VCR and eight-track tapes.

The Minolta Corporation (www.minolta.com) currently has the only portable three-dimensional digitizer; the Vivid 700 digitizer is about the size of a small portable TV. This device uses a projected laser stripe to scan an object. The object may be placed on a rotating turntable to be scanned over all surfaces. When this is done, the object can be rotated in all planes on the computer for viewing. GTI Technologies (www.genextech.com) markets a portable three-dimensional clinical camera apparatus. The x,y,z-coordinates for all visible points on the surface object can be provided by a single three-dimensional image (Figure 27.13).

When scanning a face, for example, the laser beam scans all of the facial contours and the computer software triangulates the position of the anatomy relative to the viewpoint of the observer. It then allows the user to view the three-dimensional image on a computer with the ability to rotate the

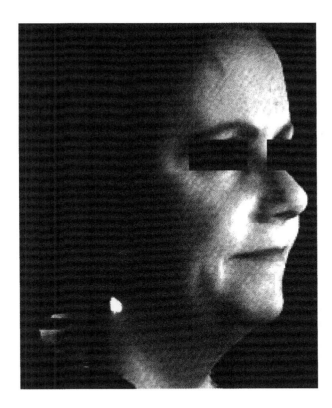

Figure 27.13 Although in its infancy, three-dimensional photography is evolving as a readily available clinical tool. The next decade will surely refine the ability to view images in all dimensions.

face through texture grids. This exciting technology will become more advanced and popular in the years to come.

The internet has affected our personal and professional lives. Telemedicine is also rapidly developing and will enable the remote diagnosis and treatment of patients, with the ability to transfer data around the world in seconds. Virtual surgery, where a surgeon at one location performs robotic surgery at a remote location, is no longer in the realm of science fiction – serious research is occurring in this arena.

Further reading

1. Delange GS, Diana M. 35-mm film vs. digital photography for patient documentation: is it time to change? Ann Plast Surg 1999;42:15; Discussion, Ann Plast Surg 1999;42:20.

2. DiBernardo BF, Adams RL, Krause J, Fiorillo MA, Gheradini G. Photographic standards in plastic surgery. Plast Reconstr Surg 1998;102:559.

3. DiSaia JP, Ptak JJ, Achauer BM. Digital photography for the plastic surgeon. Plast Reconstr Surg 1998;102:569.

4. Guy C, Guy RJ, Zook EG. Standards of photography (Discussion). Plast Reconstr Surg 1984;74:1–15.

5. Jemec BIE, Jemec GB. Photographic surgery: standards in clinical photography. Aesthetic Plast Surg 1986;10:177.

6. Morello DC, Converse JM, Allen D. Making uniform photographic records in plastic surgery. Plast Reconstr Surg 1977;59:366.

7. Nechala P, Mahoney J, Farkas LG. Digital two-dimensional photogrammetry: a comparison of three techniques of obtaining digital photographs. Plast Reconstr Surg 1999;103:1819.

8. Price MA, Goldstein GD. The use of a digital imaging system in a dermatologic surgery practice. Dermatol Surg 1997;23:31.

9. Roth AC, Reid JC, Puckett CL, Concannon MJ. Digital images in the diagnosis of wound healing problems. Plast Reconstr Surg 1999;103:483.

10. Schwartz MS, Tardy ME Jr. Standardized photodocumentation in facial plastic surgery. Facial Plast Surg 1990;7:1.

11. Zarem HA. Standards of photography. Plast Reconstr Surg 1984;74:137.

28. When and how to combine treatments

Nicholas J Lowe

This chapter will provide some guidelines on how to combine some of the available treatments. It is obviously impossible to generalize about ideal treatment combinations, as clearly every patient must be viewed individually. I have attempted in this chapter to help the reader see where and how the different treatments may be combined.

Example

Botulinum toxin plus fillers

Some patients with deep glabellar lines will still have their glabellar lines at rest after initial treatments with botulinum A toxin (BTX-A): repeat treatments are often required to achieve their eradication. In these patients, an ideal combination is to treat with BTX-A and, at the same session, a thin dermal filler such as Zyderm I (in the USA) or Fine Restylane (in Europe). This combination usually leads to an almost complete improvement of the deep lines, and the use of BTX-A gives a greater persistence of the filler.

An example of appropriate filler monotherapy would be the younger patient with atrophic lips who would benefit from only dermal filler for lip enhancement. The present author's current favourite temporary filler for lip enhancement is Perlane (see Chapter 16): it has the advantages of low risk of allergic reactions, probably < 0.1–0.2% in products since 1999.

Conversely, in the older patient who has atrophic lips plus rhytides, often due to significant lip puckering, the use of BTX-A for the upper and lower lip rhytides

injected into the obicularis oris muscle plus a longer-lasting dermal filler (e.g. Perlane) will lead to an enhanced effect and greater persistence of the filler.

Example

Lasers and combination treatments

Other patients will benefit from combinations of a variety of different lasers, e.g. the patient with skin phototype I or II and facial telangiectasia plus photodamage and lines (see Chapters 9–11). These patients often benefit from the use of a vascular specific laser (see Chapter 9) together with a skin-resurfacing laser (see Chapter 11). In addition, they may benefit from treatment with BTX-A to the crow's-feet (see Chapter 14) and forehead areas to reduce the repetitive lines, therefore enabling good collagen remodelling to occur following the laser treatment.

Non-ablative laser systems can be used successfully in combination with BTX-A in the perioral and periorbital regions, and with appropriate fillers in the glabellar, perioral and nasolabial lines. These lasers may also be combined with treatment to improve skin surface damage, e.g. glycolic acid peels, microdermabrasion plus, of course, topical retinoids and photoprotection.

Combination treatments are also extremely effective when dealing with patients who have atrophic, sunken, facial scars that are contributing to the appearance of facial skin ageing. Using only a resurfacing laser in these circumstances gives just a modest improvement. However, using a combination of scar subcision and fat transfer injections, followed by laser skin resurfacing, a greatly improved result is possible.

Example

Combined therapy for neck rejuvenation

Neck rejuvenation is an area that frequently lends itself to combination treatments. If there is significant platysmal banding then use of BTX-A is recommended; if there is poikiloderma then the use of one of the larger spot, longer pulsed vascular-specific lasers, e.g. the Sclerolaser Plus or V.Beam lasers (see Chapter 9), or non-ablative photorejuvenation (see Chapter 12) would be appropriate combinations.

If photodamage is present with skin surface problems and collagen degeneration, then a combination of chemical peels, particularly Jessner's solution plus trichloroacetic acid (TCA), together with non-ablative laser systems, such as the CoolTouch laser, is useful.

It is essential to ensure that patients being treated for facial and neck photodamage are encouraged to use more or less daily broad-spectrum sunscreen coverage. Chapter 2 details the different aspects of sunscreen use.

The concomitant use of rejuvenating topical agents, such as topical retinoids (see Chapters 3 and 4), on a routine daily or nightly basis will provide the patient with a means of reducing recurring photodamage and ageing changes following successful treatment.

There are numerous minimally invasive or non-invasive procedures that can be offered to patients who wish to undergo improvement of the ageing face and neck. Many of these treatments can be used very successfully in combination, giving an enhanced result compared to any of the treatments used alone.

The art is in the careful evaluation of patients, identification of the areas that will be responsive to the use of these treatments, and the orderly sequence and combination of these various treatments.

CHOICES OF TREATMENT IN DIFFERENT PRESENTATIONS – MILD FACIAL AGEING

Choices – upper facial region

- Fine lines: Are the lines dynamic? – consider BTX for glabellar, forehead and periorbital regions;
- Are there lines at rest? – consider temporary fillers, e.g. Zyderm I, Fine Restylane or Fine Hylaform;

- Are there lines with lines at rest and frown. – inject BTX followed immediately by temporary fillers, e.g. Zyderm I or Fine Restylane (see Chapters 13, 14, 15, 16, 17).

Moderate to severe facial ageing

All of the above options plus laser resurfacing and combination chemical peels, e.g. glycolic acid, TCA, Jessner's solution. Chapters 6, 7.

AN EXAMPLE FOR COMBINATION THERAPY *(see Fig. 28.1)*

Superficial photodamage, telangiectasia, deep glabellar lines, brow and upper lid depression.

POSSIBLE COMBINATIONS

- Botox – Corrugator and Procerus
- Pulsed dye laser, Non ablative laser

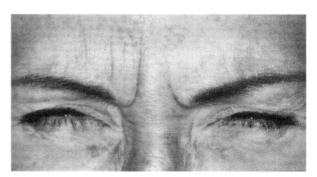

a

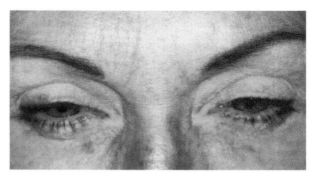

b

Figure 28.1 *(a) Severe glabellar lines, and frown and lid depression; (b) the same patient following treatment and now using tretinoin and glycolic acid creams nightly plus daily broad spectrum sunscreens.*

- Topical retinoids and glycolic acid creams alternate nights
- Daily broad-spectrum sunscreens

PERIORBITAL COMBINATION THERAPY

Botox therapy to the lateral and inferolateral aspects of the periorbital area plus superficial Erbium-YAG laser resurfacing is ideally combined.

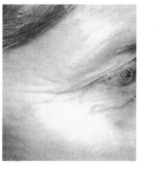
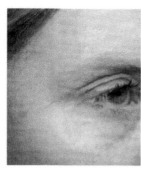

a   b

Figure 28.2 *(a) Before treatment and (b) following BTX therapy plus superficial Er:YAG laser resurfacing.*

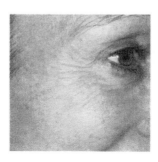
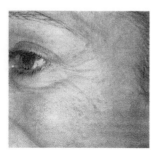

a

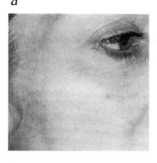
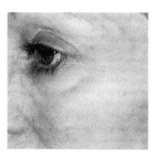

b

Figure 28.3 *(a) and (b) Two views of a patient who was a good candidate for BTX therapy in the periorbital region followed by ultrapulsed CO₂ laser resurfacing.*

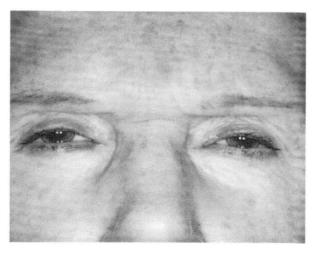

a

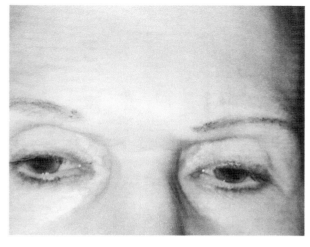

b

Figure 28.4 *Before BTX to procerus and corrugator followed by full face superficial ultrapulsed carbon dioxide laser resurfacing. (See also chapter 14.)*

Choices – central facial region

- Is there good facial structure with moderate to severe nasolabial lines? – consider BTX to zygomatic muscles (small BTX units with EMG control) plus fillers, e.g. Perlane, Hylaform, Zyplast or fat (see Chapters 16, 17, 18);
- Are there atrophic acne scars? – consider scar subcision plus fillers, e.g. Perlane, Hylaform, Zyplast, Artecoll, Dermalive or fat (see Chapters 16, 17, 18), followed by laser skin rejuvenation, either non-ablative, e.g. CoolTouch, or resurfacing, e.g. CO_2 or Er:YAG lasers (see Chapters 10, 11, 12);

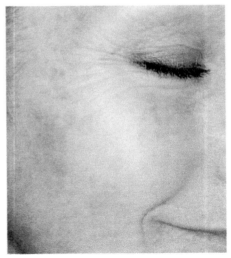
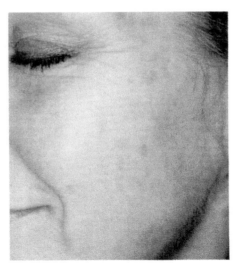

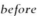
before

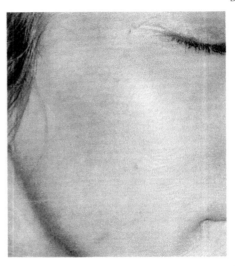
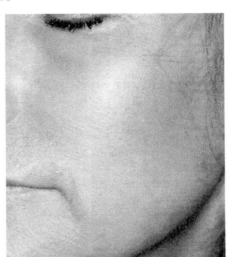

after

Figure 28.5 *Before and after combined Botox® to crows feet, ultrasoft implants to nasolabial folds and fullface ultra-pulsed carbon dioxide laser.*

• Is there severe laxity of skin and underlying structures? – consider facelift surgery then maintenance with minimally invasive options.

Choices – lower facial region (excluding lips)

• Is there good facial structure with fat migration to jowls? – consider lower facial liposuction plus non-ablative or resurfacing lasers (see Chapter 18);

• Are there prominent mesolabial folds and chin dimpling? – consider BTX to mentalis plus fillers, e.g. Perlane or Hylaform, to chin areas (see Chapters 16, 17);

• Are there severe jowls and lower facial sagging? – consider facelift surgery.

Choices – perioral region and lips

• Are there dynamic perioral rhytides? – consider BTX to obicularis oris (see Chapters 13–15);

• Is there significant lip atrophy? – consider longer-lasting dermal fillers, e.g. Perlane, Hylaform or Zyplast (see Chapters 16 and 17) and permanent implants such as Ultrasoft or Goretex (the patient must be aware of the potential need for replacement in up to 15% of implants to the lip) (see Chapters 19 and 20);

• Are there rhytides plus atrophy – consider BTX to obicularis oris, and temporary or permanent fillers/implants followed by laser resurfacing if severe (non-ablative laser if mild rhytides) (see Chapters 12–15).

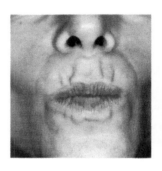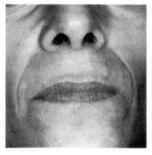

a   *b*

Figure 28.6 (a) and (b) Two views of a patient who would be a good candidate for BTX therapy in the periorbital region followed by laser rejuvenation.

PERIORAL COMBINATION THERAPY

Figure 28.6 shows a good candidate for Botox and fillers to the upper lip and nasolabial folds. Of the longer lasting temporary fillers, I now routinely use Perlane in Europe. This candidate may also be considered for nasolabial SoftForm implants. She is also a good candidate for Botox injections periorbitally and laser skin rejuvenation. She would most benefit from laser skin resurfacing but an option would be non-ablative skin resurfacing.

Choices – neck region

- Is there localized fat deposition under chin? – consider neck liposuction (see Chapter 18);
- Are there prominent neck bands and horizontal crease lines? – consider BTX (see Chapters 14 and 15);
- Is there skin surface ageing, e.g. lentigo, poikiloderma? – use pigment or vascular-specific lasers (see Chapters 8 and 9);
- Is there mild subcutaneous atrophy? – consider non-ablative resurfacing, e.g. CoolTouch (see Chapter 12);
- Is there a combination of the above? – consider BTX, Jessner's solution or TCA peel, plus non-ablative rejuvenation (see Chapters 7, 14, 15);
- Are there severe problems of neck laxity and sagging? – consider neck and facelift surgery.

SUMMARY

The patient examples in this chapter are just some of the ways in which combination therapy can be used. In patients with more severe problems such as brow and eyelid ptosis, endoscopic brow lift and/or blepharoplasty may be offered. The other topical and non-invasive treatments can then be employed to further improve and maintain facial improvement.

Appendix I
The consultation

The consultation for the patient requesting advice on facial rejuvenation is arguably one of the more difficult consultations in facial dermatology. There are some patients whose specific wishes for treatment are immediately and obviously backed up by physical evidence; for example, the patient with clearly defined glabellar lines is a candidate for botulinum toxin therapy; the patient with a comparatively small upper lip is a candidate for lip augmentation with either temporary fillers or a lip implant.

The complexity of the consultation increases when there are multiple facial ageing concerns to be addressed, for example, surface skin photodamage such as lentigo, actinic keratoses and telangiectasia, as well as redistribution of subcutaneous fat and the presence of periorbital ageing changes, for example, lid laxity.

The consultation becomes even more complex when it comes to assessing carefully the patient's (perceived) cosmetic problems. The face that the patient presents to him- or herself in the mirror may be different from the face that they themselves picture in their mind.

Patients with or without psychiatric disorders may have unrealistic expectations and may feel that a cosmetic procedure is therapeutic for underlying depression or lack of success in personal relationships or career.

The patient, therefore, who has unreasonable expectations is to be treated with caution and compassion. These patients will often be unhappy with the outcome of their procedure, regardless of the care that the physician and surgeon take in any procedure and also in the pre-treatment consultation.

We may get certain clues about unrealistic expectations by paying attention to repetitive and detailed questions about perceived problems with the patient's face and potential treatments. The patient may also be very vague about what they are trying to achieve with regard to improvement and may also exhibit an impulsiveness to have the procedures performed immediately or in the very near future. In addition, some patients will frequently have had previous procedures performed and may state dissatisfaction with prior physicians and surgeons. One must, in such cases, be aware that the patient may potentially have unrealistic expectations. In many of these instances, it is often wise for both patient and physician to advise that the patient is best served by not proceeding with a cosmetic procedure.

The next most important aspect of the consultation is to carefully document with clinical notes, drawings and photography the patient's current situation. Some of the more sophisticated Polaroid or digital photographic techniques whereby it is possible to show the patient immediately a photographic image may also assist in explaining realistic problems or lack thereof. Video presentations of the procedure(s) may be valuable for patient instruction. Patients need to be fully educated about treatment options and outcomes and this may require several patient visits.

At the initial consultation, it is essential to provide patients with written information, and a large selection of informed consent forms can be found in Appendix II of this book. The patient should be encouraged to take away and read the available literature and consent form between the first and second consultation and to make notes for the second visit of any questions for the physician. The literature and consent form should always include:

- background to the development of any procedure and rationale for treatment
- the types of patient who may benefit from a particular treatment
- the potential results, both positive and negative
- special risks and complications
- any medication that should be avoided prior to treatment, for example NSAIDs or aspirin

In most cases where photography is to be taken, consent should also be sought for this.

Finally, in view of the fact that cosmetic procedures are by their very nature elective, the patient must be made aware of all the costs they will be incurring for any procedures. The larger the treatment, the more advisable it is for the physician to obtain part-payment on reservation of the procedure(s). The balance of payment should be paid before embarking upon treatment. It may be advisable to dissuade patients from taking loans to pay for cosmetic procedures, as this may mean that either they cannot afford the procedure or may have other more pressing needs for available funds, but this is obviously up to the individual physician and patient. There have been instances of ongoing payments on a loan after treatment leading to resentment on the part of the patient and eventual dissatisfaction with the treatment.

Some of these features are summarized in the box below.

- Get to know the patient as well as possible
- Identify the (perceived) patient problem(s)
- Find out what prior procedures, if any, the patient has undergone
- What was the perception of the outcome of any prior procedures? Beware the patient unduly critical of past treatment outcomes
- What previous complications, if any, has the patient suffered?
- Explore the general medical, dermatological and, most importantly, medical history.
- What medication is the patient taking (or has taken in the past)?
- If the patient has minimal or no identifiable problem, consider suggesting counselling and strongly advise against the requested procedure.

SUMMARY

The consultation is the single most important aspect of a successful outcome to patient care in facial rejuvenation.

Appendix II
Patient information and consent forms
Pamela S Lowe, Philippa Lowe, Nicholas J Lowe

What follow are some examples of patient information and consent documents provided for my patients. These forms are always given or sent to the patient before any procedure is performed. Comprehensive information and costs of the planned treatments ensure that the patient has the full information necessary to make an informed choice about the procedures and whether to proceed.

These examples have been modified from my clinics in Santa Monica, California, and London, UK. I encourage my patients to read fully, make notes, compile questions and concerns about all the planned treatments. These can be addressed by myself or my staff at any pretreatment visit. Other practitioners will use other treatment options and will need different information and consent forms. In some countries, such consent forms may not be required to be as comprehensive as those shown here. In my opinion, nothing can help more to prepare the patient for a procedure than to be fully informed about the risks and benefits of that procedure.

All consent forms and information given here are copyright of Nicholas J Lowe.

A   Dye laser therapy of vascular skin lesions (spider veins, leg veins, vascular birthmarks, red and keloid scars)

Please read these instructions carefully and make notes on THIS sheet if you have any questions during your consultation.

You have a right to be informed about your skin condition and treatment so that you may make a decision whether or not to undergo this procedure after knowing the risks and hazards involved. This disclosure is not meant to alarm or scare; it is simply an effort to better inform you so that you may give or withhold your consent for the treatment.

Although this procedure is effective in most cases, no guarantee can be made that a specific patient will benefit from treatment.

Spider veins

Spider veins are prominent and dilated (widened) blood vessels that are frequently present on the face and neck, as well as the legs.

Treatment for spider hemangiomatas, spider veins or telangiectasia

These blood vessels frequently increase with age and a variety of treatments have been attempted, including the use of cauterization and injections of sclerosing solutions into the vessels, as well as the use of different forms of lasers.

Port wine stain or hemangioma?

A port wine stain or hemangioma is an abnormal collection or network of blood vessels present beneath a layer of otherwise normal skin. Port wine hemangiomas are present on the skin at birth and appear to grow at the same rate as the surrounding tissue.

What are the limitations of laser treatment?

It is important to realize that the laser may not completely eliminate the problem. Sometimes the laser may only cause a lightening of the area. Although extremely rare with this laser, the possibility of scarring does exist.

Finally, there is no way of predicting what long-term, undesirable, or unusual side-effects may occur as a result of laser light treatments. Every new treatment method raises the possibility that unsuspected effects may be created that will not become evident for many years following treatment. One should realize, however, that many types of lasers have been used in medicine for over 20 years, and thus far there is no evidence of unsuspected side-effects; this finding does not guarantee that they will not occur or be discovered at some time in the distant future. Some treated lesions will return years after treatment.

Costs of treatment and insurance coverage

There is no guarantee that medical insurance will cover the costs of laser treatments. Some insurance companies consider the treatment purely cosmetic. Each patient should check with the insurance carrier to determine whether treatments will be covered, especially with spider veins and leg veins.

How does the vascular laser work?

The dye laser generates a very powerful light that is yellow in color. When this light contacts the skin, the red color of the blood vessels absorbs the light, which then releases its energy as heat. The heat coagulates and reduces the small vessels under the skin. In theory, the overlying skin is not affected by this laser. However, some of the laser energy is absorbed by the outer layer of the skin (epidermis), which may result in temporary scale, crust and pigmentation. This is reduced by the skin cooling device.

What will the laser treatment feel like?

The vascular laser produces much less pain or discomfort than a needle or electrolysis lasers. However, there is a small amount of discomfort that does result from this treatment. This has been likened to the snapping of an elastic band against the skin.

A test site (small skin area) may be performed to determine the correct energy settings for each patient. The doctor will decide if this is necessary.

What else should I tell the doctor?

If you are prone to skin infections such as herpes simplex (cold sores) or impetigo (bacterial infections), tell our doctors who will prescribe a medicine for you.

PATIENTS MUST HAVE STOPPED TAKING ROACCUTANE FOR 12 MONTHS BEFORE ANY LASER TREATMENT TO THE FACE. You must tell the doctor about ALL your medicines.

What is the sequence of healing after a laser treatment?

An immediate effect of the laser treatment is that tiny blood vessels under the skin are coagulated, causing the area to turn a much darker colour. This can be disguised somewhat by using a camouflage make-up, e.g. Dermablend, Clinique Continuous Coverage. Your local pharmacy or department store may assist you prior to your treatment. Draw a red or purple biro mark on your hand and practise to determine which camouflage make-up covers the area best. Scaling, scabs, or crusts may form but can be helped by the liberal use of moisturizing cream or antibiotic ointment especially at nighttime to prevent the scab from drying out. These changes usually persist for approximately 1–2 weeks. You should attempt to keep the area as clean as possible. The scab or crust must not be picked or scratched as this may increase the chance of scarring or permanent pigment change. Do not use a cover make up until the crusts have healed.

Some patients treated over the cheek area may develop temporary swelling of the cheek and lower eye area lasting 3–4 days. This may be reduced by sleeping with extra pillows and applying ice or taking Arnica tablets for 4 days before and 4 days after treatment.

When will I see an improvement?

Initial post treatment redness should fade in 1–2 weeks. The maximum benefit from the treatment is seen after 12 weeks. This laser should not result in scarring, but some patients get increased or decreased pigment (skin colour) for several weeks or months. Rare cases of pigment changes have lasted up to 2 years. Extremely rare cases of permanent pigment change have been reported.

PATIENT POST-OP INSTRUCTIONS

What to avoid and for how long
Vigorous washing and drying to the area for 10 days. Picking and rubbing the skin for 10 days.

What to avoid doing and for how long
No restrictions on activities such as walking or exercise.

How to sleep
No sleeping pills required, no painkillers required. Sleep on your back with extra pillows to reduce swelling of the eyelids if the cheek has been treated.

What to take and for how long
Pain medications usually not required.

If you have a history of cold sores or fever blisters in the treated area, an oral anti-herpes medicine may be prescribed.

What to drink and eat
No limitations.

What to use and when
Use the ointment provided by the clinic (or Vaseline) 2–3 times a day, especially last thing at night on the treated skin until the discoloration disappears – usually for the first 7 days or until crusting, if any, disappears. No dressings are needed.

When to resume active skin care regimen
Retin A, alpha hydroxy acid creams after 30 days. Sunscreens immediately. Cosmetic camouflage make-up, e.g. Derma-blend can be used immediately if desired, unless there is crusting.

When to shower, bathe, wash, brush, comb, colour, perm hair
No restrictions, except to dry skin gently.

How to recognize when you need to call the doctor's office
If there is any sign of infection (pus, spots or crusting) or delayed healing.

What can be expected post-operatively
Some discoloration that will range from red to purple for up to 7 days, giving a bruising appearance. Swelling of treated area and the lower eyelids if the cheeks have been treated.

When can sun exposure resume
Do not sunbathe for at least 14 days. Always use SPF 15–30 sunscreen which must be started immediately after the laser especially if you are exposed to bright sunlight otherwise the treated area may become darker.

Date and time of first office visit
Clinic visits will be discussed at the time of treatment.

If there are any questions you may call the office XXX XXXX XXX during normal business hours. After hours the emergency page number is: XXX XXXX XXX

B Laser therapy for pigmented lesions and tattoos with Ruby and Alexandrite lasers (see Chapter 8)

Please read these instructions carefully and make notes on THIS sheet if you have any questions during your consultation.

You have a right to be informed about your skin condition and treatment so that you may make a decision whether or not to undergo this procedure after knowing the risks and hazards involved. This disclosure is not meant to alarm or scare; it is simply an effort to better inform you so that you may give or withhold your consent for the treatment.

Although laser surgery is effective in most cases, no guarantee can be made that a specific patient will benefit from treatment.

Introduction

Selected lasers allow safe and effective treatment for tattoos, brown birthmarks, age or (liver) spots, freckles, naevus of Ota and other benign pigmented skin lesions. The Ruby and Alexandrite lasers allow selective treatment of the melanosomes of a benign lesion, while leaving surrounding tissue relatively unharmed. The laser is more effective in treating pigmented lesions, such as age spots, than freezing (cryotherapy).

Some conditions such as melasma also known as 'mask of pregnancy' (brown, dark patches on the face in women, usually from pregnancy or contraceptive pills plus sunlight) can show unpredictable responses with any treatments including the laser. There may sometimes be a further darkening or patchy irregular lightening of the skin following laser treatment.

Questions and answers

Q. What is a benign pigmented lesion?

A. Benign pigmented lesions are caused by an excess of pigment in the skin, usually due to ultraviolet light exposure and congenital factors. In the skin there are melanin producing cells (melanocytes). An abnormal increase in either the melanosomes or melanocytes results in pigmented lesions.

Q. What is the pigmented lesion laser?

A. Ruby and Alexandrite lasers produce an intense burst of laser light that is especially optimized to treat pigmented lesions. The system's unique combination of parameters creates a thermal effect, called photothermolysis, on the excess pigment in the epidermis or dermis. The wavelengths (694 nm and 755 nm) of the lasers are optimized to be absorbed by pigment while minimally affecting the surrounding healthy tissue.

Q. What pigmented conditions are treated with this laser?

A. The most commonly treated conditions are solar lentigines, also known as 'age spots' or 'liver spots', café au lait birthmarks, freckles and naevus of Ota. What all these lesions have in common is that they are made of an over-abundance of pigment in the skin. They vary, however, in appearance. Age spots may appear as enlarged dark freckles on the face and hands. Café au lait birthmarks may appear as light-brown markings anywhere on the body and can be quite large; they are more difficult to treat and may not improve. Freckles can also be treated, if desired. Any questionable moles and brown or black skin marks or lumps require biopsy to verify that they are benign.

Q. Why should someone have a pigmented lesion treated?

A. Many people are uncomfortable with unsightly-pigmented lesions. Young adults may be embarrassed by 'age spots' and the lesions may affect their self-confidence. Young children or infants may suffer psychologically from teasing and discrimination by other children often associated with café au lait birthmarks.

Q. What does the treatment involve?

A. Treatment with the laser varies from patient to patient, depending on the type of lesion, size of the affected area, colour of the patient's skin and depth to which the abnormal pigment extends beneath the skin's surface.

If you are having your eye area treated you will be given eye protectors. Anaesthetic drops will be used prior to insertion.

The skin's reaction to the laser is usually tested during the first visit to determine the most effective treatment.

Q. Is treatment with the laser painful?

A. The laser is more comfortable and requires less recovery time than some other treatment methods, e.g. cryotherapy. As many patients describe it, each pulse feels, for a fraction of a second, like the snapping of a rubber band against the skin. Depending on the nature of the lesion and size, the physician may elect to use a local anaesthesia cream.

Q. How many treatments are necessary?

A. The number of treatments necessary is highly variable; it is difficult to predict this number in advance. Some lesions may take several treatment sessions to achieve maximum improvement. Lesions such as amateur tattoos may require 4–8 sessions. Professional tattoos may require 6–12 sessions. Some tattoos such as multi-colored ones may not clear completely.

Some lesions, such as lentigines, will require only a few pulses, while others, such as café au lait birthmarks, will require many more. Other lesions will require retreatment, necessitating multiple patient visits. Melasma may not respond at all or darken further.

What else should I tell the doctor?

If you are prone to skin infections like herpes simplex (cold sores) or impetigo (bacterial infections) tell our staff as we will prescribe a medicine for you.

Patients must have stopped taking Roaccutane for 12 months before having any laser on the face.

What is the sequence of healing after a laser treatment for tattoos?

The area will bleed slightly then crust, scab and heal to a lighter colour fading gradually over 2–6 months.

What is the sequence of healing after a laser treatment for solar lentigo?

Immediately after treatment will turn a lighter grey followed by slight scaling and reddening. It will then become darker, gradually fading to a lighter colour over 1–3 months.

Can I use make-up on the treated area?

Camouflage make-up, e.g. Dermablend, Clinique Continuous Coverage, can be used providing there is no scabbing.

LASER THERAPY FOR PIGMENTED LESIONS (ALEXANDRITE & RUBY)

Patient post-op instructions

What to avoid and for how long?
Vigorous washing and drying to the area for 10 days. Rubbing the skin for 10 days.

What to avoid doing and for how long?
No restrictions on exercise.

How to sleep?
No sleeping pills required, no painkillers required.

What to take and for how long?
Pain medications usually not required.

If you have a history of cold sores or fever blisters in the treated area, an oral anti-herpes medicine may be prescribed.

What to drink and eat
No limitations.

What is the sequence of healing?
Lesions will turn red, then a grey to dark brown colour with mild scaling. Face lesions usually heal in 3–7 days, hand and leg lesions take longer – up to 14 days.

What to use and when
Use the ointment suggested by the Clinic such as Polysporin (or a prescribed antibiotic Rx) 2–3 times a day, especially last thing at night on the treated skin until the discolouration disappears – usually for the first 7 days or until crusting, if any, disappears. No dressings are needed.

When to resume active skin care regimen
Retin A, alpha hydroxy acid creams after 10 days. Sunscreens immediately. Cosmetic camouflage make-up e.g. Derma-blend can be used immediately if desired, unless there is crusting.

When to shower, bathe, wash, brush, comb, colour, perm hair
No restrictions.

How to recognize when you need to call the doctor's office
If there is any sign of infection or delayed healing.

What can be expected post-operatively?
Some discoloration that will range from red to brown scaling for between three to 14 days.

When can sun exposure resume?
Do not sunbathe for at least 14 days. Always use SPF 15–30 sunscreen which must be started immediately after the laser especially if you are exposed to bright sunlight otherwise the treated area may become darker.

Date and time of first post surgery visit
Clinic visits will be discussed at the time of treatment

RUBY LASER FOR TATTOO REMOVAL

Patient post-op instructions

What to avoid and for how long?
Vigorous washing and drying to the area for 10 days. Rubbing the skin for 10 days.

What to avoid doing and for how long?
No restrictions.

How to sleep
No sleeping pills required, no painkillers required.

What to take and for how long
Pain medications usually not required.

   If you have a history of cold sores or fever blisters in the treated area an oral anti herpes medicine may be prescribed.

What to drink and eat
No limitations.

What is the sequence of healing after a laser treatment for tattoos
The area will bleed slightly then crust, scab and heal to a lighter colour fading gradually over 2–6 months.

What to use and when
Use the ointment advised by the Clinic (or Vaseline) until crusting, if any, disappears. Keep the area covered for 3 days. Change dressing after a shower or bath.

When to resume active skin care regimen
Retin A, alpha hydroxy acid creams after 10 days. Sunscreens once crusting has gone. Cosmetic camouflage make-up e.g. Derma-blend can be used immediately if desired, unless there is crusting.

When to shower, bathe, wash, brush, comb, colour, perm hair
No restrictions.

How to recognize when you need to call the doctor's office
If there is any sign of infection or delayed healing.

When can sun exposure resume
Do not sunbathe for at least 14 days. Always use SPF 15–30 sunscreen, which must be started immediately after the laser especially if you are exposed to bright sunlight, otherwise the treated area may become darker.

First office visit after laser
Clinic visits will be discussed at the time of treatment.

If there are any questions you may call the office XXX XXXX XXX during normal business hours. After hours the emergency page number is: XXX XXXX XXX

C Laser hair removal (see Chapter 22)

Please read these instructions carefully and make notes on THIS sheet if you have any questions
during your consultation.

You have a right to be informed about your skin condition and treatment so that you may make a
decision whether or not to undergo this procedure after knowing the risks and hazards involved. This
disclosure is not meant to alarm or scare; it is simply an effort to better inform you so that you may give
or withhold your consent for the treatment.

Although laser hair removal is effective in most cases, no guarantee can be made that a specific patient
will benefit from treatment.

Introduction

For many men and women, unwanted hair can be an emotional disfigurement. Getting rid of it can be painful.
Until recently, the only options for removing unwanted hair were unpleasant-smelling hair removal creams,
sharp razors, stinging wax or painful electrolysis needles.

What is the laser hair removal process?

Laser hair removal uses a laser to remove unwanted hair, reducing the need for routine shaving and waxing.
This advanced technology transcends the older, painful hair removal treatments to deliver long-lasting results.
Because the laser treats more than one hair at a time, it is possible to treat larger areas such as the back, shoulders, arms, legs and face.

What are the benefits of laser hair removal?

Larger areas may be treated using lasers than with electrolysis or tweezing.

It combines the speed of shaving with lasting results.

Laser hair removal is effective on almost any area of the body where smoother, hair-free skin is desired.

How many treatments will I need?

The number of treatments you may require for optimal long-term benefits depends on the area you wish to
have treated, your skin type and your hair's growth cycle. We treat until the hair is gone. Several treatments
are often necessary for a significant reduction in hair growth: however, your hair grows in cycles and many
factors influence its growth. Age, ethnicity, weight, hormones, diet, medication and metabolism all play a part
in your hair's location, thickness and resilience.

The laser slows the growing capacity of follicles in the growth cycle at the time of the treatment. Since
some hair follicles may enter their growth cycle after your treatment, many treatments may be required to
deliver optimal results. Treatment results will vary from patient to patient depending on skin and hair color.

N.B.: Removing hair does not make it grow back thicker, darker or quicker. The opposite is usually the
case. Laser treatment should cause the hair to grow back slowly, finer, sparser and lighter in color.

How is laser hair removal different from electrolysis?

Electrolysis is a much slower process. With electrolysis, a needle is actually inserted into each hair follicle one
at a time. Once inserted, an electric current burns the follicle to retard hair growth. Laser hair removal uses
the non-invasive, cool light of the laser to scan the treatment area, and within seconds all the hairs in the laser's
beam are treated. Most patients who have had both procedures say that laser hair removal is less painful, faster,
convenient and more effective.

Can anyone have hair removal?

No, certain skin color and hair colouring do not respond favorably to hair removal using lasers, e.g. skin type
4 (black or very dark brown) often will hypopigment (lighten) following treatment and skin that has tanned
previously may burn. Different lasers can be used in these situations. Very light or red hair may not respond
at all to treatment.

Certain medications that cause sensitivity to light are contraindicated. During the laser treatment it is important you let the laser operator know if you are on *any* medications or herbal remedies such as acne medications, anticancer drugs, antidepressants, antihistamines, anti-inflammatories, antimicrobials, antipsychotic drugs, diuretics, hypoglycemics, herbal/organic or hormonal.

Is this laser safe?

Observations in patients at our research centre and other centres have suggested that this is a safe form of treatment. Side-effects that may occur include temporary redness and scaling around the areas of laser treatment, especially around the hair follicle. Other possible side-effects include decreased or increased pigmentation. These pigment changes may be more noticeable in darker skin and to date have been temporary.

Occasionally the treatment site may burn, causing temporary swelling, blistering and scabbing, particularly if the skin has been tanned recently (within the last 2 months). Changes of skin color from sunlight or tanning beds can alter the amount of potential skin damage from laser.

It is essential that you tell the doctor and/or his staff if you have had any sun exposure or tanning bed exposure since your last treatment with the laser. We can then lower the laser energy or repeat a small test area prior to treatment.

Our current laser has a cooling spray that reduces the heat on the skin surface, so allowing a greater effect on the hair follicles with much less skin surface damage.

What will the laser feel like?

It will feel like an elastic band being snapped against the skin. Local anesthesia cream can be prescribed if wanted but is usually unnecessary.

How will I receive treatment and how often?

Usually you will have a small test area treated and observed for colour change. Following this test, treatment will be determined; however, despite having a test area some patients (especially darker skin types) may still have an adverse reaction after a complete treatment. Most patients require a further treatment between 2–6 weeks depending on the body area and continue with treatments until they have their desired reduction of growth.

We are unaware of any long-term side-effects but every new treatment method raises the possibility that unexpected effects may be created that will not become evident for many years following treatment.

What else should I tell the doctor?

Patients must have stopped taking Roaccutane for 12 months before having any laser on the face.

What are the laser treatments like?

Laser hair removal is a three-step process. The area is cleansed, shaved if necessary and treated with the laser. The laser energy passes through the skin and is absorbed by the pigment in the hair follicle. The darker the skin or hair, the more absorption.

Treatments can last from a few minutes to an hour or more, depending on the size of the area to be treated.

What will I look like after the treatment?

The area treated will look red and possibly feel hot. The hair follicles may also appear swollen. Hydrocortisone cream can be applied to help reduce the redness.

Following treatment

After your treatment, the area is cleansed and you can return to your normal activities immediately. Your physician may recommend that you apply Hydrocortisone cream for a few days. You must use sunscreen if you are to be exposed to the sun and avoid sunbathing, sun exposure and tanning prior to any treatments.

Hirsutism (excessive hair growth): questions and answers

What is hirsutism?
Hirsutism is the increased growth of body hair in areas outside the usual female pattern. The hair type is thick and dark instead of the usual fine body hair. It usually affects the beard area of the face, the chest, stomach, back and thighs.

What causes hirsutism?
It is normal for a woman's body to make male sex hormones (androgens) as well as female sex hormones (estrogens and progestogens). An androgen is a male sex hormone that makes the skin and body hairs grow. If your body makes too much androgen, or if your body hairs are very sensitive to androgens, this may cause more hair to grow on the face and the body (hirsutism).

Hirsutism can also be caused by some medicines. Your doctor can advise you whether any medicines you are taking are likely to make your hirsutism worse.

How many women have hirsutism?
In a study in Great Britain of women aged 18–38, 10 in every 100 had some form of hirsutism.

Does race affect hirsutism?
Women from different races have different amounts of body hair. Also, different cultures have different ideas of what are normal and abnormal amounts of body hair.

Does hair grow faster in the summer?
It is not true that hair grows faster in the summer than in the winter. However, if you have hirsutism, the summer can be a more upsetting time when the skin is less covered by clothing.

How can hirsutism be treated?
Most of the cosmetic treatments for hirsutism are only temporary. Therefore, in more severe cases, treatment with drugs may be necessary. Medical treatment can be with a combined oral contraceptive (contraceptive pill). In a combined oral contraceptive there are two hormones called estrogen and progestogen (female sex hormones). These help by decreasing the amount of androgens that are in the blood and made by the ovaries (female sex organs that produce eggs).

Treatment with an oral contraceptive containing an antiandrogen or with an antiandrogen on its own is also used for hirsutism. An antiandrogen is a type of proestrogen that blocks the effects of androgen hormones. The antiandrogen will attach itself to androgen receptors in the hair follicles (but it does not unlock them), and it blocks the receptors (like the wrong key jammed in a lock), so that the androgens cannot affect the hair.

Drugs called glucocorticoids can also be taken for the treatment of hirsutism. They treat hirsutism by lowering the amounts of a hormone in the blood, which stops the adrenal gland (a gland above the kidney that makes hormones) from making androgens.

When will I notice an improvement in my hirsutism with medical treatment?
To see a definite improvement in your hirsutism you may have to wait a few months, possibly longer.

Can I use a combination of cosmetic and medical treatments?
Cosmetic hair removal may be needed while waiting for the medical treatment to take effect and for hair already grown. The Alexandrite laser hair removal method may complement medical treatment by slowing down the rate of hair growth. There is now a new prescription cream available in the USA that slows the rate of hair growth. This is sometimes advised after laser hair removal.

D　Skin rejuvenation using Cool Touch and Vascular lasers

Please read these instructions carefully and make notes on THIS sheet if you have any questions during your consultation.

You have a right to be informed about your skin condition and treatment so that you may make a decision whether or not to undergo this procedure after knowing the risks and hazards involved. This disclosure is not meant to alarm or scare; it is simply an effort to better inform you so that you may give or withhold your consent for the treatment.

Although this procedure is effective in most cases, no guarantee can be made that a specific patient will benefit from treatment.

Introduction

Two main types of laser are now routinely used to rejuvenate skin by stimulating new collagen formation below the skin surface. The skin surface itself is not damaged.

Cool touch laser

These laser for skin rejuvenation may be useful for some patients who do not wish to have laser resurfacing.

How does it work?

The new Cool Touch laser (1320 nm laser) is designed to be absorbed in the dermis (the supporting deeper layers of the skin).

The outer skin is protected by precision cooling of the skin layers so there is no visible wounding or trauma to the surface.

The laser is absorbed by the connective tissue (collagen and elastic tissue in the dermis), producing new collagen formation, improving the skin appearance and reducing fine lines and wrinkles. In a recent research study a group of patients treated once monthly over a 4-month period of time had visible improvement in the appearance of the lines and wrinkles.

What patients may be treated?

Patients with all skin types may be treated with the Cool Touch laser. Facial skin lines, wrinkles and some acne scars are suitable for treatment.

How many treatments will I need?

We advise a course of four treatments over a 6-month period, at 4–6-weekly intervals and maintenance treatments every 6–12 months.

How long do the benefits last?

In a recent study of patients followed for 6 months after their final treatment the improvement lasted during that time.

Because the laser has not been used for longer than this time period we do not know how long-lasting or permanent these improvements will be. Patients may require further treatment sessions to maintain the initial improvement. It is not, at this time, possible to predict how frequently these re-treatment sessions will be needed, and will vary from patient to patient.

Will I need any pre-treatment with Cool Touch laser?

You will have some anaesthetic cream applied before the treatment. Please arrive 20 minutes before your appointment time for this to be put on.

No other pre-treatment is needed unless you have a history of cold sores (herpes simplex) in the areas to be treated.

What else should I tell the doctor?

If you are prone to skin infections such as herpes simplex (cold sores) or impetigo (bacterial infections) tell our staff and we will prescribe a medicine for you.

What areas can be treated?

Lines around the eyes and mouth, lax skin of the face and neck, certain stretch marks and some types of scarring.

What can I expect to feel during the treatment?

You should feel cool spray and then a stinging sensation. The area may feel hot after treatment for up to 15 minutes.

If you are having your eye area treated you may have to wear eye protectors. Anaesthetic drops will be used prior to insertion.

What will I look like afterwards?

The majority of patients will have temporary (up to 1 hour) skin redness which will fade and can be covered with light make-up.

How long will my appointment be?

From 15 to 30 minutes, depending on the size of the area to be treated.

Can I return to work immediately?

Yes, if you are red this can be covered with make-up.

Will I need further treatment?

You may need future courses of treatment to maintain improvement.

What are the possible complications?

The laser could cause skin blistering particularly over areas where scars are present. Blisters may lead to scarring and changes in skin colour and pigment.

Other long-term side-effects have not been reported but since this is a new form of technology, further research may report more side-effects.

Vascular laser

This type of laser has been available for treatment of spider veins and some birthmarks for over 20 years. It was noticed that the skin quality and structure improved in some patients following the use of this laser on the face and neck for birthmarks and spider veins. Research has also shown skin rejuvenation and new collagen formulation.

This laser for skin rejuvenation may be useful for some patients who do not wish to have laser resurfacing.

How does it work?

The laser is absorbed by the blood vessels under your skin and releases growth factors that stimulate new collagen and elastin formation in your skin.

What patients may be treated?

Patients with lighter skin types and the presence of some pinkness or spider veins on the cheeks or around the eyes.

How many treatments will I need?

We advise a course of four treatments over a 6 month period, at 4–6 weekly intervals and maintenance treatments every 6–12 months.

How long does the treatment last?

We do not know the duration of benefits as yet because the laser has not been used for long time periods for skin aging and we do not know how long-lasting or permanent your improvements will be. Patients may require further treatment sessions to maintain the initial improvement. It is not, at this time, possible to predict how frequently these re-treatment sessions will be needed and will vary from patient to patient.

What else should I tell the doctor?

If you are prong to skin infections such as herpes simplex (cold sores) or impetigo (bacterial infections) tell our staff and we will prescribe a medicine for you.

Will I need any pre-treatment with Pulsed Vascular laser?

You will not need any anaesthesia before the laser treatment.

No pre-treatment is needed unless you have a history of cold sores (herpes simplex) in the areas to be treated. Please advise the doctor/nurse and you will be prescribed anti-cold sore medication to start the night before treatment and to be continued for at least 7 days.

What areas can be treated?

Lines around the eyes and mouth, lax skin of the face and neck, certain stretch marks and some types of scarring.

What can I expect to feel during the treatment?

You should feel a cool spray and then a stinging sensation. The area may feel hot after treatment for up to 15 minutes.

If you are having the treatment around the eyes it may be necessary to use metallic protective lenses which require local anaesthetic eye drops.

What will I look like afterwards?

You may see some redness that will fade over a few days; however, some areas may occasionally go a darker red. These may last for up to one week. Camouflage make-up can be used, e.g. Dermablend.

Lower eyelid swelling can occur in some patients lasting up to 2 days. This may be reduced by applying iced water soaks or an ice pack to the eyelids and sleeping with the head elevated with additional pillows.

How long will my appointment be?

For 15 to 30 minutes, depending on the area to be treated.

Can I return to work immediately?

Providing you can cover the area with camouflage make-up, you may return to work immediately.

Will I need further treatment?

You may need future courses of treatment to maintain improvement.

What are the possible complications?

The laser could cause skin blistering, particularly over areas where scars are present. Blisters may lead to scarring and changes in skin colour and pigment.

Other long-term side-effects have not been reported but as this is a new form of technology, further research may report more side effects.

Some doctors are now using a high-intensity light instead of vascular or CoolTouch™ lasers. There is also another variation on the CoolTouch laser called the V-Beam, which works in a similar way.

E Laser skin resurfacing for wrinkles, lines, scars and other skin lesions (see Chapters 10 and 11)

Please read these instructions carefully and make notes on THIS sheet if you have any questions during your consultation.

You have a right to be informed about your skin condition and treatment so that you may make a decision whether or not to undergo this procedure after knowing the risks and hazards involved. This disclosure is not meant to alarm or scare; it is simply an effort to better inform you so that you may give or withhold your consent for the treatment.

Although laser surgery is effective in most cases, no guarantee can be made that a specific patient will benefit from treatment.

History of CO_2 lasers

These lasers have been used effectively by dermatologists to destroy or excise conditions such as warts, superficial skin cancers and acne scars. The advantages of treating these conditions with a laser rather than a knife have been less bleeding, more control for the doctor, less infection and in some cases faster surgery. However, these old lasers have the potential to scar as heat builds up in the surrounding healthy tissue which may be damaged.

How does the laser differ from chemical peels or dermabrasion?

During a chemical peel, areas such as deeper wrinkles may be masked by the frosting effect of the chemical on the skin. Some skin surfaces may absorb the chemical peel at different rates and the depth of the peel may be unpredictable, leading to a risk of scarring and some discoloration.

During dermabrasion, the blood produced by the sanding effect reduces visibility. These missed areas will only become apparent after healing. Dermabrasion also carries a risk of infection from blood-borne diseases. The surgery is virtually bloodless, because the high-energy laser seals blood vessels as it goes.

Will I need an anesthetic?

One hour prior to laser treatment, a topical anesthetic cream may be applied to the area. This will numb the skin. Ice may also be applied. Some patients prefer to have a local injection of anesthesia.

For full-face laser peels, you will need sedational anesthesia administered by a consultant anesthetist. If you have any type of sedational anesthesia, it will be necessary for someone to collect you and take you home.

What problems can be treated?

Lines around the mouth, eyes, deeper scars and frown lines, as well as some acne or surgical scars.

Will I need to have any pre-treatment?

You may be prescribed Retin A or a bleaching gel some weeks prior to the laser treatment. The day before the procedure you will begin taking an antibiotic and Acyclovir by mouth (to prevent cold sores or fever blisters). These will be continued for 7 days after the laser treatment. The night before you may take a sleeping tablet to help you sleep. Photographs will be taken before treatment.

Anti-inflammatory drugs may thin your blood, increase bruising and bleeding. These must be stopped 4 days before your treatment and for 4 days afterwards. Advise the doctor/nurse if you are taking: Aspirin, Advil, Arthrotec, Brufen, Clinoril, Diclofemac, Feldene, Ibuprofen, Indocid, Ketcid, Mobic, Motrin, Naprosen, Orudis, Porstan, Voltarol and Vioxx.

What happens during the laser resurfacing treatment?

The doctor will map out the area to be treated. He will then evenly treat those areas with the laser. Deeper lines will be re-treated if needed. This laser provides good depth control even for deeper lines and wrinkles. The wrinkles are reduced by peeling down the high points or 'shoulders' of the wrinkle. Some deeper areas may need three or four passes. Other areas may be feathered and blended in, using less power. With the CO_2 laser the surgery is virtually bloodless as the laser seals the walls of the surrounding vessels. If there is a lot of sun damage to the soft part of the lip (vermilion border), there may be some bleeding. Deeper lines may need a repeat laser after 6 months.

The procedure takes 15–30 minutes for areas around the mouth or eyes, and 60–90 minutes for a full-face laser.

How will I look and feel after treatment?

Immediately after laser treatment, the skin will look raw with an occasional yellow-brown area. The skin may feel hot for 1–2 hours, and this hot feeling may persist for some days, similar to a sunburn. If you had intravenous sedation, you will be drowsy for at least 6–8 hours and sometimes the next day. In the next few days as healing occurs, a thin scab will appear which will be gradually replaced by scaling and peeling. Camouflage make-up, e.g. Dermablend, Clinique Continuous Coverage, can be used within 10 days for local areas and approximately 14 days for a full-face peel. Your local department store may assist you prior to your treatment.

The area will initially be red, fading to a light pink. This pink color sometimes lasts for up to 4 months and represents a new blood supply.

The improvement of your skin is a gradual process and will take up to 6 months or longer before the final results of the treatment can be assessed.

Risks and discomforts

The most common side-effects and complications of this type are:

Hyperpigmentation (increased skin color): this is more common in those with dark complexions but may occur with any skin type; it is usually temporary but can be permanent. It should respond to the use of Hydroquinone cream, lotions and sunscreens post-operatively. Exposure to the sun without sunscreens must be avoided.

Hypopigmentation (decreased skin color): this is uncommon and appears to be related to the depth of the laser. It can occasionally be permanent.

Erythema (redness of skin): the laser-treated areas have a distinctive redness which may well last 1–4 months beyond the time normally required to heal the skin surface (usually 7–10 days). This redness is thought to represent increased blood flow during healing. Exposure to the sun, alcohol consumption and perspiring may prolong the erythema.

Scarring: any procedure in which the surface of the skin is removed can heal with scarring. This usually occurs because of some secondary factor which interferes with healing, such as infection, irritation, scratching, poor wound care or exposure to the sun. This scarring usually disappears in a few months, but some scarring may be permanent. Hypertrophic reactions or keloids in susceptible people may appear. These may improve with injections or laser treatment.

Allergic reactions: irritations to some of the medications or creams may develop, especially to the antibiotic creams or ointments. This manifests itself as a redness and/or an itchy rash and/or with small white spots that may be painful to touch. An increased sensitivity to wind and sun may occur, but is temporary and clears as the skin heals.

TREATMENT OF SCARS

Despite claims to the contrary, we cannot eliminate scars, but with the latest treatments, you can diminish them. You will not get 100% improvement with any treatment for scarring and it is important you realize this. Scarred skin will never return to the original smooth surface. Two or three treatments may be needed over a 2-year period to achieve your maximum improvement. It is not possible to predict how a patient will respond. You do not want to overtreat a scar and cause any more damage.

Frequently used treatments for scar reduction:

Cortisone injections and tape

Best for: hypertrophic (red, raised) scars, but also effective in shrinking and flattening very firm scars (keloids).
Problems: over time, cortisones can cause a chronic thinning of the skin.

Shaving

The area around the scar is numbed, then the scar is removed with a scalpel. Usually followed by cortisone injections for a few weeks.
Best for: larger, raised scars.
Problems: may leave skin discoloration, and scar may return.

Freezing

The upper layers of the skin are frozen, causing blistering and peeling, which reveals new skin underneath.
Best for: reducing the size of raised acne scars.
Problems: may lighten skin.

Collagen, Hylaform, Perlane and Restylane

Injected into the scar site.
Best for: raising soft, sunken scars such as those from acne.
Problems: not for people with rheumatic or autoimmune diseases as it may lead to allergic skin swellings. Results only last 4–6 months; repeat treatment is required.

Artecoll

Combination of collagen and methacrylate.
Best for: elevating depressed scars. Can be permanent.
Problems: over corrections. Low risk of allergy and bumps.

Fat injections

Best for: sunken acne scars on cheeks and lower face. No allergy risks, as it is your own fat.
Problems: repeat treatments required.

Laser resurfacing

The laser removes the top layers of skin.
Best for: improving minor skin irregularities, such as sunken acne scars. 100% improvement is not to be expected and the results for each patient vary considerably, as do the number of treatments needed.
Problems: several treatments may be needed for deeper scars.

Surgical revision

The scar is cut away and the skin is rejoined in a less noticeable fashion.
Best for: wide or long scars, and scars that are the product of plastic surgery procedures.
Problems: yet more surgery.

Scar subcision and elevation

Best for: saucer-shaped sunken scars.
Problems: risk of temporary bruising. Often needs to be repeated.

Chemical peels

An acid solution is applied to the skin, removing the top layer.
Best for: small superficial scars only, not deeper scars, diminishing smooth, sunken scars and making skin tone more even.
Problems: peels may require up to 2 weeks to heal and cause redness and irritation.

Pulsed dye lasers

This process targets blood vessels feeding the scar, leading to flattening and lightening of the scar.
Best for: hypertrophic red, raised scars.
Problems: can lead to bruising and discoloration that usually lasts 1–2 weeks.

PATIENT INSTRUCTIONS

Patient must be seen the day after their laser resurfacing procedure. This is mandatory.

Please inform us of any medications you are taking on a regular basis. It may be necessary to stop these prior to the resurfacing but we must be informed.

I am/not taking medication for ....

The last medication I took was .... for ....

I have not taken Roaccutane for 12 months ....

YOUR PRESCRIPTION CHARGES ARE SEPARATE. IT IS VERY IMPORTANT THAT YOU TAKE YOUR ANTIBIOTICS AND ACYCLOVIR AS PRESCRIBED. PLEASE COMPLETE THE ENTIRE COURSE OF ANTIBIOTICS EVEN IF YOU HAVE NO INFECTION.

In order to accommodate individual tolerances, you will be given a prescription for 5 sleeping tablets (full-face only). Only use these if you have trouble sleeping.

You will be given a prescription for antibiotics (full-face and mouth only): please take one the night before, then as advised by the doctor's prescription.

You will be given a prescription for anti-fever blister (cold sore) medication (full-face and mouth only). Please take one the night before, then as advised by the doctor's prescription.

If you are having sedation from the anaesthetist you must be driven to and from the clinic. If you are having valium on the day of your laser, you must have someone drive you home. *You will not be allowed any sedation unless you have designated a driver. The doctor will discuss and advise you at your pre-operative visit.*

Please arrive about 15 minutes before your appointment.

Please do not drink coffee, alcohol or strong tea for 24 hours prior to the resurfacing. Avoid all caffeine.

IF YOU HAVE ANY FURTHER QUERIES PRIOR TO YOUR RESURFACING, PLEASE TELEPHONE 000 000 000 OR PAGER 0000 0000. IT IS IMPORTANT TO US THAT ALL YOUR QUESTIONS HAVE BEEN ANSWERED.

Laser resurfacing–after treatment instructions

THE AREA TREATED BY THE LASER WILL BE CRUSTED AND WEEP FOR UP TO 7 DAYS. IT MAY ALSO FEEL TENDER. SMALL AREAS OF SKIN MAY BLEED SLIGHTLY FOR A FEW DAYS, ESPECIALLY AROUND THE LIPS AND EYELIDS. AS HEALING OCCURS, THE SKIN WILL FEEL TIGHT AND HOT.

You will be supplied with a cream to massage into your skin as often as possible. The mouth dries out rapidly owing to movement and careful attention should be paid to keep this moisturized. If there is any sign of infection, call the doctor immediately: 00 0000 000 (office) or 0000 00000 (pager).

It is very important that the patient be seen the day after surgery for ice-cold soaks and application of cream. On this day, the areas should be soaked twice a day, once in the morning and once at night. **You must be available to see the doctor for up to 7 days post surgery**. You are encouraged to soak your face as often as you wish using iced water, and only leave on for 3 minutes at a time. It is important that you wash the cloths between soaks. You must moisturize immediately after the soaks. Your skin may feel hot like a sunburn for 6–10 days.

Avoid any strenuous activity that may cause perspiration and excessive alcohol consumption for 7 days. Apply the cream provided to the treated area until all signs of scabbing or peeling have disappeared. Apply at least 6 times a day, *once every hour*, and after every soak. DO NOT LET THE SKIN DRY OUT as this may increase the risk of infection and scarring. Whenever the face feels tight or a crust is forming, moisturize and/or soak. If there is any sign of infection call the doctor immediately: tel: 000 0000 0000 (office) or 0000 00000 (pager). During healing, the skin may itch: you can have antihistamine pills prescribed and a mild sleeping pill. Stop using any other creams and lotions such as glycolic acid or tretinoin until the doctor advises you to continue. Resurfacing patients will be given a prescription for sleeping pills. You do not have to use them, but we advise it for the first few nights post-laser.

Make-up/moisturiser

Make-up and moisturizers can be applied after all of the crusting has resolved. The most effective approach is the use of a green colour stick that can be complemented by your normal foundation.

Excess skin pigment

Should you notice any new skin pigmentation or browning 2 weeks or more after resurfacing call us the next business day. Your doctor will probably suggest that you begin using an anti-pigment gel.

DO NOT GO OUT IN THE SUN UNTIL ALL SIGNS OF SCABBING HAVE GONE. ONCE THE SCABBING HAS GONE COMPLETELY, START USING THE RECOMMENDED SUNSCREENS DAILY, AVOIDING ALL SUNBATHING.

We must stress how imperative it is that the patient is seen on the immediate 2 days after the ultrapulse procedure, so please plan accordingly.

Some patients are extremely sensitive to various creams and lotions which may manifest itself as an itchy rash and/or small white spots. Do not be alarmed as the normal skin barrier will return after healing is complete. If you think you have a sensitivity rash or are having any problems, please telephone: 000 0000 0000 (office), 00000 000000 (pager).

Post-operative follow-ups relating to the surgery for 3 months after the procedure are at no charge.

DO NOT PICK OR SCRATCH. THIS WILL CAUSE SCARRING OR DISCOLORATION. MOISTURIZE.

Questions and answers

Q. What to avoid and for how long

A. Planning any social or professional activities for the first 10 days. Avoid alcohol for 7 days alter the procedure.

Q. What to avoid doing and for how long

A. Social and work activities for the first 10 days, although some patients may heal more rapidly.
Avoid any strenuous activity which may cause perspiration.

Q. How to sleep

A. Elevate head with extra pillows – sleep on back.
If you wake in the night reapply the ointment provided by the clinic.

Q. What to take and for how long

A. Sleeping pills for three to seven nights if you cannot sleep.
Pain medications for example; Paracodol as needed. You'll be given antibiotics and anti herpes simplex treatments. Take these for the total duration of the prescription, usually 7–10 days.

Q. What to drink and eat

A. Plenty of fluids. Avoid excessive alcohol consumption for 7 days.

Q. What to use and when

A. Use the moisturising ointment provided by the clinic as often as possible, e.g. up to 10 times daily and during the night if you wake up.

Q. When to resume active skin care regimen

A. Retinoids, alpha hydroxy acids after 2 weeks. Sunscreens maybe started after 10 days. The doctor may give further advice on when to restart these products.

Q. When to shower, bathe, wash, brush, comb, colour, perm hair

A. You may shower from the first day using warm not hot water. Avoid soaps and shampoos on the face.
You may find that ice cold water soaks, using clean face cloths soothe the hot skin. This can be done as often as you want. Be sure to reapply the creams afterwards.

Q. How to recognize when you need to call the doctor's office

A. If you get any blistering, infected spots or severe pain and itching. If you have any skin browning starting after 2 weeks.

Q. When to wear make-up, mascara, earrings

A. Delay for 14 days.

Q. What can be expected post-operatively

A. Weeping oozing, with swelling and crusting for the first 2 days. Hot skin similar to a sun burn, for up to 10 days. After that, scaling and itching during the healing.

Q. When can sun exposure resume

A. Within 2 weeks but only using sunscreens and sun protection hats.

Q. First office visit after surgery

A. Usually every day for the first week. Specific times will be given at the time of your visit. If there are any questions you may call the office telephone number during normal hours.

If there are any questions you may call the office XXX XXXX XXX during normal business hours. After hours the emergency page number is: XXX XXXX XXX

ARTECOLL FOR SCARS

Questions and answers

Q. What are the side effects?

A. If the injection lies close to the skin surface. The implant may appear as light coloured. This colour difference can even prove to be of a permanent nature, in which case surgical removal may be necessary. Artecol is not recommended for patients with thin/transluscent skin.

Although never reported, an anaphylactic shock could occur.

Anti-inflammatory drugs may thin your blood, increase bruising and bleeding. These must be stopped 4 days before your treatment and for 4 days afterwards. Advise the doctor/nurse if you are taking: Aspirin, Advil, Arthrotec, Brufen, Clinoril, Diclofemac, Feldene, Ibuprofen, Indocid, Ketcid, Mobic, Motrin, Naprosen, Orudis, Porstan, Voltarol and Vioxx. Panadol or Tylenol is permissible.

The theoretical possibility of the formation of foreign body granulomas reaction to this implant, must be taken into account. These would show as red lumps under the skin.

Q. Have there been any reported cases of allergic reactions to Artecoll?

A. A small risk of allergic reactions (granulomas) have been reported. These may respond to a dilute cortisone injection. In rare occasions granulomas need to be surgically excised.

Q. How does Artecoll differ from other filler materials such as Zyplast or hyaluronic acid fillers?

A. It is a pennanent implant rather than a temporary filler.

The goal of Artecoll is to reduce wrinkles or scars, not to eliminate them.

Please read these instructions carefully and make notes on THIS sheet if you have any questions during your consultation.

You have a right to be informed about your skin condition and treatment so that you may make a decision whether or not to undergo this procedure after knowing the risks and hazards involved. This disclosure is not meant to alarm or scare: it is simply an effort to better inform you so that you may give or withhold your consent for the treatment. Although this procedure is effective in most cases, no guarantee can be made that a specific patient will benefit from treatment.

What is ARTECOLL?

It is a mixture of collagen, polymethyl and methacrylate microspheres (PMMA).

The substance used as a carrier for the microspheres is collagen 3.5%. The allergizing ends of the collagen molecules have been removed, which minimizes the risk of allergic reaction. The gel-like properties of the collagen is the carrier for Artecoll. Under normal conditions the gel prevents microsphere sinkage, whereas under pressure it becomes liquid thus enabling injection.

The collagen is absorbed by the skin leaving the methacrylate microspheres as a permanent filler for scars.

Because it is a permanent implant, you may have to return for several injections to obtain the correction you desire.

Questions and answers

Q. What is the skin test?

A. The skin test is a way to determine if you are an appropriate candidate for Artecoll implantation. Because a small number of people may have an existing allergy and antibodies for bovine collagen (the carrier) it is necessary to determine this prior to an Artecoll injection, using double skin testing, i.e. two skin tests.

Q. How is the skin test performed?

A. A small amount of collagen used in Artecoll will be injected into the skin of your inner arm near the elbow joint. The skin around the injected area should be watched closely for signs that would indicate a reaction.

Watch the area around the injection site. Observe it frequently for the first 6 hours after the injection, then check it daily for the next 4 weeks (usually when you get dressed in the morning or get ready for bed at night). A second injection will be given at least 4 weeks after the first and examined 2 weeks later.

Q. What do I look for?

A. Positive skin test   The skin test is considered positive when you can see one or more of the following signs.

- redness
- hardening around the injection site (induration)
- fishing (pruritus)
- tenderness
- swelling

If you see any of these please call your doctor who may ask you to come into the office so that the area can be observed.

Negative skin test   When there is no skin reaction and the skin appears normal after the injection, the test is considered to be a negative skin test. A negative skin test is a strong indication, but not a guarantee, that you do not have an allergy to the collagen in Artecoll.

Q. What are the appropriate uses for Artecoll?

A. Depressed scars on the face.

Q. Does the Artecoll procedure hurt?

A. Your skin will be made numb using an anaesthetic cream and ice before injections of a local anaesthetic. You will feel a pin prick with these injections.

Q. How will I look and feel following the procedure?

A. The implantation is sually followed by slight swelling, reddening and occasional bruising. This normally lasts for 1-2 days, though it can be of longer duration in some cases.

  As it is permanent, Artecoll will probably always remain palpable as a thickening beneath the skin. After absorption of the collagen the implant may feel somewhat hard at first, although it will soften up in the following months with the growth of connective tissue around the microspheres.

Q. How long will it take to see results?

A. Immediately, but you may have to return for further injections to obtain the desired correction over a period of time.

Q. Can patients be allergic to Artecoll?

A. There have been some patients reporting an allergic reaction. These can appear as red raised lumps or scars which may be permanent. Injections of cortisone may reduce the allergic reaction.

Q. How often is re-injection needed?

A. As you will lose approximately half the volume injected over a period of 2–3 months, plan on two to three injections to achieve the desired result.

  Where too little growth of connective tissue occurs the scar treated may well appear again. This phenomenon is especially noticeable in patients who previously absorbed collagen injections quickly. In such cases, a further injection(s) at the foundation of the first implant might prove desirable depending on the doctor's advice.

Q. Who should not use Artecoll?

A. Anyone allergic to collagen or Artecoll.

Q. What are the alternatives to Artecoll?

A. Despite claims to the contrary, you cannot eliminate scars, but with the latest treatments, you can diminish them. You will not get 100% improvement with any treatment for scarring and it is important you realize this. Scarred skin will never return to the original smooth surface. It is not possible to predict how a patient will respond. You do not want to overtreat a scar and cause any more damage. Here are some of the most frequently used methods of scar reduction:

ARTECOLL FOR SCARS – PATIENT CONSENT FORM

Patient name:..

Kindly ensure that this questionnaire is completed before receiving an Artecoll treatment. Please discuss any questions you may have with your physician.

1. Have you ever had an Artecoll skin test? YES ☐ NO ☐
   If yes, when?..
2. Did you have an allergic reaction to the skin test? YES ☐ NO ☐
3. Have you ever had a skin test for collagen products? YES ☐ NO ☐
   If yes, when?..
4. Did you have an allergic reaction to that skin test? YES ☐ NO ☐
5. Do you have a history of allergies? If yes, please list:

   ....

   ....

6. Do you have a history of multiple severe allergies or
   Anaphlaxis (i.e. severe or allergic exaggerated reaction)? YES ☐ NO ☐
7. Have you ever had a reaction to lidocaine or other
   local anaesthetics? YES ☐ NO ☐
8. Do you have a history of allergies to any bovine (cow)
   collagen products (i.e. collagen-based sutures,
   haemostatic sponges or collagen implants)? YES ☐ NO ☐
9. Are you undergoing or planning to undergo desensitization
   injections to meat products? YES ☐ NO ☐
10. Do you have a history of dietary beef allergies? YES ☐ NO ☐
11. Do you have a history of connective tissue diseases? YES ☐ NO ☐
12. Do you have any skin inflammation, infection or other skin
    conditions in the area to be treated (i.e. cysts, pimples, rashes
    or hives)? YES ☐ NO ☐
    If yes, specify:..
13. Do you have or have you previously had facial herpes
    simplex in the area to be treated? YES ☐ NO ☐
14. Are you on immune-suppressive therapy (i.e. steriods or
    other therapies aimed at reducing the responsiveness of
    the immune system?) YES ☐ NO ☐
15. Are you taking anticoagulants (i.e. asprin or
    anti-inflammatory drugs?) YES ☐ NO ☐
16. Could you be or are you pregnant or nursing? YES ☐ NO ☐

(The safety of ARTECOLL during pregnancy or in children has not been established)

17. Please indicate any drugs you are currently taking including
    non-prescription over the counter drugs

    ....

    ....

POST-TREATMENT INFORMATION FOR PATIENTS

After you have received an Artecoll implant, some pain, swelling itching or redness at the site of injection may occur. If the pain is uncomfortable, use Panadol following the directions on the bottle. Cold compresse or ice packs can also be used to reduce any swelling, itching or discomfort. Redness may last from 1–7 days and, in some patients, longer.

If you have adhesive tape over the implant site, try to leave it in place at least overnight. The tape is used to minimize movement of your facial muscles to avoid dislocation of the implant. In order to allow the implant to stabilize, try to avoid excessive movement of your facial muscles for the next few days.

The implant may feel somewhat hard at first, however it will soften over time as your body produces its own collagen and new connective tissue.

Keep in mind that the implant acts by stimulating your body to produce new collagen and connective tissue to surround each microsphere, so the complete effect of the implant may not be apparent for up to 3 months. It is possible that after the swelling has gone down your scar may temporarily return after a few weeks. You may need several injections over a period of time, depending on your doctor's advice.

TEMPORARY SKIN FILLERS

A   Hyaluronic acid (HA) for facial lines (see Chapter 16)

Please read these instructions carefully and make notes on THIS sheet if you have any questions during your consultation.

You have a right to be informed about your skin condition and treatment so that you may make a decision whether or not to undergo this procedure after knowing the risks and hazards involved. This disclosure is not meant to alarm or scare; it is simply an effort to better inform you so that you may give or withhold your consent for the treatment.

Although this treatment is effective in most cases, no guarantee can be made that a specific patient will benefit from treatment.

Hyaluronic acid (HA)
HA has been used for the correction of facial wrinkles, folds and scars (e.g. acne and chicken pox scars).

Description
Hylaform®, Restylane® and Perlane® are sterile, elastic-like, clear, colourless, transparent gels composed of HA. HA is a naturally occurring chemical in human tissues, including skin. HA is chemically, physically and biologically identical in the tissues of all species. It serves to produce collagen and skin support.

Indications and usage
HA is indicated for the correction of wrinkles, folds and scars in the skin. Hylaform® or Restylane® are less viscous (thick) than Perlane® and are usually used in finer lines.

The procedure
Prior to your HA injection you will be given a local injection (similar to a dental block) to numb the area. After HA has been injected, the skin will be lightly massaged to smooth to the contour of the surrounding tissue.

After the first treatment, one or more additional injections (at least 1 week apart) of HA may be necessary to achieve the desired level of correction and fullness.

To sustain correction, repeat injections over time may be necessary (i.e. after 5–12 months). The need for re-injection may vary from site to site and is dependent upon a variety of factors, including anatomic location and the cause of the problems.

The patient will be charged for each HA syringe used at each injection.

Precautions
Some HA (Hylaform) is produced from materials of avian origin and contains trace amounts of avian protein. Patients with known allergies to materials of chicken origin should not be treated with Hylaform, but may receive Restylane or Perlane, which are synthetically produced.

As in any procedure into the skin, the injection of HA is associated with an inherent risk of infection. HA should not be used in areas where inflammatory processes or infections are present, e.g. active acne.

Problems with HA
In some patients HA injections or the HA may cause transient pain or bruising at the site of injection. Injection sites are frequently associated with pinpoint bleeding which usually resolved soon after injection.

Patients with known bleeding and/or coagulation disorders those who are on anticoagulant therapy or those taking the anti-inflammatory drugs listed below are at greater risk from this complication.

Anti-inflammatory drugs may thin your blood, increase bruising and bleeding. These must be stopped four days before your treatment and for four days afterwards. Advise the Dr/Nurse if you are taking: Aspirin, Advil, Arthrotec, Brufen, Clinoril, Diclofemac, Feldene, Ibuprofen, Indocid, Ketcid, Mobic, Motrin, Naprosen, Orudis, Porstan, Voltarol and Vioxx.

Local redness, swelling and itching may occur. It usually resolves within approximately one month. On occasions, some patients have experienced prolonged erythema (redness).

A small group of patients reported acne like lesions that formed at the injection site between the time of injection and up to two months after treatment.

In some patients an allergic reaction may occur – red or discoloured, sometimes lumpy bumps in the skin may be seen which can last for several months and in some cases may be permanent. The exact incidence of allergy is currently being investigated.

Patients with a suspected reaction to HA may be given test injections to forearm skin to see if it is safe to receive HA.

HA may last between 3 months to over a year, depending on the site of the injection.

It is not possible to accurately predict how many HA syringes will be needed to meet each patient's desired improvement. Only an estimate of the amounts needed can be given. Some patients may choose to have further injections after the initial treatment and will be charged for these.

Patient post-op instructions

What to avoid and for how long
Anti-inflammatory drugs may thin your blood, increase bruising and bleeding. These must be stopped 4 days before your treatment and for 4 days afterwards. Advise the doctor/nurse if you are taking: Aspirin, Advil, Arthrotec, Brufen, Clinoril, Diclofemac, Feldene, Ibuprofen, Indocid, Ketcid, Mobic, Motrin, Naprosen, Orudis, Porstan, Voltarol and Vioxx. Excessive alcohol and vitamin E supplements may all increase bruising.

What to avoid doing and for how long
No restrictions.

How to sleep
No sleeping pills required.
    If you have had lips and mouth area injected elevate head with pillows

What to take and for how long
Pain medications, e.g. Paracodol as needed. Iced water soaks or ice packs to reduce the swelling. Arnica tablets may be taken for approximately 4 days before and 4 days after treatment. If you have a history of cold sores or fever blisters in the treatment areas an oral anti-herpes simplex medicines may be prescribed.

What to drink and eat
No restrictions.

When to shower, bathe, wash, brush, comb, colour, perm hair
No restrictions.

How to recognize when you need to call the doctor's office
Painful swelling, bruising, blistering. Any lumpy redness occurring after 2 weeks.

What can be expected post-operatively?
Bruising and swelling for up to 3 days particularly with lip fillers.

When can sun exposure resume?
Immediately, with sunscreen.

Date and time of first office visit
Usually not required until further injections are needed unless complications occur.

If there are any questions you may call the office XXX XXXX XXX during normal business hours. After hours the emergency page number is: XXX XXXX XXX

B   Zyderm and Zyplast collagen (see Chapter 17)

Please read these instructions carefully and make notes on THIS sheet if you have any questions during your consultation.

You have a right to be informed about your skin condition and treatment so that you may make a decision whether or not to undergo this procedure after knowing the risks and hazards involved. This disclosure is not meant to alarm or scare; it is simply an effort to better inform you so that you may give or withhold your consent for the treatment.

Although this procedure is effective in most cases, no guarantees can be made that a specific patient will benefit from treatment.

What is collagen?

Collagen is a natural protein that provides structural support. It is found throughout the body – in skin, muscle, tendon and bone. Fibres of collagen are woven together like threads in fabric to form a framework into which new cells can grow. In the skin, collagen provides texture, resiliency and shape.

The collagen in human skin is very similar to the collagen found in certain animals. As a result, animal collagen has had many medical applications; for example, animal collagen has been used in sutures for over a century. Heart valves used during surgery are also made of collagen.

Injectable Zyderm and Zyplast collagen are made of collagen from cow skin that has been highly purified. This material is so similar to your own collagen that it is accepted by your body and becomes an integral part of your skin.

How was injectable collagen developed?

In the early 1970s a group of biochemists and physicians at Stanford University were researching alternatives to skin grafts. In the course of this work they developed the concept of purifying animal collagen so thoroughly that it could be used to replace lost skin tissue. Further research by Collagen Corporation led to the development of Zyderm collagen and Zyplast collagen.

How long has injectable collagen been used?

Injectable collagen was first used to treat patients in 1976.

How do Zyderm and Zyplast collagen work?

Both Zyderm and Zyplast collagen lend additional support to the collagen network within the skin. When a physician injects small amounts of either material directly into the areas where the body's own collagen has been weakened, depressions can be raised to the level of the surrounding skin. Thus, lines and scars can be minimized. Injectable collagen supplements the body's own collagen and raises depressions to the level of surrounding skin.

How does Zyderm collagen differ from Zyplast collagen?

Zyderm collagen was formulated especially for people with small or superficial contour problems. It can be particularly effective in smoothing delicate frown and smile lines, as well as the fine creases that develop at the corners of the eyes and above and below the lips. It can also help correct certain kinds of shallow scars.

Zyplast collagen was designed to treat depressions requiring a stronger material. It is used for more pronounced contour problems (such as deeper scars, lines, and furrows) and for areas upon which more force is being exerted, such as the corners of the mouth or 'smile' lines.

Zyderm and Zyplast collagen may be used alone or in conjunction with one another. Your physician will determine the potential benefits of each and an appropriate course of treatment.

Which skin depressions cannot be helped by either material?

Depressions with sharp edges and narrow 'ice pick' acne scars do not usually respond to these materials.

Can injectable collagen take the place of surgical procedures such as face-lifts and dermabrasion?

No, injectable collagen treatments are not meant for people who have excess facial skin or for those who want a major resurfacing of the skin. However, doctors often use Zyderm or Zyplast collagen in conjunction with surgery to fill in depressions not amenable to surgery. By using injectable collagen following a face-lift or dermabrasion, surgical results can be enhanced.

How do collagen creams differ from injectable collagen?

Regardless of the ingredients, moisturizers work only on the skin's surface as a temporary cap to help retain water. Zyderm and Zyplast collagen, however, are medical products that are injected below the skin's surface where contour problems begin and where collagen replacement can help.

Can anyone be treated with Zyderm collagen or Zyplast collagen?

No. Your doctor will inquire about your medical history in order to determine if you are an appropriate candidate for treatment. If you have a personal history of auto-immune diseases, you cannot receive injectable collagen: these would include (but are not limited to) rheumatoid arthritis, psoriatic arthritis, scleroderma (including CREST syndrome), systemic or discoid lupus erythematosus, or polymyositis, a dietary allergy to beef, or if you have recently been on corticosteroid or immunosuppressive therapy, your physician may want to administer additional skin tests before deciding if you should be treated.

Also ineligible for treatment are people with a history of an anaphylactic reaction and those who are sensitive to lidocaine (a small amount of this anaesthetic is contained in both Zyderm and Zyplast collagen). Furthermore, people who have had a previous allergic reaction to either Zyderm or Zyplast collagen may not be treated. Neither Zyderm nor Zyplast collagen should be used for breast augmentation, and neither material should be injected into bone, tendon, ligament or muscle.

If you have any questions about these medical conditions, be sure to discuss them with your doctor. You will also be skin tested prior to treatment. Anyone who exhibits a sensitivity to the material, as demonstrated by the skin test, cannot proceed with treatment.

What is involved in injectable collagen treatment?

There are three steps: a skin test, the treatment series, and periodic touch-ups.

How does the skin test work?

To determine if you are eligible for treatment with either Zyderm or Zyplast collagen, your doctor will inject a small amount of collagen into your forearm, just below the skin's surface. Both you and your doctor should observe the test site closely for 4 weeks for any signs of sensitivity to the material such as redness, swelling, or itching. Pay special attention to your test site during the first 3 days since the majority of test reactions occur during this period. At the first sign of any of these problems, contact your doctor. A second skin test will be performed after 4 weeks.

Your collagen injection treatments can begin 2 weeks later, provided that your skin tests are normal (negative).

Only about three out of every 100 tested patients show a sensitivity to the test and cannot be treated with injectable collagen; 97% of all test patients can be treated.

Is the treatment painful?

You may find that the injections are somewhat uncomfortable, particularly around the nose or lips. However, both Zyderm and Zyplast collagen contain a small amount of lidocaine that helps numb the area temporarily, and most people report that the injections are relatively painless.

How will my skin look and feel immediately after treatment?

Most patients feel comfortable in resuming their normal activities following treatment. Temporary puffiness of the treated areas, however, should be expected, especially with Zyderm collagen.

How common are treatment reactions?

With more than 500,000 people treated to date, only a small number of patients (approximately 1–2%) have developed an allergic reaction after one or more treatment injections. These reactions may consist of prolonged redness, swelling, itching and/or firmness at some or all injection sites. Most have lasted between 3 and 4 months, but in some cases have exceeded 1 year.

In less than 1% of treated patients, formation of a scab and sloughing (shedding) of the tissue at the treatment site have been noted, which can result in a shallow scar. On rare occasions, abscess formation has occurred at implantation sites. These reactions develop weeks to months following injections, and may result in induration and/or scar formation.

Of the patients who have developed an allergic reaction after treatment 50% had an unreported or unrecognized response to the skin test. **With proper monitoring of the skin test, many of these reactions could have been prevented.** The remaining 50% of this group developed allergic reactions despite a response-free skin test.

An additional 1% of individuals experience symptoms similar to those of an allergic reaction that may, however, occur periodically. Recent research has shown that some of these patients are allergic to bovine collagen.

If you observe any symptoms such as redness and/or swelling, please inform your physician. He or she will determine if you should discontinue treatment; no further injectable collagen can be administered to anyone who has experienced an allergic reaction to the material.

Are there any other types of reactions I should be aware of?

Yes. There is a possibility that you could experience a reaction related to the injection process itself. However, this does not mean it is necessary to discontinue treatment. For instance, mild bruising or slight blush could occur at the injection site. If you have previously had facial herpes simplex at the site of injection, there is a chance that the injection process itself could provoke another herpes simplex eruption. Anti-inflammatory drugs may thin your blood, increase bruising and bleeding at injection sites. These must be stopped four days before your treatment and for four days afterwards. Advise the Dr/Nurse if you are taking: Aspirin, Advil, Arthrotec, Brufen, Clinoril, Diclofemac, Feldene, Ibuprofen, Indocid, Ketcid, Mobic, Motrin, Naprosen, Orudis, Porstan, Voltarol and Vioxx. In addition, any injection carries a small risk of infection.

Some physicians have reported the occurrence of connective tissue diseases such as rheumatoid arthritis, systemic lupus erythematosus, dermatomyositis (DM), and polymyositis (PM) subsequent to collagen injections, in patients with no previous history of these disorders. Statistical analysis, comparing the number of collagen treated patients who were diagnosed with the two rare connective tissue diseases (PM and DM) with the expected number of these diseases, suggests that the rate of occurrence of these two rare diseases appears to be higher than expected in the collagen-treated population. However, a causal (cause and effect) relationship between collagen injection and the onset of auto-immune disease or systemic connective tissue disease has not been established.

Also, an increased incidence of cell-mediated and humoral immunity to various collagens have been found in systemic connective tissue diseases such as rheumatoid arthritis, juvenile rheumatoid arthritis, and progressive systemic sclerosis (scleroderma). Patients with these diseases may thus have an increased susceptibility to an allergic response and/or accelerated clearance of their implants when injected with bovine dermal collagen preparations. If you have any of these diseases, you should discuss this specifically with your doctor.

It is possible that, during the process of administering injectable collagen, the needle could be accidentally placed into or through a blood vessel. This could result in blockage of the blood flow and loss of circulation to nearby sites, which in one case resulted in loss of vision in one eye.

There have been infrequent reports of the injectable collagen being visible in the skin, in the form of a small raised or white area at the treatment site, which may persist from a few weeks to several months. In addition, some areas (such as compressed scars) resist precise placement of the material, resulting in a slight elevation beside the defect.

Does the correction last forever?

No. Touch-up injections are usually needed to maintain maximum correction. Because both Zyderm and Zyplast collagen implants are similar to your own skin, they will be altered by the same ongoing mechanical forces such as smiling or other muscle activity and biochemical processes – such as aging and active acne – that caused the original skin depressions. It has been reported that the body may deposit its own collagen at the site of collagen implantation. You should therefore be aware that part or all of the correction may last for 2 years or longer.

How often will I need a 'touch-up' injection?

Most patients who choose to receive touch-up injections for lines or furrows do so within 3–12 months of the original treatment series. For scars, and perhaps those depressions treated with Zyplast collagen, the time between touch-up injections may be longer.

Without touch-up injections, how will my skin look?

Correction may subside gradually until your skin looks like it did before treatment.

Patient post-operative instructions

What to avoid and for how long

Anti-inflammatory drugs may thin your blood, increase bruising and bleeding. These must be stopped 4 days before your treatment and 4 days afterwards. Advise the doctor/nurse if you are taking: Aspirin, Advil, Arthrotec, Brufen, Clinoril, Diclofemac, Feldene, Ibuprofen, Indocid, Ketcid, Mobic, Motrin, Naprosen, Orudis, Porstan, Voltarol and Vioxx. Excessive alcohol and vitamin E supplements may all increase bruising.

What to avoid doing and for how long

No reslriclions.

How to sleep

No sleeping pills required.

If you have had lips and mouth area injected elevate head with pillows.

What to take and for how long

Pain medications, e.g. Paracodol as needed. Iced water soaks or ice packs to reduce the swelling. Arnica tablets may be taken for approximately 4 days before and 4 days after treatment. If you have a history of cold sores or fever blisters in the treatment areas an oral anti-herpes simplex medicine may be prescribed.

What to drink and eat

No restrictions.

When to shower, bathe, wash, brush, comb, colour, perm har

No restrictions.

How to recognize when you need to call the doctor's office

Painful swelling, bruising, blistering. Any lumpy redness occurring after 2 weeks.

What can be expected post-operatively
Bruising and swelling for up to 3 days particularly with lip fillers.

When can sun exposure resume
Immediately, with sunscreen.

Date and time of first office visit
Usually not required until further injections are needed unless complications occur.

If there are any questions you may call the office XXX XXXX XXX during normal business hours. After hours the emergency page number is: XXX XXXX XXX

PERMANENT FACIAL IMPLANT (see Chapter 19)

SoftForm (or UltraSoft) facial implants

Please read these instructions carefully and make notes on THIS sheet if you have any questions during your consultation.

You have a right to be informed about your skin condition and treatment so that you may make a decision whether or not to undergo this procedure after knowing the risks and hazards involved. This disclosure is not meant to alarm or scare; it is simply an effort to better inform you so that you may give or withhold your consent for the treatment.

The appearance of your skin is affected by the strength and elasticity of the natural collagen support layer beneath it. Over time, this support layer weakens and facial creases and furrows appear. SoftForm facial implant is a subdermal implant which helps to eliminate these creases and furrows by providing structure and support underneath the skin.

What are SoftForm and UltraSoft facial implants?

The SoftForm facial implant is a soft, tube-shaped implant made of a biocompatible polymer called ePTFE (expanded polytetrafluoroethylene). The ePTFE polymer is a proven material that has been used for more than 20 years in a variety of medical applications that includes the replacement of deteriorated blood vessels in over 3.5 million people, hernia repair, abdominal wall reinforcement and, subsequently, soft tissue augmentation of the face.

How do SoftForm and UltraSoft facial implants work?

The SoftForm implant helps to eliminate deep facial creases and furrows by providing structure and support beneath the skin. The SoftForm facial implant helps to reduce the depth of the crease or furrow by raising the crease or furrow to the level of the surrounding skin.

What are the appropriate uses for facial implants?

Deep facial creases such as nasolabial folds, oral commissures, deep glabellar furrows and vermilion borders may be appropriate indications for SoftForm implant.

How do SoftForm and UltraSoft differ from other filler materials such as collagen replacement therapy or fat injections?

SoftForm is a subdermal implant which helps to eliminate deep furrows by providing structure and support underneath the skin. It is a persistent material which is not absorbed or broken down by the body over time.

Filler material, such as collagen, Hylaform, Restylane and fat injections, reduce wrinkles by 'filling in' the lines and wrinkles just under the surface of the skin. Collagen replacement therapy and fat are gradually absorbed by the body and need to be re-injected.

Who is a candidate for SoftForm and UltraSoft?

SoftForm implant is best suited for someone with pronounced facial creases or furrows who is seeking lasting results. SoftForm implant is not an appropriate treatment for fine, superficial lines. Prior to treatment you will discuss, in consultation with your physician, whether you are an appropriate candidate for the SoftForm facial implant procedure.

What is involved in the procedure?

Treatment consists of a simple in-office procedure done under a local anaesthetic. The implant is inserted below the surface of the skin through two small incisions which can be camouflaged if needed. Small sutures will hold the implant in place and should be removed in 7–10 days. The procedure generally takes less than 30 minutes, but will vary depending on the number of implants used.

Does the procedure hurt?
Each person will respond differently to the procedure. You may feel discomfort when the doctor injects a local anaesthetic. However, you should not feel discomfort during the actual procedure.

How will my face look and feel following the procedure?
You may experience some swelling or bruising, which usually lasts for a few days up to 2 weeks following treatment. Many patients return to normal activities the day after treatment as these effects may be partially camouflaged with cosmetics.

Some patients experience a sensation of tightness in the implanted area for approximately 5–7 days. You will always be able to 'feel' the implant under your skin, although this should decrease over time.

Can the procedure leave a scar?
As with any surgical procedure, there are associated risks and benefits and the possibility of scarring. In order to place each implant, two small incisions approximately 1/4 inch (5 mm) in size must be made in the skin. Although there will be scars at these incision sites, over time they usually become unnoticeable.

How long will it take to see results?
While you will see results immediately, swelling does occur and final healing takes approximately 3–4 months. Usually, within 5–7 days following the implantation, most people will not be able to tell that you have had a procedure.

How long will results last?
The SoftForm facial implant is a permanent material. It will remain in the area in which it was placed unless you choose to have it removed. As you age, furrows may slowly reappear over time.

Will treatment with the implants take the place of other surgical procedures such as face-lifts and/or laser resurfacing treatment of fine, superficial wrinkles?
People who have excess facial skin or those who want a resurfacing of their skin or who have fine, superficial lines may be appropriate candidates for SoftForm facial implant in combination with the above other procedures to fill in deep creases or furrows.

Can patients be allergic to SoftForm and UltraSoft?
While it is possible to have an allergic reaction to almost any material, there have been no reported cases of an allergic reaction to the SoftForm material.

Problems that may occur with SoftForm and UltraSoft implants
Infection may occur at implant sites – you will be routinely treated with antibiotics to help prevent this occurring.

The implant may become too close to the undersurface of the skin and produce lumpiness. The implant may need to be removed. If an implant is to be removed, you will not be charged for surgery to remove this.

Nasolabial folds are caused by the action of the lower facial muscles. SoftForm implants will offer a good improvement but may NOT completely fill these lines and folds.

The implant may move and need to be removed. If an implant is to be removed, you will not be charged for surgery to remove this.

It may shrink and shorten and need to be removed. If an implant is to be removed, you will not be charged for surgery to remove this.

The implant may protrude out through the skin. The implant will need to be removed; you will not be charged for surgery to do this.

Problems with lip SoftForm

Between 15% and 20% of all lip implants have one or more of the above problems. This seems to occur because of the extra movement of the lips during eating, speaking, etc.

If the implant has to be removed, you will not be charged for the surgery to remove it. However, we do not reimburse any fees if the SoftForm has to be removed. If you choose to replace the implant, you will be charged for the second operation.

Summary of SoftForm and UltraSoft

1. There may be skin discolouration over the implant for a period of time.
2. The material may become infected or tender after implantation requiring its removal. A significant infection may result in damage or loss to the overlying skin. A haematoma seroma (collections of blood or serum) could form, requiring surgical drainage.
3. SoftForm implant is used for subdermal soft tissue augmentation of the face. It is implanted into areas surrounded by arteries and blood vessels. There is a chance that during the procedure one of these arteries or blood vessels may be punctured, causing bleeding and/or bruising.
4. The body may have a hypersensitivity or allergic reaction to the material that would require its removal. This may result in inflammation, and possibly infection.
5. Bruising and/or swelling can occur, as with any bruise.
6. Irregularity of the implant associated with lumping may occur. This may require a surgical procedure to adjust or remove the implant.
7. Occasionally doctors or patients may not be pleased with the placement of the implant and it may require replacement or removal. If an implant is to be removed, you will not be charged for surgery to remove this.
8. The implant may protrude out of the incision sites, especially the lips, and this will require removal.

Patient post-operative instructions

What to avoid and for how long

Anti-inflammatory drugs may thin your blood, increase bruising and bleeding. These must be stopped 4 days before your treatment and for 4 days afterwards. Advise the doctor/nurse if you are taking: Aspirin, Advil, Arthrotec, Brufen, Clinoril, Diclofemac, Feldene, Ibuprofen, Indocid, Ketcid, Mobic, Motrin, Naprosen, Orudis, Porstan, Voltarol and Vioxx. No alcohol for 2 days. Avoid vitamin E supplements for 4 days, this may increase bruising.

What to avoid doing and for how long

Vigorous exercise for 4 days, e.g. jogging, yoga, aerobics and riding. Walking is pemitted. Avoid rapid or vigorous movements of the mouth and lips.

How to sleep

Sleep on your back with extra pillows. No sleeping pills required.

What to take and for how long

Pain medications, e.g. Paracodol as needed. Iced water soaks or ice packs to reduce swelling. Arnica tablets may be taken for approximately 4 days before and 4 days after treatment. If you are prescribed antibiotics and anti-herpes simplex medicines take for the full course.

What to drink and eat

No restrictions on diet. Limit alcohol for 2 days.

When to resume active skin care regimen

Avoid retinoids, alpha hydroxy acid creams, sun block around the sites of the stitches and for one week after the stitches are removed. You can continue to use on the rest of the skin.

When to shower, bathe, wash, brush, comb, colour, perm hair

No restrictions.

How to recognize when you need to call the doctor's office

Redness, pain, bleeding, weeping fluid and pus.

What can be expected post-operatively

Bruising and swelling particularly with lip implants for up to 7 days.

When can sun exposure resume?

Immediately, with sunscreen.

Date and time of first office visit

Usually not required until further injections are needed unless complications occur.

If there are any questions you may call the office XXX XXXX XXX during normal business hours. After hours the emergency page number is: XXX XXXX XXX

CHEMICAL PEELS (See also Chapters 6–7)

A   Alpha-hydroxy acid peel

> Please read these instructions carefully and make notes on THIS sheet if you have any questions during your consultation.
>
> You have a right to be informed about your skin condition and treatment so that you may make a decision whether or not to undergo this procedure after knowing the risks and hazards involved. This disclosure is not meant to alarm or scare; it is simply an effort to better inform you so that you may give or withhold your consent for the treatment.
>
> Although this procedure is effective in most cases, no guarantee can be made that a specific patient will benefit from treatment

Introduction

Glycolic acid is an alpha-hydroxy acid derived from sugar cane and is non-toxic. It is not absorbed into the body and will not cause any systemic side-effects like chemicals used in some other chemical peels.

Glycolic acid loosens dead surface cells to reveal softer, smoother, younger skin beneath. After just a few weeks, your skin looks brighter and clearer and dry skin becomes hydrated and smooth.

Glycolic acid helps reduce cell accumulation at the upper levels of the skin. It promotes a healthy, youthful glow by reducing the visible signs of aging, smoothing complexions, balancing irregular skin tones and softening the skin.

Studies confirm glycolic acid increases skin thickness and reduces abnormal skin pigmentation.

The depth of the peel is controlled by three factors: the preparation of the skin, the concentration of the solution, and the length of time it is applied.

The skin peel should be repeated once a week for 4–6 weeks, with a minimum four peels advised, followed by a maintenance peel once a month. If you have sensitive skin you will be advised to reduce the peels to once every 2 weeks over an 8–12 week period. Glycolic acid peels gradually improve your skin with repeated peels.

What should I avoid before treatment?

You should avoid any change in your normal face care routine 1–2 weeks prior to the peel treatment, such as facial hair bleaching, electrolysis, an exfoliating facial or exfoliating scrubs, recent laser treatments, sunbathing, tanning beds or use of any new creams. Please inform your therapist if you change your routine at any time as this may alter your response to the peeling agent.

The procedure

1. The face is cleansed with the appropriate cleansing solution. These cleansers temporarily strip the skin of its natural oils and allow for deeper penetration of the glycolic acid.
2. Application of glycolic acid; the patient will experience a mild stinging sensation. The acid is left in place for 2–10 minutes before it is washed off. The strength, type and time of peel will be decided at the time of your treatment.
3. The face may become pink after the solution is applied. There may also be a faint whitish discoloration in some areas, especially along the upper cheek. Occasionally, small blisters may occur with crusting.
4. Occasionally, the face will have a blotchy appearance following the peel. This will fade within 1–2 hours.
5. Make-up may usually be applied immediately after the peel.
6. Some patients do not peel at all except with longer application times and higher concentrations. However, there is still a beneficial effect to the skin without any obvious peeling and redness.
7. If you have comedones (blackheads) and milia you may need acne surgery during the course of peels. (See acne surgery and milia consent form).

Post-peel care

1. The face should be cleansed gently with a soap-free cleanser such as cetaphil or aquanil and lukewarm water twice a day.
2. Moisturizers may be applied to the face twice a day.
3. The skin may shed and peel, especially in oily areas such as the chin and side of the nose.
4. Under no circumstances should the patient pick off any dead peeling skin. This may cause bleeding and discoloration of the area.
5. You must not expose yourself to the sun without a sunscreen for at least 6 weeks; to do so incurs the risk of pigmentation of the area. A minimum of SPF 15 (UVA rating) sunscreen should be used daily to protect the skin.

Potential complications

1. Some patients may experience more pain and stinging than others, especially sensitive skin types. This should resolve once the glycolic acid is washed off. If stinging persists, please call the office.
2. Hyperpigmentation (brown spots) may occur in some patients, despite their best efforts to avoid sunlight, as it is impossible to avoid all ambient light. Bleaching creams can help.
3. Some acne lesions may initially be more red and noticeable. These lesions usually improve following the procedure.
4. Fine blood vessels of the face are not relieved by peeling and may appear more vibrant. Cosmetics can be used to camouflage these. They may also be treated by electrocautery or with the tunable dye laser.
5. Rarely, bacterial infections may occur and if a patient has a predisposition towards herpes simplex (cold sores), these lesions may be precipitated by the glycolic acid peel. Both these conditions, if they develop, can be treated with antibiotic or antiviral medications.

GLYCOLIC ACID PEELS

Patient name ....

Date ....

I hereby authorize Dr xxx xxx or Dr xxx xxx and whomever they may designate as their assistant(s), if any, to perform upon the above-named patient the following surgical procedure(s) at xxxx on this occasion and all similar procedures in the future as specified below:

....GLYCOLIC PEELS ....

We do not guarantee results; we only guarantee that the physicians in this office will use their best efforts and best judgements on your behalf.

I have read the information in this package, pages x–x.

I agree this constitutes full disclosure and that it supersedes any previous verbal or written disclosures. I certify that I have read and fully understand the above paragraphs, and that I have had sufficient opportunity for discussion and to ask questions.

I agree to allow Dr xxx and his staff to photograph or videotape me before, during or after the procedure. These photographs and videotapes shall be the property of Dr xxx and may be used for teaching publication or scientific research.

Patient signature .... Date ....

Witness signature .... Date ....

B Jessner's peels (See Chapters 6 and 7)

Please read these instructions carefully and make notes on THIS sheet if you have any questions during your consultation.

You have a right to be informed about your skin condition and treatment so that you may make a decision whether or not to undergo this procedure after knowing the risks and hazards involved. This disclosure is not meant to alarm or scare; it is simply an effort to better inform you so that you may give or withhold your consent for the treatment.

Although this procedure is effective in most cases, no guarantee can be made that a specific patient will benefit from treatment.

Introduction

A light peel may be performed with Jessner's solution, which is a mixture of resorcinol, salicylic acid and lactic acid, and is stronger than glycolic acid.

These chemical peels work by producing a separation and shedding of the upper layers of the skin, which is then replaced by new skin. This activity of new skin formation is thought to stimulate the production of your own collagen. With Jessner's solution, you may need two peels over a 6- or 12-month period. These peels are usually effective for mild sun-damaged skin, mild acne, fine acne scarring, sallow skin, fine lines and irregular pigmentation.

These superficial peels cause the skin to become pink or red and sometimes flaky and scaly. Light cosmetic camouflage is sometimes needed.

These peels can be repeated to achieve the desired results.

Procedure

1. The face is cleansed with soap, sebanil or acetone. These cleansers temporarily strip the skin of its natural oils and allow even deeper penetration of the Jessner solution.
2. The acid solution is then applied. You will experience a mild stinging sensation.
3. The solution will be reapplied several times and allowed to dry between applications.
4. To relieve some of the stinging during the peel, a cooling fan is directed at the face. Following the peel, application of iced water and gentle washing helps in soothing.
5. The face may become pink or red after the peel and there may be a faint white discoloration in some areas. Mild swelling may also be noted. These are normal reactions to the acid solution and will disappear rapidly.

Potential complications

1. Some patients may experience more pain and stinging than others. This should resolve once the acid is washed off. If the stinging persists, please call the office.
2. Hyperpigmentation (brown spots) may occur in some patients despite their best efforts to avoid sunlight, as it is impossible to avoid all ambient light. Bleaching creams can help.
3. Some acne lesions may initially be more red and noticeable. These lesions usually improve following the procedure.
4. Fine blood vessels of the face are not relieved by peeling and may appear more vibrant. Cosmetics can be used to camouflage these. These may also be treated with the tuneable dye laser.
5. Mild swelling of the face may appear the day after the peel. This can be treated with cold compresses and should resolve quickly.
6. It is important to tell the doctor if you have a prior history of cold sores or fever blisters (herpes simplex) or if you have **active** herpes simplex. The doctor can then prescribe an oral medicine that will prevent the risks of getting new lesions.
7. Some patients do not peel until longer application times and higher concentrations are used. However, there may still be a beneficial effect without any obvious peeling and redness.

8. Occasionally, the face will have a blotchy appearance following the peel. This will fade with time. Sometimes crusting occurs, especially around the sides of the face and on the cheeks.

9. Because temporary swelling may occur, some wrinkles may be initially hidden and then subsequently recur as the swelling subsides. However, the overall look will be smoother.

10. There are no dietary restrictions with this treatment. If minor swelling around the mouth occurs, the initial diet (day 1–2) may be soft foods or liquids only.

Pre-peel instructions

IT IS NOT WORTH YOUR WHILE HAVING A JESSNER'S PEEL UNLESS YOU ARE WILLING TO USE DAILY SUNSCREEN PROTECTION AND AVOID SUNBATHING.

You may be recommended to apply a skin preparation with or without a skin lightening cream prior to treatment. You must apply sunscreen every morning and avoid the sun.

Tell the doctor or staff about any prior problems such as:

Scarring

Abnormal skin pigment/color

Previous cold sores or fever blisters (herpex simplex) or **active** herpes simplex – you may be given antibiotics or Zovirax to pervent a recurrence of this problem

Previous skin infections, such as hair follicle infections and acne.

Patients taking Roaccutane must have discontinued usage for 6 weeks prior to the Jessner's peel.

We recommend that you avoid direct sunlight, abrasive scrubs and keratolytic topicals such as AHA, BPO, sulfur and salicylic acid for a day or two pre-peel.

The peel will not be performed if you are sunburnt.

Two days prior to the peel, try to avoid any alcohol, aspirin or ibuprofen as these may alter the response to the peels.

We recommend that you discontinue smoking a week before and after the peel as cigarette smoking can affect skin blood flow and the rate of healing.

On the day of the peel, do not wear any make-up or jewelry. Choose clothing that has buttons or zips at the front and does not go over your head. Do not wear contact lenses on that day.

Men should shave.

If you have noticed any skin infections, cold sores or fever blisters (herpes simplex) or have **active** herpes simplex on the morning of the peel, please let the doctor or staff members know as the peel may be postponed.

Post-peel homecare

Your skin may be red and slightly swollen after the peel and will feel tight. You will have an antibiotic moisturizing ointment applied and you may apply light make-up over that ointment on the day of the peel. Do not use make-up on any crusted areas until these are healed.

During the first evening post-peel, the skin may feel hot and feverish, which can be relieved by aspirin or ibuprofen every 4 hours.

As whiteness diminishes, redness appears like a sunburn and slowly darkens. The next day the skin colour ranges from a dark brownish-red to a golden or deep brown as the dead skin cells get ready to slowly separate from the epidermal layers. The skin will exfoliate in sheer dark sheets on its own.

You must adhere to strict sun avoidance post-peel, and sunblock must be used if there is to be any sun exposure at all.

You must re-apply the moisturizing antibiotic ointment 5–6 times a day or whenever the skin feels tight or dry, especially on crusted areas.

Wash your face with water only for the first few days; then you may use mild soap such as Cetaphil, Neutrogena Foaming Wash or Oil of Olay Foaming Wash. You may apply a clean face flannel soaked in ice water any time as a soothing application.

Avoid products containing fragrances and sunscreens.

Avoid strenuous activity that may cause perspiration for 2 days.

If there is any crusting, apply a soothing balm or light moisturizing cream (without fragrance) to keep the crusts moist, 4 or 5 times per day. DO NOT PICK OR SCRATCH – this will cause scarring. Skin must not be pulled off before it is ready; this can cause bleeding, rawness, redness, scabbing, a risk of infection and a slowing of the healing process.

Some patients notice slight peeling or crusting in certain areas of the face. This may appear immediately or within 2–3 days. Sometimes you may not notice this – this does not mean that the peel has not worked. It means that the turnover of the skin has not increased to such a state that you can see it with the naked eye.

Blackheads and whiteheads already formed deep in the follicle are normal and may surface. Acne should not be picked. Topical exfoliants, medications and scrubs should be delayed for 1–3 weeks and re-introduced gradually. Daily use of sunblock is especially important now.

It is permissible to take showers with water at body temperature (i.e. avoid hot water). Gently wash the skin with a soothing cleanser such as Cetaphil.

Do not rub your face dry; pat it dry with a soft towel.

It is also beneficial to the healing process to drink plenty of water.

If you have been given oral antibiotics or anti-viral antibiotics such as Zovirax, it is most important to continue to take these each day until the course is finished.

Your peel may be repeated every 6–12 months to continue to achieve a steady improvement of your skin complexion and appearance.

C   Trichloracetic acid (TCA) peels (see Chapters 7 and 8)

Please read these instructions carefully and make notes on THIS sheet if you have any questions during your consultation.

You have a right to be informed about your skin condition and treatment so that you may make a decision whether or not to undergo this procedure after knowing the risks and hazards involved. This disclosure is not meant to alarm or scare; it is simply an effort to better inform you so that you may give or withhold your consent for the treatment.

Although this procedure is effective in most cases, no guarantee can be made that a specific patient will benefit from treatment.

Introduction

A chemical peel is a surgical procedure performed at the clinic with solutions of trichloracetic acid (TCA) of strengths from 20% to 40%. This acid is not absorbed into the body and will not cause any systemic side-effects, unlike chemicals used in some other chemical peels. The upper layer of skin is 'killed' and is shed or peels off when it is replaced by new skin. The depth of the peel is controlled by the concentration and the amount of acid applied. This procedure is especially good for sun-damaged skin, small wrinkle lines, irregular pigmentation, and very small scars. A deep chemical peel takes about 1 week to heal and will remove most of the abnormalities listed above. A superficial peel may be done, which does not require staying home during the healing time. The skin peels as after sunburn in 4–5 days. This can be repeated at 2-week intervals to get the desired results.

Repeat peeling of the skin with TCA, up to 25%, results in a freshening of the skin with a decrease in subtle lines and pigmentation and improvement in skin texture. Repeated application is made until the desired effect is achieved. Deeper 40% TCA peels, with or without occlusion, result in a far greater depth and resulting necrosis, yielding much greater improvement but a greater risk of complications.

The procedure

1. The face is first cleansed with acetone or sebanil.
2. The physician then applies the peeling agent. The patient will experience a stinging sensation to that area. This may last for 30–60 minutes.
3. The face may swell shortly after the solution has been applied and turn pink. Over the next few days, the face will turn a dark brown color. Streaks of white may show amidst the dark brown. This is normal and the patient should not be concerned. Freckles and pigmentation will seem larger than before, owing to the swelling.
4. An antibiotic ointment (polysporin) may be applied to the face twice daily. The face can be gently splashed with warm water and patted dry. Mineral oil may be used with cotton to gently cleanse the skin.
5. Under no circumstances should the patient peel off the dead skin. To do so will cause recurrence of pain and possible bleeding areas. If the skin is curling off, the dead skin can be cut off with scissors. It should never be stripped off the skin. As the skin begins to peel, the face is in the healing phase, and may begin to itch. If the itching is severe, medication will be prescribed to alleviate it.
6. After peeling, the face will be bright red. This redness will fade toward a fresh pink tone in 3–6 weeks in the average individual. However, make-up may be worn 1 week after the entire face has peeled. In the areas that have been peeled, apply antibiotic ointment to keep these areas soft.
7. The patient must not expose themselves to the sun for at least 6 weeks following the facial peeling. To do so incurs the risk of pigmentation of the face. A minimum of SPF 15 sunscreen must be used to protect the skin.
8. There are no dietary restrictions with this treatment; however, as the swelling may make it difficult to open the mouth during the first day or two, the initial diet may consist of liquids only. Restrict talking and mouth movements so as not to disrupt the crust. During the entire time of the process (5–7 days), activity should be restricted. No exercise or undue physical motions.
9. Occasionally, the face will have a blotchy appearance following the peel. This generally fades with time.

10. Because of the swelling that occurs, residual wrinkles are hidden and the face may present a smoother appearance initially than subsequently. The face overall, however, will be smoother and more youthful-looking.

11. During the process of the peel (5–6 days), it is helpful if the patient has someone with them to aid in the recuperative period.

Complications

1. Some patients may experience more pain and throbbing than others. If prescribed analgesics do not relieve this, call our office for instruction.

2. Although infrequent, some patients may develop scars from the peel. These generally occur around areas of movement, such as the mouth and jaw. Therefore, it is imperative to limit talking and chewing until ointment is applied to the crust, generally on the fourth or fifth day.

3. Hyperpigmentation may occur in some patients despite their best efforts to avoid sunlight, for it is impossible to avoid all ambient light. Bleaching creams can help.

4. Fine blood vessels of the face are not relieved by peeling and may show up even more vibrantly. Cosmetics may be used to cover them up. They may also be treated by light electrocautery or laser surgery.

5. Redness of the face may persist in some patients longer than 2–3 months; with time, it should disappear. Most make-up will cover the erythema (redness).

What chemical peels can do

1. Correct sun damage (actinic degeneration).
2. Flatten mild scarring.
3. Remove rhytides (wrinkles).
4. Improve irregular hyperpigmentation.

What chemical peels cannot do

1. Chemical peels cannot change pore size. They might increase pore size temporarily.
2. Chemical peels cannot improve lax skin which may require a face lift.
3. Chemical peels cannot improve deep scarring.
4. Chemical peels cannot always remove dark pigmentation in dark-skinned individuals.

What to do before the chemical peel

1. Wash your face with soap and water.
2. Pull your hair back off your face.
3. Do not wear any jewelry.
4. Wear a top which you do not have to pull over your head.
5. Eat a light breakfast or lunch.
6. Have someone with you to drive you home.

Before the appointment, purchase a large tube of polysporin ointment and white vinegar.

After the peel

1. Soak your face for 15 minutes four times a day in a solution of one tablespoon of white vinegar in one quart of water.
2. You may be given a prescription for a mild painkiller.
3. Apply a thin layer of the ointment supplied several times daily.
4. Sleep on your back with your head on a few pillows.
5. Return to the office in 2 days and in 1 week for a follow-up appointment.
6. Avoid strenuous exercise for 2 weeks.
7. Start using your sunscreen about 14 days after the peel. Avoid direct sun exposure for 6 weeks (unprotected), then only with sunscreen.
8. Call this office if you have unexpected problems or questions.

BOTULINUM TOXIN (BOTOX, DYSPORT, NEUROBLOC): FACIAL EXPRESSION LINES (See Chapters 13–15)

Please read these instructions carefully and make notes on THIS sheet if you have any questions during your consultation.

You have a right to be informed about your skin condition and treatment so that you may make a decision whether or not to undergo this procedure after knowing the risks and hazards involved. This disclosure is not meant to alarm or scare; it is simply an effort to better inform you so that you may give or withhold your consent for the treatment.

Although this treatment is effective in most cases, no guarantee can be made that a specific patient will benefit from treatment.

Botulinum toxin

Botulinum toxin (BTX) is a medicine produced by the bacterium that very rarely causes botulism food poisoning. Botox is not alive but is a protein, which weakens and inactivates muscles. BTX is a potent toxin that blocks neuromuscular transmission in the area into which it is injected. In other words, it can stop messages from being sent from a neuron to a muscle, or a sweat gland and, therefore, it can stop the muscle or gland from performing tasks. This is another example where 'natural' products are used for medicinal purposes: fungi produce penicillin, cowpox virus protects against smallpox, and the foxglove plant produces the 'poison' digitalis which millions of patients take daily for heart disease. With current bioengineering it is common for bacteria to produce the necessary medicine for a specific disease.

First clinical uses of BTX

In 1973 BTX was used as a treatment for patients with crossed eyes. By weakening the overactive eye muscles, this medicine provided an alternative to surgery. After this 'breakthrough' BTX quickly gained acceptance for other ophthalmologic disorders, including nystagmus and blephospasm (involuntary spasm of the eyelids), to name a few.

Other specialists use BTX for their patients

Neurologists have explored possible indications for BTX therapy for their patients. It has now become the mainstay of non-surgical therapy for spasmodic neck muscles, spasmodic laryngeal muscles, writer's cramp, certain tremors, tics, multiple sclerosis, cerebral palsy, post-stroke states, spinal cord injuries, nerve palsies, Parkinson's disease and facial spasms. Other indications include swallowing problems and speech impediments. Genitourinary disorders of spastic bladder and other disorders have also been studied. Congenital muscular disorders or acquired nerve injuries have been improved by balancing muscles with BTX.

Safety

While BTX is very potent in a high concentration, it is used in very small quantities with high margins of safety. After a muscle is injected, its first effects are not seen for 48 hours and the complete effect on the muscle may not be seen for 2 weeks. A safety feature of BTX is that complete recovery of the muscle occurs with time. This is possible owing to the body's ability to repair itself with the formation of new transmitters that allow reactivation of the muscle.

Background to the cosmetic use of BTX

BTX injections for facial lines were pioneered in 1988 by Doctors Jean and Alastair Carruthers, a Vancouver ophthalmologist and her husband, a dermatologist. The ophthalmologist noted that the wrinkles disappeared in her patients with eyelid spasms who were treated with BTX. This led to further research that confirmed the effectiveness and safety of the BTX vaccine for improving wrinkles due to overactive muscles of the face.

In 1996 at the annual meeting of the American Academy of Dermatology in Washington, a research presentation by Dr Nicholas Lowe confirmed that BTX was effective for facial expression lines. Significant improvement was noted in both forehead frown lines and crow's feet. No significant side-effects were noted beyond the expected injection discomfort. The length of effective improvement for the forehead frown lines was approximately 17 weeks. In 2001 another type of BTX (Neurobloc) became available.

BTX for frown lines

Crease lines and wrinkles are a natural process of aging due to a combination of aging, sun damage, gravity, and the muscle action of laughing, talking, frowning and crying. Filling agents including Collagen, Fibrel, autologous fat and Gortex are the mainstay of non-surgical treatments. Surgical options include face, forehead, neck and eyelifting operations, dermabrasions, laser resurfacing, and deep chemical peels.

Between the eyebrows, the vertical frown lines result from over-active muscles. These muscles are also used when concentrating. By drawing the eyebrows inward, one expresses anger, confusion or anxiety. Repeated often enough, permanent skin creases develop and, even when relaxed, these frown lines remain. Neutralization of these overactive brow muscles helps eliminate these negative appearances.

BTX for crow's feet

Wrinkles radiating from the corner of the eyes caused by smiling, laughing or squinting are especially distressing to some individuals. Previously, no reasonable medical or surgical solution improved this problem due to the strong underlying muscles. Even with the deepest chemical peels or laser resurfacing techniques, rapid recurrence of these lines around the eyes is inevitable. BTX has now proved to be effective at preventing the recurrence of wrinkles by inhibiting the underlying muscles.

Horizontal forehead lines

Some individuals use different muscles for raising the brows; others 'talk' with their forehead. A more dilute toxin is used when treating the horizontal forehead lines. Another alternative for this area is a forehead lift, which is now increasingly being performed endoscopically in order to leave minimal surgical scars. Unfortunately, longevity has not been established with this particular procedure.

Lower face and neck lines

Some people may be suitable for treatment with BTX. This area is most dynamic when talking, smiling and eating. As one ages, muscle activity leads to some lines, and fat is lost from this area. Replacement of fat is now possible with the newer, longer-lasting techniques. One recent advance has been the development of a permanent filling agent called SoftForm, used for lip enhancement and some lower facial lines. BTX may be used to improve some lower face and vertical neck lines or neck bands.

Commonly asked questions

How painful are the injections?

The smallest needles are used and the medicine itself does not sting as much as the usual local anaesthetic. Most patients feel it less than a collagen injection. Pain can be minimized by the use of ice cooling the skin just prior to injections.

What should be expected after BTX therapy?

BTX is a safe therapeutic agent for wrinkles. Complications have been minor and only transient. Bruising may occur at the injection site especially around the eye area and a brief pain or headache may follow. Bruising may be greater in patients who are taking aspirin or any blood thinning medicines. Bruising may be reduced by taking Arnica tablets for approximately 4 days before and 4 days after treatment. These products should be avoided, if possible, prior to the injection. Ice helps to prevent bruising. Anti-inflammatory drugs may thin your blood, increase bruising and bleeding. These must be stopped 4 days before your treatment and for 4 days afterwards. Advise the doctor/nurse if you are taking: Aspirin, Advil, Arthrotec, Brufen, Clinoril, Diclofemac, Feldene, Ibuprofen, Indocid, Ketcid, Mobic, Motrin, Naprosen, Orudis, Porstan, Voltarol and Vioxx. Panadol or Tylenol is permissible.

How long does BTX last?

Successful therapy is not immediate but is signaled by muscle weakness that may begin several days after injection, with a peaking weakness at 10 days. Paralysis after the initial injection lasts between 3 and 7 months for most patients.

How often is re-injection needed?

Re-injection is suggested every 3–4 months to keep the muscles paralysed and allow the furrows to completely smooth out. Once an area is smooth, patients are instructed to return for therapy only when they notice a return of muscle movement which may not occur for 4–12 months; even longer has been reported.

Who should not use BTX?

Although there have been no reports of birth defects with this medicine, no pregnant patients will be treated. It is also our policy not to inject BTX in nursing mothers.

Patients with a history of neuromuscular disease (multiple sclerosis and myasthenia gravis) or other types of disease involving neurotransmission should avoid this medicine.

Patients taking the following medicines may experience increased effects of BTX on the injected muscles; aminoglycoside antibiotics (Streptomycin, Tobramycin and Garamycin injections), penicillamine, quinine and calcium channel blockers (Calan, Cardizem, Dilacor, Norvasc, Procardia, Verelan).

What are the alternatives to BTX?

Filling agents including fat, collagen, Fibril and Gortex; resurfacing procedures with acids or lasers; and lifting operations of the forehead, temporal, neck and mid face regions.

What unexpected benefits have come from BTX?

Tension headaches for some patients have disappeared. These occurred in patients who were using forehead and brow muscles during periods of stress and tension. When these muscles were relaxed, the headaches faded.

How exactly does BTX inactivate the muscle?

BTX inhibits the release of acetylcholine (a nerve transmitting chemical) at the joining site of the nerve to the muscle so that the muscle never gets the message to contract. Remember muscles only have the ability to contract; an opposing muscle contracts to produce movement in the opposite direction. To rejoin the nerve to the muscle, the body organizes and produces new motor endplates which re-establish the connection.

Does the body make antibodies to the BTX protein?

Yes, especially if enough toxin is injected often enough. The crucial amount is several hundred units (much more than the usual cosmetic dosage) and perhaps booster injections placed within 1 month of the initial injections. Antibodies have been more of a problem for neurological disorders where larger amounts of BTX are required. When sufficient amounts of antibodies are formed, the therapeutic effects of BTX are greatly reduced. A very small number of people have antibodies that inactivate the BTX (probably from foods eaten previously). They will not improve significantly, if at all.

Have there been any reported cases of allergic reactions or hives to BTX?

No reported cases of a true allergic reaction have been reported. People who are known to be allergic to botulism toxin or albumin should avoid BTX.

What happens if a female patient becomes pregnant shortly before or after treatment?

A number of neurological and ophthalmological patients have delivered normal children after receiving their injections. For safety reasons no pregnant or nursing females will be treated.

What can be done for the drooping eyelid if this occurs?
Temporary drooping of one or both eyelids is the most significant complication and occurs in well below 1% of all injections. This is a result of the local dissemination of the toxin in the injection site and can be minimized by accurate dosing, as well as keeping the patient in an upright position for 3–4 hours after injection. If drooping eyelids occur, it is usually minimal and is usually resolved by 2 weeks. Special eyedrops may temporarily reduce eyelid droop.

As a patient, after receiving my injections how can I help BTX be more effective and avoid side-effects?
Use the muscle: intentionally making the muscle contract helps localize the protein to the selected muscle for ablation.

Can BTX be used to weaken – not totally paralyse – a muscle?
Yes, in fact this is done so that the face will not be left expressionless. It can also be used to balance a weak muscle on the opposite side. By injection of the medicine into the subcutaneous tissue, not the muscle, and by using a smaller dosage, a weakening of the muscle is more likely to occur.

What is the best method for getting deepest frown furrows to disappear?
In our study, improvement after the initial injection lasted about 17 weeks. Re-injection every 3–4 months is recommended, rather than waiting for the muscle to recover. This keeps the muscle paralysed and allows the skin to smooth out over the next 12 months.

Also an infection of a skin filler, e.g. Restylane plus BTX will give greater improvement in deep furrow lines.

NOTE
Some individual patients require two or more courses of injections of BTX to see optimum effect. A very small percentage of people are resistant (non-responsive) to BTX.

If you do not see **any results after 10 days** we will repeat the injection at no cost to yourself. However, you must have contacted this office and informed us **within 14 days** of your original injection in order to be given this top-up injection at no charge. If you have received a top-up injection and the muscle is still active after 10 days, please note we will not do a further injection. You may be building up antibodies to BTX and a further injection to the area will be of no benefit.

BTX may not stop all muscular activity, especially in those patients with deeper lines and/or stronger muscles. Occasionally other muscles close to the paralysed muscle will become stronger as they try to compensate for the paralysed area (e.g. the muscles at the outer eyebrow area may eventually take over the frowning action of the eyebrows). You may need an additional injection to the area that is over-compensating. After the crow's feet are injected you may notice a deeper crease under the eyes as the muscles at the sides relax. This may require further injection.

Results may vary with different treatments, i.e. one treatment may be better than the next – this does not mean it has not worked, rather that your muscle activity may vary from time to time.

Patient post-op instructions

What to avoid and for how long
Anti-inflammatory drugs may thin your blood, increase bruising and bleeding. These must be stopped 4 days before your treatment and for 4 days afterwards. Advise the doctor/nurse if you are taking: Aspirin, Advil, Arthrotec, Brufen, Clinoril, Diclofemac, Feldene, Ibuprofen, Indocid, Ketcid, Mobic, Motrin, Naprosen, Orudis, Porstan, Voltarol and Vioxx. Excessive alcohol and vitamin E supplements may all increase bruising.

What to do
Do use the muscles that were injected repetitively for up to 1 hour if possible, e.g. smile or frown a lot – it may help with the 'take' of BTX.

What to avoid doing and for how long
Avoid rubbing the injected sites. Avoid vigorous exercise for four hours.

How to sleep
No restrictions.

What to take and for how long
You should not need any pain medications but, if you do take paracetamol or paracodol. Avoid anti-inflammatory drugs (see above). Bruising may be reduced by taking Arnica tablets for approximately four days before and 4 days after treatment.

What to drink and eat
No restrictions.

When to resume active skin care regimen
Retinoids, alpha hydroxy acid creams and sun block may be resumed immediately.

When to shower, bathe, wash, brush, comb, colour, perm hair
No restrictions.

How to recognize when you need to call the doctor's office
Severe swelling or bruising, or if your face or eyebrows start to droop.

When to wear make-up, mascara, earrings
Immediately.

What can be expected post-operatively?
Bruising and swelling are possible, particularly at the crow's feet area which can cause a black eye. The effect of the injection is not immediate and may take several days to work with maximum effect after 10 days.

When can sun exposure resume?
Immediately. with sunscreen.

Date and time of first office visit
Usually not required until further injections are needed unless complications occur.

If there are any questions you may call the office XXX XXXX XXX during normal business hours. After hours the emergency page number is: XXX XXXX XXX

LIPOSUCTION AND FAT HARVEST/FAT INJECTION (See Chapter 18)

Please read these instructions carefully and make notes on THIS sheet if you have any questions during your consultation.

You have a right to be informed about your skin condition and treatment so that you may make a decision whether or not to undergo this procedure after knowing the risks and hazards involved. This disclosure is not meant to alarm or scare; it is simply an effort to better inform you so that you may give or withhold your consent for the treatment.

Although this treatment is effective in most cases, no guarantee can be made that a specific patient will benefit from treatment.

Liposuction

Liposuction – also called liposculpture, lipoplasty, or suction lipectomy – is a cosmetic surgery technique developed by cosmetic dermatologic surgeons and plastic surgeons to remove fat deposits that do not respond to dieting and exercise. These fatty bulges are most commonly found in the thighs, hips, abdomen, buttocks, knees, ankles, calves and arms. They are also found in the facial areas such as the chin, cheeks, jowls and neck.

This information sheet will provide you with a basic understanding of liposuction, including who are the best candidates, what to expect, what the procedure entails, and likely results. It is important that you understand the procedure, so be sure to ask any questions you may still have.

Are you a good candidate?

The best candidates for liposuction are healthy men and women with good skin elasticity and realistic expectations for liposuction. 'Realistic' means that improvement, not always perfection, is the goal. The fatty bulges should be localized to a few areas and the individual should be near their ideal body weight. Cellulite, or waffled skin, may not be cured by liposuction.

It is natural for women, in particular, to accumulate fatty deposits on the hips, buttocks and abdomen; and fat in men tends to accumulate around the mid-section. Some men experience gynecomastia, or enlarged breasts.

Liposuction can enhance the appearance of men and women of all ages while boosting self-esteem. This procedure is not for obese people. It is not meant to replace good eating and exercise habits, or to counter obesity; however, liposuction *can* offer help to remove unwanted fatty deposits in many areas of the body.

Your cosmetic surgeon will discuss your condition to see if liposuction is right for you.

What are the complications?

Liposuction is a popular procedure that is a normally safe (when using local anaesthetic methods) and effective method of removing excess fat. Like all surgery, any cosmetic surgery involves some level of risk.

Variations from the ideal result are possible. Complications could include uneven skin surface, depression in the skin, especially in patients with poor skin elasticity, lumpiness, bleeding, infection, discoloration, fluid accumulation beneath the skin, numbness and scarring. Although complications with this type of liposuction surgery are extremely rare, they can include severe infections and death.

Before surgery

During your consultation, we will discuss the areas of your body you would like to change. You may undergo an examination to thoroughly assess your fat storage, skin elasticity, and review your medical and health history. We can discuss the placement of incisions and what other procedures may need to be performed to achieve the proper result. Anti-inflammatory drugs may thin your blood, increase bruising and bleeding. These must be stopped 4 days before your treatment and for 4 days afterwards. Advise the doctor/nurse if you are taking: Aspirin, Advil, Arthrotec, Brufen, Clinoril, Diclofemac, Feldene, Ibuprofen, Indocid, Ketcid, Mobic, Motrin, Naprosen, Orudis, Porstan, Voltarol and Vioxx. We advise you to stop smoking 2 weeks before and after surgery as healing can be impaired. Excessive alcohol and vitamin E supplements also may increase bruising. This bruising may be reduced by taking Arnica tablets for approximately 4 days before and 4 days after treatment, and by having ultrasound post-operatively.

Although you will be mobile immediately following your liposuction, you may want to arrange for someone to drive you home after surgery.

Liposuction: how it is done

Liposuction is performed on an outpatient basis. The latest liposuction techniques involve injecting the area to be suctioned with a special dilute fluid plus anaesthesia prior to suctioning. This is called **tumescent liposuction**. The fluid constricts the surrounding blood vessels, making the procedures nearly bloodless, while minimizing the pain. The rest of the procedure is performed in the same way as traditional liposuction.

Liposuction begins with small incisions, approximately 1/4 inch (5 mm) in length, near the area where fat is to be removed. A thin, hollow tube, called a *cannula*, is inserted and is attached to a machine or syringe that creates a strong vacuum; we then manipulate the cannula under the skin to remove the unwanted fatty deposits.

With local tumescent anaesthesia, you may feel pressure, movement, or an occasional stinging sensation during the procedure, but rarely actual pain. Your dermatologic surgeon will determine the amount of fat to remove by feeling and pinching the skin throughout the surgery.

After your surgery

Most patients are mobile immediately after liposuction, although an extra day or two of rest may be needed when large amounts of fat are removed. Keep in mind that healing is a gradual process and varies from patient to patient. You begin normal activity as soon as possible to reduce post-operative complications, but in some cases you may be advised to avoid strenuous activity for a few days.

Airplane flying can increase bleeding and drainage due to pressure changes following the liposuction; this is not usually dangerous, but may be embarrassing or distressing for you. We therefore recommend you avoid flying, if possible, for 5–7 days. A blood-coloured drainage from the liposuction entry-holes is normal for up to 5 days.

We recommend that a tight-fitting garment, similar to a girdle or biking shorts, be worn after surgery to reduce swelling. Your stitches will be removed within 7–10 days if they are not dissolvable.

You have been given fluids into the skin during the procedure, and you will experience swelling and some bruising, but this is only temporary. You may feel a little bruised and sore as if you had over-exercised that part of the body, but you should be able to resume work in a few days. Some patients bruise more extensively than others, but this will fade in 2–3 weeks. This bruising may be reduced by taking Arnica tablets for approximately 4 days before and 4 days after treatment, and by having ultrasound postoperatively.

Liposuction is a surgical procedure, and your body has to heal before you see the full benefits. Your results will likely be visible within 2 or 3 weeks, but the full effect may not be fully evident for 6–12 months after surgery in some cases.

You should maintain a balanced diet and exercise regularly to fully enjoy the new you for many years to come. With realistic expectations, most patients are pleased with the improvements from their liposuction procedure. The goal is for you to be more comfortable with your body and happy with your new shape.

Lumpiness and unevenness of the fat may occur, which can last several weeks or months. This usually resolves itself but may be permanent. It may be helped by post-operative ultrasound or further liposuction.

If too much fat is removed from some areas this may lead to depressions in the skin surface. Bruising may be reduced by taking Arnica tablets for approximately 4 days before and 4 days after treatment, and by having ultrasound postoperatively.

LIPOSUCTION AND FAT HARVEST/FAT INJECTION
INFORMED CONSENT

I UNDERSTAND THATY IF I DO NOT FOLLOW THE INSTRUCTIONS GIVEN TO ME AND/OR IF I DO NOT ADVISE DR. XXXX OR DR. XXXX OF ANY QUESTIONABLE OR UNUSUAL CONDITIONS THAT MAY ARISE DURING MY RECOVERY PERIOD, THERE COULD BE COMPLICATIONS AND/OR ADDITIONAL RISKS AND CONSEQUENCES.

WE DO NOT GUARANTEE RESULTS, WE ONLY GUARANTEE THAT THIS OFFICE AND DOCTORS WILL USE THEIR BEST EFFORTS AND BEST JUDGEMENTS ON YOUR BEHALF.

I HAVE READ THE INFORMATION IN THIS PACKAGE PAGES X–X

I AGREE THIS CONSTITUTES FULL DISCLOSURE AND THAT IT SUPERSEDES ANY PREVIOUS VERBAL OR WRITTEN DISCLOSURES. I CERTIFY THAT I HAVE READ AND FULLY UNDERSTAND THE ABOVE PARAGRAPHS, AND THAT I HAVE HAD SUFFICIENT OPPORTUNITY FOR DISCUSSION AND TO ASK QUESTIONS.

I AGREE TO ALLOW DR. XXXX AND HIS STAFF TO PHOTOGRAPH OR VIDEO TAPE ME BEFORE. DURING OR AFTER THE PROCEDURE. THESE PHOTOS AND VIDEOS SHALL BE THE PROPERTY OF DR. XXXX AND MAY BE USED FOR TEACHING PUBLICATION OR SCIENTIFIC RESEARCH.

PATIENT SIGNATURE... DATE............................

FAT INJECTIONS (LIPOTRANSFER)

A new technique for improving deep facial lines of the lower face, as well as facial features such as 'hollow' cheeks and nasolabial lines is fat harvesting. Your own fat is collected during liposuction or fat harvesting using the local tumescent anaesthesia method (see above). It is then frozen and may be used for 18 months and injected, ideally every 2–3 months.

Patients may need a nerve block around the area similar to a dental injection.

Recent experience with this procedure suggests that after several (4–6) fat injections improvement may last up to 2–3 years. There is no risk of allergy as it is your own fat that is being injected.

Complications

Temporary swelling and bruising may last for some days after the injection. Each patient's response is different and some patients may have more swelling and bruising than others.

Post-operative instructions

What to avoid and for how long

Anti-inflammatory drugs may thin your blood, increase bruising and bleeding. These must be stopped 4 days before your treatment and for 4 days afterwards. Advise the doctor/nurse if you are taking: Aspirin, Advil, Arthrotec, Brufen, Clinoril, Diclofemac, Feldene, Ibuprofen, Indocid, Ketcid, Mobic, Motrin, Naprosen, Orudis, Porstan, Voltarol and Vioxx. Vitamin E supplements may all increase bruising. Alcohol for 4 days before the procedure and 4 days after the procedure.

What to avoid doing and for how long

Flying for 5 days. Avoid running and vigorous exercise until you feel comfortable. Walking after the first day is allowed.

How to sleep

Sleep on your back if you have had stomach, chin or thigh liposuction.

What to take and for how long

Pain medications, e.g. Paracodol as needed. Antibiotics that have been prescribed for the full course. Arnica tablets may be taken to reduce swelling for approximately 4 days before and 4 days after treatment.

What to drink and eat

Plenty of fluids. Normal diet.

What to use and when

You will need to replace the absorbent dressings provided after 2–3 days, sooner if weeping is heavy or if you shower/bath. You should wear support garments, e.g. lycra biking shorts for abdominal and thigh liposuction. Neck garments or bandages will be provided for neck and jaw liposuction. Weeping may last between 2 and 7 days.

When to resume active skin care regimen

No restrictions.

When to shower, bathe, wash, brush, comb, colour, perm hair

You can start showering and bathing the day following the procedure.

How to recognize when you need to call the doctor's office

If you develop any fevers, painful red swellings or bleeding at the site of the liposuction.

When to wear make-up, mascara, earrings

If you have liposuction on the neck and lower face make-up can be applied immediately to camouflage any bruising.

What can be expected post-operatively

Bruising, swelling, weeping and discomfort. You may experience some thickening and lumpiness under the skin. This is fibrous tissue that usually goes away over several weeks.

Date and time of first office visit

You will be seen 7 days following the liposuction unless you have concerns.

If there are any questions you may call the office XXX XXXX XXX during normal business hours. After hours the emergency page number is: XXX XXXX XXX

PERMANENT HAIR REPLACEMENT: TRANSPLANTATION OF HAIR TO CORRECT BALDNESS (See Chapter 21)

Please read these instructions carefully and make notes on THIS sheet if you have any questions during your consultation.

You have a right to be informed about your skin condition and treatment so that you may make a decision whether or not to undergo this procedure after knowing the risks and hazards involved. This disclosure is not meant to alarm or scare; it is simply an effort to better inform you so that you may give or withhold your consent for the treatment.

Although this procedure is effective in most cases, no guarantee can be made that a specific patient will benefit from treatment.

The principle

The success of hair transplantation depends on the fact that transplanted hair follicles (roots removed from their original location, usually from the rear and sides of the scalp, to a bald or balding area) will behave as they did in their original site. For example, even in the most advanced cases of common male pattern baldness (MPB), a horseshoe-shaped fringe of hair persists. Hair follicles moved from this hairy fringe to a bald area on the same patient's scalp will take root and grow. It is believed that these grafts will continue to grow for a lifetime. Some less common types of hair loss, in addition to ordinary MPB, can be helped by this procedure.

The procedure

Anti-inflammatory drugs may thin your blood, increase bruising and bleeding. These must be stopped 4 days before your treatment and for 4 days afterwards. Advise the doctor/nurse if you are taking: Aspirin, Advil, Arthrotec, Brufen, Clinoril, Diclofemac, Feldene, Ibuprofen, Indocid, Ketcid, Mobic, Motrin, Naprosen, Orudis, Porstan, Voltarol and Vioxx.

At the beginning of each session, the patient is given a mild tranquilizer (valium) orally. This minimizes anxiety, reduces discomfort and helps to prevent or decrease any side-effects that might be caused by the anaesthetic. A pain-killing injection may be used.

Lines of hair in the donor area (the area from which the hair follicles will be taken) are clipped to a 2-mm length, separated by rows of hair that are not cut. The hair above the donor area, together with the rows of hair left intact, are then used to completely camouflage the donor sites immediately after the procedure. In order to ensure better coverage, it is recommended that the hair in this area be left at least 1.5–2.0 inches (4–5 cm) long.

The donor area and the recipient area (the bald area into which hair will be grafted) are anaesthetized by injecting a local anaesthetic with a very small gauge needle that is about the size of an acupuncture needle. Anaesthetizing the areas is the only painful part of the session and the above technique usually causes less discomfort than a visit to the dentist.

After anaesthetizing the donor area, grafts are then removed from the scalp and prepared for transplanting. A variety of graft types is now used in the recipient area.

'Micrografts' are obtained by slicing the grafts into tiny pieces, each of which contains only 1–2 hairs. These are then placed into tiny holes made by a needle in front of the larger slit grafts to achieve the look of a natural hairline, or they are used in between the larger grafts to fill in any hairless gaps.

The grafts may be sliced into sections, each containing approximately 3–4 or 5–6 hairs, which are placed into small 'slits' made into the recipient area. These slit or minigrafts may be used to produce natural-looking hair with gradually increasing hair density. They are also used in areas such as the crown. Slit grafts are an important new resource for those patients who only want (or need) light coverage, have or will have very large bald areas, or have very little hair in the donor areas; a limited supply of donor grafts produces a sprinkled type of hair growth that is far more natural-looking than the clumpy or 'barbie-doll' look for those who have fine textured and/or light-coloured hair, or those who have (or will have) sparse temple hair, in whom densely transplanted hair would look unnatural.

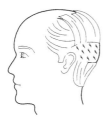

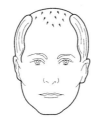

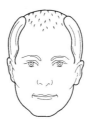

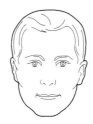

Donor site

Recipient site

Small strips (2–3 mm in width) are 'harvested' from hair-bearing sections of the scalp.

Micrografts are implanted in carefully plotted patterns. Grafts must be placed so that nourishment from blood vessels is unimpeded.

After shedding the original hair from the grafts within 3 weeks, new lasting hairs grow from grafts in 8–12 weeks.

The result, while it cannot achieve the density of hair growth before the balding process began, is cosmetically pleasing.

In general, slit grafts and micrografts produce more natural-looking results than an equivalent amount of donor tissue transplanted as round plug grafts. However, because no bald skin is actually removed (hair is only added), slit grafts and micrografts cannot ultimately produce the same density of hair as round grafts. Each case must be considered on an individual basis. There are a number of factors that influence the decision as to which type of grafts will be used and where they will be placed; these include the texture and colour of hair, hair density, the size of the donor areas, the size of the site to be transplanted, and the patient's goals. In most patients, a combination of the graft types will be used in order to achieve the most natural-looking results.

Grafts are held in place by congealed blood. To keep the grafts secure and properly oriented, a turban-like bandage is applied after the operation and left in place overnight. The following day, the bandage is removed and the area is cleansed.

Number of sessions of transplant procedures needed

If slit grafts are used, often only two and a half to three and a half sessions are necessary to produce satisfactory and natural-looking coverage in any given area.

Slit grafts have the advantage of not removing any existing hair as the 'slits' can be made between them. With round plug grafting, the patient will temporarily have less hair than before the operation. Each time a hole is made in the recipient area, some hair will be removed. The round graft put in each hole will not have any hair for the first 3 months, so during that period of time there will actually be less hair present than prior to surgery. On the other hand, as indicated earlier, ultimately more density will be produced by round grafts than slit grafts.

It is becoming more common for patients to have one or two 'early' transplanting sessions, before hair loss has reached an advanced stage. The benefit of these early sessions is threefold: the remaining hair provides natural camouflage for the initial sessions; the transplanted hair (once it has grown) will persist, thus providing additional coverage for any later sessions; and sessions can be spaced further apart, thus spreading the inconvenience and cost over a longer period of time.

Note 'Area to be transplanted' refers to either the front one-third or one-half of the head or the crown. To transplant both the front and crown areas usually requires 3–6 sessions.

Transplant sessions may be as far apart as the patient wishes; however, they are not done in any given area without several weeks' interval between the first two sessions, and a wait of 3–4 months between following sessions. If entirely separate areas are being transplanted at the same time (e.g. the front and the crown), sessions can be much closer (e.g. the crown can be done the day after the front).

The number of grafts that should be transplanted at one session and the frequency of transplant sessions depend on the characteristics of each individual case; this can be planned out in advance for each patient.

What to expect after each session

A crust or scab will form over each graft shortly after the procedure, and will remain attached for 7–14 days. When the area is healed, the crusts will then separate from the scalp and fall off, leaving a clean pinkish area to indicate the site of each graft. Although these crusts are plainly visible during the 1-week healing period, most patients can easily cover these by combing the adjacent hair over the transplanted site. If a hairpiece is normally worn, it may be used to conceal the crusts after the first week (and should be worn as little as possible for an additional week). The slit grafts leave much less visible marks, and are virtually undetectable within 7–10 days. The holes made for micrografts disappear within a few days to a week.

The hairs in the transplanted grafts are shed between the second and eighth week after the procedure. Sometimes many of these hairs fall out attached to the separate crusts; occasionally they persist longer. Rarely, one or two of the transplanted follicles does not shed its hair at all, but continues to grow immediately after the procedure. With these expectations, the grafts are usually bare for a period of 10–14 weeks after the operation, during which time the hairs are shed and the follicles recuperate to produce new hair. A new generation of hair is usually visible at the surface of the scalp by the twelfth week after transplanting, but this may occur slightly earlier, or up to 8 weeks later in individual patients. These hairs grow at the same rate as they did in their original location. Slit grafts usually show regrowth 2–4 weeks earlier than standard round grafts.

When a large area is transplanted, swelling of the forehead frequently occurs. While this swelling is usually mild, and lasts only 2–4 days, it occasionally can be severe enough to cause a large amount of puffiness around the eyes (approximately 1 out of 50 patients has swelling bad enough to cause 'black eyes').

Generally the swelling begins 2–3 days after the procedure and is most noticeable after the first session; with subsequent treatment it usually occurs in a milder form or not at all. In view of this, if possible, it is advisable to schedule a holiday to coincide with the first session. Please be assured that the swelling is **always** temporary and has no harmful effect on the healing transplants. Contrary to what many patients have been told, the scalp (hairy or bald) has an excellent blood supply. A certain amount of bleeding during the transplant procedure is expected and is simply controlled by applying pressure. The donor areas are stitched closed to produce better scars and to minimize bleeding. The stitches are removed 5–7 days later.

The scalp may be gently shampooed on the second or third day after transplanting. Patients from out of town should stay nearby overnight, after the transplant procedure, so the bandage can be removed and the area properly cleansed the day following surgery.

Final results

After a period of 4–6 months, the skin surface of the grafts has usually blended in with the surrounding scalp. In some patients, however, the grafts may be a shade lighter initially. The grafts are usually level with the surrounding scalp, but are occasionally slightly elevated. Such grafts are flattened down with an electric needle without interfering with hair growth. This is only necessary in approximately 1 out of every 100 patients.

The final appearance is that of 'early thinning', which is not meant to imply 'thin' but rather to convey the idea that you cannot expect to look like you did when you were a teenager.

In summary, with the new techniques of micrografting and slit grafting, the front hairline no longer appears as abrupt or dense as was the case with traditional round grafts. Micrografts create a very natural-looking hairline, enabling patients to wear their hair in virtually any style, including combing the hair straight back. Slit grafts create a more feathered, less tufty appearance, thus avoiding the 'barbie-doll' look that sometimes is present with round grafts before the area has been densely transplanted. They also do not result in the removal of any existing hair in the recipient area and are therefore advantageous for transplanting in patients with 'early' baldness.

PROPECIA (FINASTERIDE) TABLETS – PROPECIA IS FOR USE BY MEN ONLY (See Chapter 21)

What is PROPECIA used for?

PROPECIA is used for the treatment of male pattern hair loss on the vertex and the anterior mid-scalp area.

PROPECIA is for use by **MEN ONLY** and should **NOT** be used by women or children.

What is male pattern hair loss?

Male pattern hair loss is a common condition in which men experience thinning of the hair on the scalp. Often, this results in a receding hairline and/or balding on the top of the head. These changes typically begin gradually in men in their 20s.

Doctors believe male pattern hair loss is hereditary and is dependent on hormonal effects. Doctors refer to this type of hair loss as androgenetic alopecia.

Results of clinical studies

For 12 months doctors studied over 1800 men aged 18–41 with mild to moderate amounts of ongoing hair loss. All men, whether receiving PROPECIA or placebo (a pill containing no medication) were given a medicated shampoo. Of these men, approximately 1200 with hair loss at the top of the head were studied for an additional 12 months. In general, men who took PROPECIA maintained or increased the number of visible scalp hairs and noticed improvement in their hair in the first year, with the effect maintained in the second year. Hair counts in men who did not take PROPECIA continued to decrease.

In one study, patients were questioned on the growth of body hair. PROPECIA did not appear to affect hair in places other than the scalp.

Will PROPECIA work for me?

For most men, PROPECIA increases the number of scalp hairs, helping to fill in thin or balding areas of the scalp. Men taking PROPECIA noted a slowing of hair loss during 2 years of use. Although results will vary, generally you will not be able to grow back all the hair you have lost. There is not sufficient evidence that PROPECIA works in the treatment of receding hairline in the temporal area on both sides of the head.

Male pattern hair loss occurs gradually over time. On average, healthy hair grows only about half an inch each month. Therefore, it will take time to see any effect.

You may need to take PROPECIA daily for 3 months or more before you see a benefit from taking PROPECIA. PROPECIA can only work over the long term if you continue taking it. If the drug has not worked for you in 12 months, further treatment is unlikely to be of benefit. If you stop taking PROPECIA you will likely lose the hair you have gained within 12 months of stopping treatment. You should discuss this with your doctor.

How Should I Take PROPECIA?

Follow your doctor's instructions:

- Take one tablet by mouth each day.
- You may take PROPECIA with or without food.
- If you forget to take PROPECIA, do not take an extra tablet. Just take the next tablet as usual.

PROPECIA will not work faster or better if you take it more than once a day.

Who should not take PROPECIA?

- PROPECIA is for the treatment of male pattern hair loss in MEN ONLY and should not be taken by women or children.
- Anyone allergic to any of the ingredients.

A warning about PROPECIA and pregnancy
- Women who are or may potentially be pregnant:
  - must not use PROPECIA
  - should not handle crushed or broken tablets of PROPECIA.

If a women is pregnant with a male, the baby absorbs the active ingredient in PROPECIA, either by swallowing or through the skin, which may cause abnormalities of the male baby's sex organs. If a women who is pregnant comes into contact with the active ingredient in PROPECIA, a doctor should be consulted. PROPECIA tablets are coated and will prevent contact with the active ingredient during normal handling, provided that the tablets are not broken or crushed.

What are the possible side-effects of PROPECIA?
Like all prescription products, PROPECIA may cause side-effects. In clinical studies, side-effects from PROPECIA were uncommon and did not affect most men. A small number of men experienced certain sexual side effects. These men reported one or more of the following: less desire for sex; difficulty in achieving an erection; and a decrease in the amount of semen. Each of these side-effects occurred in less than 2% of men. These side-effects went away in men who stopped taking PROPECIA. They also disappeared in most men who continued taking PROPECIA.

The active ingredient in PROPECIA is also used by older men at a five times higher dose to treat enlargement of the prostate. Some of these men reported other side-effects, including problems with ejaculation, breast swelling and/or tenderness and allergic reactions such as lip swelling and rash. In clinical studies with PROPECIA, these side-effects occurred as often in men taking placebo as in those taking PROPECIA.

PARTICLE RESURFACING (PR) (See Chapter 8)

Please read these instructions carefully and make notes on the THIS sheet if you have any questions
during your consultation
You have a right to be informed about your skin condition and treatment so that you may make a
decision whether or not to undergo this procedure after knowing the risks and hazards involved. This
disclosure is not meant to alarm or scare: it is simply an effort to better inform you so that you may give
or withhold your consent for the treatment.

Why is particle resurfacing (PR) different from other microdermabrasion machines?

PR was developed more than 20 years ago in Italy. In this clinic we use Sodium Bicarbonate Medical Grade
Class 1™ microcrystals or aluninium oxide. This PR machine uses a unique push–pull system which allows
the crystals to move along the surface of the skin by either vacuum power or pressure assist. Vacuum forces
pull the crystal and pressure assist pushes the crystal along the skin surface.

Other microdermabrasion machines only work on vacuum power. As the skin is 'sucked' the top and middle
layers of the skin arc separated. Without the pressure assist system pushing these layers back together the skin
may become swollen and damaged. Our machine can only be used in a doctor's office.

How does PR differ from chemical peels or dermabrasion?

The PR machine has the ability to achieve epidermal (skin) regeneration results similar to those obtained with
traditional mechanical dermabrasion or various chemical peels, but without the discomfort or down-time
patients can expect from the latter procedures.

The procedure may be good for patients who have 'maxed out' on superficial chemical peels and who may
not be ready for medium depth peeling or for laser resurfacing.

It is usually bloodless, non-invasive and, in contrast to chemical peels, chemical-free.

An advantage of PR is that it can be used on any skin type, including fair and very dark skin.

Will I need an anaesthetic?

Treatment is usually painless and well tolerated.

Some patients have described the sensation as being similar to a cat licking your skin.

It is associated with a minimum of down-time, therefore, patients can have lunch-time treatments and return
to work without problems.

What problems can be treated?

We can remove dead and flaking skin to create an immediate improvement in your skin's appearance. This
unique approach stimulates the production of fresh young skin cells and collagen.

Fine lines and wrinkles can be diminished or reduced by the procedure, as can scars resulting from acne,
chicken pox, and hypertrophy. Acne related problems such as closed and open comedones; blackheads and
whiteheads may respond.

A variety of relatively superficial abnormalities such as stretch marks can be improved. It is also effective
for removal of permanent make-up.

Dull, thickened and sallow skin can be rejuvenated with one or more treatments improving skin texture,
consistency, and colour. It may diminish brown age spots and mottled red skin (hyperpigmentation).

Difficult to treat areas such as the neck, décolleté and the back of the hands can be treated successfully.

Deep rhytides (wrinkles). dermal melasma (deep brown marks), deep scars, telangiectases (red veins) or
actinic keratosis (sun damage) will not disappear with PR. Deep defects can be better treated by procedures
such as carbon dioxide laser or deep chemical peels.

Micro-particle reurfacing (PR) is ideal for:

- Patients who cannot afford to take time off for healing from chemical or lasers.
- Active patients who do not want to put off outdoor or social activities such as tennis, golf or skiing.
- Skin that is sensitive to chemicals or make-up.
- Acne-prone skin that has not responded well to acne remedies.
- Young patients with early skin changes who wish for softer, smoother skin.
- Stretch marks, fine lines, brown spots.

Will I need to have any pre-treatment?

You will be instructed to discontinue all alpha hydroxy acid-containing products – as well as Retin A cream and benzoyl peroxide preparations, 2 days prior to the PR appointment. Please discuss any other prescription creams you may have been given with the nurse. Do not discontinue their use without checking first. If you have a history of recurrent herpes simplex infections within the past year, you will be offered the choice of taking low dose preventative anti-viral agent for the duration of the course, starting 1 day before treatment starts.

Anti-inflammatory drugs may thin your blood, increase bruising and bleeding. These must be stopped 4 days before your treatment and for 4 days afterwards. Advise the doctor/nurse if you are taking: Aspirin, Advil, Arthrotec, Brufen, Clinoril, Diclofemac, Feldene, Ibuprofen, Indocid, Ketcid, Mobic, Motrin, Naprosen, Orudis, Porstan, Voltarol and Vioxx. Excessive alcohol and vitamin E supplements may all increase bruising.

Accutane treatment has to be stopped for least 6 months before starting PR.

What happens during PR treatment?

PR treatments usually last about 10–30 minutes. Stretch marks can take as long as 2 hours.

The procedure is analogous to a gentle sandblasting of the skin.

The treatment area is thoroughiy cleansed with water. The skin surface is then prepared with alcohol to remove make-up residue and oil. The patient's eyes are covered with goggles or tape to prevent irritation from the crystals. If a patient uses contact lenses, he/she removes them prior to the treatment.

The crystals are projected from the reservoir via a tubing system and handpiece onto the patient's skin. At the same time, the crystals and loosened skin debris are evacuated from the treated surface into a second tubing system, and finally deposited in another closed container, thereby preventing contamination.

How will I look and feel after treatment?

All patients experience some erythema. This is in fact the desired effect and usually lasts an hour or two. In some cases patients with deeper blemishes or thicker skin the erythema may last for several hours and, occasionally, a few days. Broken capillaries may temporarily appear to be more obvious.

Patients often develop streaking which usually fades within a day or two.

Transient odema (swelling), especially in the periorbital (eye) areas, has been observed. Cool compresses (such as frozen peas) help resolve it within a few days.

Expect the treated skin to feel tight temporarily, such as after exposure to sun or wind.

Deep treatments, aimed at scar tissue or stretch marks may produce some spotting of blood; healing generally takes at least 3–4 days.

Post treatment care

Make-up should be avoided for a day after the procedure if any bleeding has occurred. Otherwise make-up can be applied after treatment although it is preferred that you avoid it to allow the pores to flush out and close.

Use a bland moisturizer and liberal amounts of chemical-free sunscreen.

Deep treatments for scars and stretch marks may require an antibiotic ointment for a few days while healing.

Scientific Study

In a recent scientific study, patients completed a PR questionnaire. The overall initial satisfaction among the patients was predominantly rated as very good to excellent. More than 85% would recommend the procedure to a friend or family member. PR was experienced as pleasant in the majority of patients.

Patients with finer rhytides, mottled discoloured skin, and photoaging achieved the greatest benefit. Results were not dramatic, but subtle, appearing after the second or third treatment. Patients usually reported that their make-glided on better because of the overall improved smoothness of their skin, and that their skin was also more radiant. Compliments from relatives and friends further emphasized the overall improved appearance. Patients reported satisfaction with the smoothness and 'healthy glow' of their skin.

How often will I need treatment?

A series of five to 10 sessions performed 1 week apart can improve the appearance of acne scars and fine wrinkling, and treat sun-damaged skin as well as enhance the blending of post-laser skin.

What are the risks and discomforts?

Wound healing – This is generally not an issue as no open wound exists. After a deep treatment, an animation may occur.

Bruising/swelling/infection – Bruising and swelling generally are non-existent.

Skin infection – This is a possibility any time a skin procedure is performed. However, the epidermis (outer layer) has only been partially removed, and is unlikely to occur.

Pigment changes (skin colour) – As the outer portion of skin is removed, there is a small risk of the treated area becoming somewhat altered in colour to the surrounding skin. This usually resolves within 1 month.

Scarring – Scarring is a rare occurrence, but it is a possibility where the skin's surface is disrupted. To minimize the chances of scarring, it is important that you follow all post-operative instructions carefully.

Eye exposure – Protective eyewear (shields) will be provided. It is important to keep those shields on at all times during the treatment in order to protect your eyes from accidental particle exposure. It would feel as if grit or sand had got into your eye.

Lines/streaking – You may have temporary lines or streaking of the skin which could last several days.

Herpes simplex blisters/cold sores – If you have a history of herpes simplex or cold sores, a reactivation of this condition can occur over the treated area. Please advise the doctor/nurse if you have this condition and you will be given a prescription prior to any treatment.

PATIENT QUESTIONNAIRE

PATIENT NAME.. DATE ....

In order to have us tailor the treatment to your needs, please answer the following questions.

	YES	NO
Have you had micro Particle Resurfacing (PR) or similar treatments in the past?	☐	☐

If so, how many...

Have you ever had a laser peel?	☐	☐

When?..

Have you had a herpes or cold sore infection?	☐	☐

With what frequency?..

Have you taken Accutane for acne treatment?	☐	☐

When did that treatment end?..

Are you currently using any of the following prescription?
or over-the counter products?

	YES	NO
Retin A	☐	☐
Renova	☐	☐
Tretmom	☐	☐
Zorac Gel (Tazarotene)	☐	☐
Differin gel	☐	☐
Alpha Gly products	☐	☐
Beta Hydroxy	☐	☐
Glycolic/Alphahyoxy Acid	☐	☐
Antioxidants,e.g. vitamin E, Ginko Bioba	☐	☐
anticoagulants, Aspirin, anti-inflammatories	☐	☐

*Do not discontinue prescription creams without checking first

Have you ever had a glycolic acid peel?	☐	☐

Where...

Are you wearing contact lenses?	☐	☐

ROSACEA (See Chapter 9)

Rosacea, (ro-za'she-ah) is a skin disease that causes redness and swelling on the face. Often referred to as 'adult acne,' rosacea may begin as a tendency to flush or blush easily, and progress to persistent redness in the centre of the face that gradually involves the cheeks, forehead and chin. As the disease progresses small blood vessels and tiny pimples begin to appear on and around the reddened area.

Unlike acne, there are no blackhead or whiteheads. This disease affects mainly the forehead, cheeks, chin and lower half of the nose.

When it first develops, rosacea may come and go on its own. When the skin doesnot return to its normal colour and when other symptoms, such as pimples and enlarged blood vessels, become visible, it is best to seek advice from a dermatologist. The condition rarely reverses itself and may last for years. It can become worse without treatment.

How do I recognize rosacea?

Pimples of rosacea appear on the face as small, red bumps some of which may contain pus. These may be accompanied by the development of many tiny blood vessels on the surface of the skin. Rosacea may also be accompanied by oily skin, and possibly dandruff.

In more advanced cases of rosacea, a condition called *rhinophyma* (re'no-fi'mah) may develop. The oil glands enlarge causing a bulbous, enlarged red nose and puffy cheeks. Thick bumps can develop on the lower half of the nose, and nearby cheeks. *Rhinophyma* rarely occurs in women.

The eyes may also become involved. Some rosacea patients experience burning and grittiness of the eye – a condition commonly known as conjunctivitis. If this condition is not treated, it can lead to even more serious complications for the eyes.

At risk for rosacea?

Rosacea is rare in childhood, and usually develops over a long period of time. It may first seem like a tendency to blush easily, a ruddy complexion, or an extreme sensitivity to cosmetics. Those most likely to develop rosacea are fair-skinned adults, especially women, between the ages of 30 and 50, although it may affect men or women of any age. For some unknown reason, women get rosacea more often than men, and some cases of this disorder have been associated with menopause. An occasional embarrassment or a tense moment may also trigger flushing.

Drugs that dilate the blood vessels can make rosacea worse. Strong cortisone-containing creams may also cause or aggravate rosacea.

Dos and don'ts for rosacea patients

The exact cause of rosacea is still unknown. The best prevention may be to avoid things that make the face red or flushed.

- Avoid hot drinks, spicy foods and alcoholic beverages. Caffeine does not cause flushing but stopping caffeine intake after heavy use can make rosacea worse. It's important to note that alcohol may worsen a case of rosacea, symptoms may be just as severe in someone who does not drink at all. This condition has been unfairly linked to alcoholism, harming many innocent people.
- Practise good sun protection. This includes limiting exposure to sunlight, using sunscreens and avoiding extreme hot and cold temperatures which may help relieve the symptoms of rosacea.
- Avoid rubbing, scrubbing or massaging the face. Rubbing will tend to irritate the reddened skin.
- Avoiding irritating cosmetics and facial products. Use hair sprays properly.

Treatment options

Many people with rosacea are unfamiliar with it and do not recognize it in its early stages.

Identifying the disease is the first step to controlling it. Self-diagnosis and treatment are not recommended, as some over-the-counter skin applications may make the problem worse.

Dermatologists often recommend a combination of treatments tailored to the individual patient. Together, these treatments can stop the progress of rosacea and sometimes reverse it.

Gels and creams may be prescribed by a dermatologist or general practitioner. A slight improvement can be seen in the first 3–4 weeks of use. Greater improvement will be noticed in 2 months.

Oral antibiotics tend to produce faster results than topical medications.

Cortisone creams will often heal the bumps and help reduce the redness of rosacea. However, they should not be used for a long period of time and strong preparations should be avoided. Only use these creams under the direction of your dermatologist or general practitioner.

The persistent redness may be treated with a small electric needle or by laser surgery to close off the dilated blood vessels. Cosmetics may offer an alternative to the more specific treatment.

It is important to eliminate the factors that cause additional skin irritation. Daily facial products such as soap, moisturizers and sunscreens should be free of alcohol or other irritating ingredients. Moisturizers used along with topical medications should be applied very gently after the medication has dried. When going outdoors, especially on warm sunny days, sunscreens with a SPF of 15 or higher are necessary.

Other treatments

Rhinophyma is usually treated with surgery. The excess tissue that has developed can be carefully removed with a scalpel, laser or through electrosurgery. Dermabrasion, a surgical method that smooths the top layer of the skin, will then help improve the look of the scar tissue. Sometimes regrowth may occur in spite of treatment.

The key to a successful recovery from rosacea is early diagnosis and treatment. It is also important to follow all of your dermatologist's instructions. Rosacea can be treated and reversed if medical advice is sought in the early stages. When left untreated, rosacea will get worse and may be more difficult to treat.

SCAR TREATMENTS

Despite claims to the contrary, you cannot eliminate scars altogether but, with the latest treatments, you can reduce them significantly. You should not overtreat a scar and cause any more damage.

Some of the most frequently used methods of scar reduction are

Cortisone injections and tape
One of the most common ways to reduce a scar.
Best for: hypertrophic (red, raised) scars, but also effective in shrinking and flattening very firm scars (keloids).
Disadvantages: over time, cortisone can cause a chronic thinning of the skin.

Shaving
The area around the scar is numbed, then the scar is removed with a scalpel. Usually followed by cortisone injections for a few weeks.
Best for: larger, raised scars.
Disadvantages: may leave skin discoloration, and scar may return.

Freezing
The upper layers of the skin are frozen, causing blistering and peeling, which reveals new skin underneath.
Best for: reducing the size of raised acne scars.
Disadvantages: may lighten skin.

Collagen or hylan injections
Collagen is injected into the scar site.
Best for: raising soft, sunken scars such as those from acne.
Disadvantages: not for people with rheumatic or auto-immune diseases as it can lead to allergic skin swellings. Results last only 4–6 months; repeat treatment is required.

Fat injections
Best for: sunken acne scars on cheeks and lower face. No allergy risks, since it is your own fat.
Disadvantages: may need repeat treatments.

Laser resurfacing or dermabrasion
A machine removes the top layers of skin.
Best for: improving minor skin irregularities, such as sunken acne scars. If the defect is minor, only one treatment may be needed.
Disadvantages: several treatments may be needed for deeper scars.

Surgical revision
The scar is cut away and the skin is rejoined in a less noticeable fashion.
Best for: wide or long scars, and scars that are the product of plastic surgery procedures.
Disadvantages: further surgery.

Scar subcision and elevation
Best for: saucer-shaped sunken scars.
Disadvantages: risk of temporary bruising. Often needs to be repeated. Further surgery.

Chemical peels

An acid solution is applied to the skin, removing the top layer.

Best for: small superficial scars, diminishing smooth, sunken scars and evening out skin tone.

Disadvantages: light peels require very little healing time, but deeper ones may require 1–2 weeks to heal and cause redness and irritation. Not for deeper scars.

Pulsed dye lasers

This process targets blood vessels feeding the scar, leading to flattening and lightening of the scar.

Best for: works best on hypertrophic red, raised scars.

Disadvantages: can lead to bruising that usually lasts 1–2 weeks. May need multiple treatments.

Silicon patches

Small Band-Aid-like cushions that supply silicon (said to accelerate the healing of thick scars) to the scar site.

Best for: raised scars, according to manufacturers.

Disadvantages: experts have not seen much evidence that they work very well ('But they can't hurt and compared to something costly like laser surgery they are cheap enough to try out for yourself').

Vitamin E and lotions

There are more studies saying that vitamin E does not work than those saying it does. Other special scar solutions, such as topical gel, claim to soften and smooth scars, but results are mostly anecdotal.

Best for: minor scars.

Disadvantages: some people may experience skin irritation, and results can be subtle.

Adrenocorticosteroids (e.g. prednisone, prednisolone, kenalog, decadron, triamcinolone) are cortisone-like substances. These medicines are anti-inflammatory agents and are effective at reducing inflammation and thickening of the skin.

They are used to reduce the inflammation of acne, keloid (thickened) scars and inflammation associated with skin conditions such as psoriasis, pyoderma gangrenosum or lupus erythematosus.

The medicine is injected directly into the skin lesion. A decrease in redness and swelling is usually seen within 24–48 hours.

Possible side-effects include lack of response to the injection and atrophy of the skin. This is seen as a small depression or 'pit' in the injection site. This side-effect can be minimized by using the appropriate concentration of corticosteroid for the skin lesion and body part.

Other rare side-effects may include a rebound worsening of psoriasis, skin fragility or easy bruising at the injection site.

We do not guarantee results; we only guarantee that physicians at this office will use their best efforts and best judgments on your behalf.

I have read the information in this letter and I have discussed it with my physician. I understand the information provided.

Patient signature .... Date ....

Witness signature .... Date ....

HOW TO USE THE CREAMS RECOMMENDED BY YOUR PHYSICIAN

Wrinkling, rough skin texture, age spots and patchy skin pigmentation are largely the result of chronic sun exposure (UV radiation). Unfortunately, your skin has an excellent memory and shows the damage it acquired even 30–40 years ago. Even if you obediently use sunscreens daily now, your skin may still suffer the damaging effects of sunbathing as a teenager. Fortunately, there are many things you can do to help correct or improve these sun-induced effects.

There are several main types of creams: tretinoin (vitamin A), glycolic acid, lightening creams and antioxidants.

Tretinoin (similar to Retin-A and Retinova)

How does it work?
Tretinoin is a vitamin A cream that has been well established in its treatment for acne and some forms of abnormal pigmentation. However, more recently, it has been shown to help reverse sun damage. It helps to accelerate the normal turnover time of the superficial layers of the skin, thereby improving skin texture and color and imparting a more youthful look. Additionally, it helps to stimulate new collagen production in the deeper layers of the skin (the dermis). This may help to correct fine-line wrinkling. You may start seeing improvement after 3 months but maximum effects may not be seen for about 6 months.

What problems can occur?
1. Itching and excessive scaling. If this happens, stop using it for 2–3 days, then restart, but reduce the frequency to every second or third night or day.
2. Apply moisturizer the other nights and, if required, during the day. Restart daily or every other night or day once the itching/scaling has diminished.
3. Use sunscreen every morning – at least SPF 15 for maximum protection.

USE THIS CREAM

Every night	☐	Every third night (then, if tolerated, every other night	☐

APPLY TO THE

Face	☐	Eyelids (upper and lower)	☐
Neck	☐	Chest	☐
Arms	☐	Hands	☐

Continue using this cream until the doctor tells you otherwise.

HOW TO APPLY
1. Apply in small-sized blobs to each part of the skin and rub in.
2. Do not get cream in the eyes; if you do, rinse with running warm or cold water and wash hands.
3. Always test a small area of skin with the cream first. If it stings excessively or itches excessively, please call the clinic.

Glycolic acid creams

They are also called alpha-hydroxy acids (AHA).

How do they work?

Many of the formulations contain the AHA glycolic acid, a constituent of sugar cane. Sensitive skin formulations may contain gluconolactone, a gentler AHA: this is an antioxidant agent, which helps prevent, as well as reverse, the oxidative aging process of the skin. Glycolic acid in general alters the outer skin by increasing the shedding of the skin. This leads to a smoother skin surface and, secondly, a stimulation of collagen to support tissues of the skin, leaving the skin healthier looking.

This cream may cause a sensation of tingling when applied to the skin.

What problems can occur?

1. Itching, scaling and drying: if this happens, stop using it for 2–3 days, then restart, but reduce the frequency to every second or third night or day.
2. Apply moisturizer the other nights and if required during the day. Restart daily or every other night once the itching/scaling and/or drying has diminished.

USE THIS CREAM

Every night	☐	Every other night	☐
Every morning	☐	Every third night	☐

APPLY TO THE

Face	☐	Eyes	☐
Neck	☐	Chest	☐
Arms	☐	Hands	☐

Continue using this cream until the doctor tells you otherwise.

HOW TO APPLY

1. Apply in small-sized blobs to each part of the skin.
2. Do not get cream into the eyes; if you do, rinse with running water and wash hands.
3. Always test a small area of skin with the cream first. If it stings excessively or itches excessively, please call the clinic.

Skin 'lightening' creams (hydroquinone mixed with other ingredients)

How do they work?

These creams reduce the amount of pigment (melanin) that your skin produces. They usually contain hydroquinone or kojic acid.

These creams take 3–6 months to show an effect: be patient.

You must use a sunscreen every morning, SPF 15 (UVA****).

What problems can occur?

1. If you *do not* apply a sunscreen every day, your skin will respond to the sun and go darker, even reacting to sunlight through window glass (for example when driving).
2. Itching, scaling and drying: if this happens, stop using it for 2–3 days, then restart, but reduce the frequency to every second or third night or day.
3. Apply moisturizer the other nights and, if required, during the day. Restart daily or every other night once the itching/scaling and/or drying has diminished.

USE THIS CREAM

Every night	☐	Every other night	☐
Every morning	☐	Every third night	☐

APPLY TO THE

Face	☐	Eyelids (upper and lower)	☐
Neck	☐	Chest	☐
Arms	☐	Hands	☐

Continue using this cream until the doctor tells you otherwise.

HOW TO APPLY

1. Apply in small-sized blobs to each part of the skin.
2. Do not get cream into the eyes; if you do, rinse with running water and wash hands.
3. Always test a small area of skin with the cream first. If it stings excessively or itches excessively, please call the clinic.

Vitamin C and other antioxidant creams

How does it work?

Vitamin C is a major antioxidant in the body, as well as being important in collagen synthesis. It may help to 'mop up' damage from sunlight and irritancy from chemicals. New types of topical vitamin C may give more efficient help to improve skin tone and elasticity.

Vitamin C and related ingredients have the following effects:

1. They protect us from free radical damage.
2. They fight free radical attack.
3. They prevent future signs of aging.
4. They are thought to provide a stimulus for new collagen in the skin.
5. They diminish the appearance of aging skin.

What problems can occur?

1. Sometimes these creams can sting after they are applied, rather like lemon on a cut: this is normal.
2. Try gentle washing with soap free cleansers (such as cetaphil, pH 5.5).
3. If necessary, stop using the cream and call the office.

USE THIS CREAM

Every night	☐	Every other night	☐
Every morning	☐	Every third night	☐

APPLY TO THE

Face	☐	Eyelids (upper and lower)	☐
Neck	☐	Chest	☐
Arms	☐	Hands	☐

Continue using this cream until the doctor tells you otherwise.

HOW TO APPLY

1. Apply in small-sized blobs to each part of the skin and rub in.
2. Do not get cream in the eyes; if you do, rinse with running warm or cold water and wash hands.

3. Always test a small area of skin with the cream first. If it stings excessively or itches excessively please call the clinic.

Sunscreens

Please use sunscreens *every day* with an SPF of 15; they should have a three (***) or four (****) UVA star rating in Europe. Every morning after washing or showering, apply the sunscreen to the sun-exposed skin of the face, neck and hands.

Summer and outdoor days
In the summer, on outdoor days, or snow skiing in the winter, please use a waterproof sunscreen with an SPF of 25–30 (a three (***) or four (****) UVA star rating) in Europe.

Some suggested sunscreens (Europe)
Ambre Solaire
La Roche Posay
Neutrogena
Nivea
Piz Buin
Soltan
Vaseline
Vichy

These sunscreens are available at most pharmacists.

Some suggested sunscreens (USA)
UVA star ratings do not apply in the USA; look for sunscreens that contain Avobenzone (Parasol 1789). Mexoryl is another UVA screen ingredient from Europe that may become available in the next few years.
Presun
Ombrelle
Uvaguard (shade)

Index

Note: Page numbers in **bold** indicate patient information/consent documents.

Note: references to figures are indicated by 'f' and references to tables are indicated by 't' when they fall on a page not covered by the text reference.